Resounding Praise for
FOOD FIX

'Dr Hyman is a leader in the food world, building bridges between disparate viewpoints, creating connections between different worlds, and using this to construct an original plan to move toward better health for ourselves and the planet.'

Nina Teicholz, author of *The Big Fat Surprise*

'An influential read.' **Dr Mehmet Oz**

'The revolution starts with what we put on our plates and into our bodies. But even before that, it starts with *Food Fix*. Read this book to change the world.' **Tim Ryan, US representative (OH)**

'A wake-up call. Dr Hyman has not just the diagnosis but the remedies we need.' **Daniel Goleman, author of *Focus***

'Dr Hyman's voice is at once fresh, powerful, informed, passionate, and encouraging.'

Walter Robb, former co-CEO, Whole Foods Market

'Our food system went to Dr Hyman for a checkup. He diagnosed chronic influence-peddling, inflammation of the profit motive, sclerosis of the lower politician, and a severely ruptured public interest. Read this. Take two actions and tweet him in the morning.'

**Ken Cook, president and cofounder,
Environmental Working Group**

'An authoritative, illuminating account. Profoundly disturbing and vitally important.' **Dr James Gordon, author of *Transforming Trauma***

'Highlights the need to focus on what we put on our plates as a way to improve our diets, our health, and our planet.'

Barry M. Popkin, PhD, professor of nutrition, University of North Carolina

'Mark Hyman encourages us to think about how our food is produced, prepared, and purchased. Highly recommended.'

Ann M. Veneman, former US secretary of agriculture

'Dr Hyman's diagnostic skills are on display in this brilliant book. *Food Fix* gives hope for personal and planetary healing. Thank you, Mark, for shining your light on our path forward.'

Tom Newmark, chairman, The Carbon Underground

FOOD
FIX

How to Save Our Health, Our Economy,
Our Communities and Our Planet –
One Bite at a Time

DR MARK HYMAN

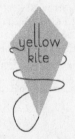

First published in the United States in 2020 by Little Brown Spark
An imprint of Little, Brown and Company
A division of Hachette Book Group, Inc

First published in Great Britain in 2020 by Yellow Kite
An Imprint of Hodder & Stoughton
An Hachette UK company

This paperback edition published in 2021

1

A CIP catalogue record for this title is available from the British Library

Paperback ISBN 978 1 529 39163 3
eBook ISBN 978 1 529 38814 5

Printed and bound in Great Britain by Clays Ltd, Elcograf S.p.A.

Hodder & Stoughton policy is to use papers that are natural, renewable
and recyclable products and made from wood grown in sustainable forests.
The logging and manufacturing processes are expected to conform
to the environmental regulations of the country of origin.

Yellow Kite
Hodder & Stoughton Ltd
Carmelite House
50 Victoria Embankment
London EC4Y 0DZ

www.yellowkitebooks.co.uk

To the farmers, eaters, communities, advocates, activists, scientists, businesses, and policy makers who are working to fix our food system

Contents

FOOD
FIX

FOOD
FIX

Introduction

It is a wonderful feeling to recognize the unity of a complex of phenomena that to direct observation appear to be quite separate things.

— ALBERT EINSTEIN

It is . . . our apparent reluctance to recognize the interrelated nature of the problems and therefore the solutions that lies at the heart of our predicament and certainly on our ability to determine the future of food.

— PRINCE CHARLES

There is one place that nearly everything that matters in the world today converges: our food and our food system—the complex web of how we grow food, how we produce, distribute, and promote it; what we eat, what we waste, and the policies that perpetuate unimaginable suffering and destruction across the globe that deplete our human, social, economic, and natural capital.

Food is the nexus of most of our world's health, economic, environmental, climate, social, and even political crises. While this may seem like an exaggeration, it is not. The problem is much worse than we think. After reading *Food Fix* you will be able to connect the dots of this largely invisible crisis and understand why fixing our food system is central to the health and well-being of our population, our environment, our climate, our economy, and our very survival as a species. You will also understand the forces, businesses, and policies driving the catastrophe, and the people, businesses, and governments that are providing hope and a path to fixing our dysfunctional food system.

3

But why would a doctor be so interested in food, the system that produces it, and food policy?

As a doctor, my oath is to relieve suffering and illness and to do no harm. As a functional medicine physician, I was trained to focus on the root causes of disease and to think of our body as one interconnected ecosystem.

Our diet is the number one cause of death, disability, and suffering in the world. Our food has dramatically transformed over the last 100 years, and even more radically over the last 40 years, as we have eaten a diet of increasingly ultraprocessed foods made from a handful of crops (wheat, corn, soy). If poor diet is the biggest killer on the planet, I was forced to ask, what is the cause of our food and the system that produces it? This led to a deep exploration of the entire food chain, from seed to field to fork to landfill, and the harm caused at each step of the journey. The story of food shocked me, frightened me, and drove me to tell this story and to find the possibility of redemption from the broken system that is slowly destroying the people and things we love most.

Our most powerful tool to reverse the global epidemic of chronic disease, heal the environment, reverse climate change, end poverty and social injustice, reform politics, and revive economies is food. The food we grow, how we grow it, and the food we eat have tremendous implications not just for our waistlines but also for our communities, the planet, and the global economy.

Chronic disease is now the single biggest threat to global economic development. Lifestyle-caused diseases such as heart disease, diabetes, and cancer now kill nearly 50 million people a year, more than twice as many as die from infectious disease. Two billion people go to bed overweight and 800 million go to bed hungry in the world today. One in two Americans and one in four teenagers have pre-diabetes or type 2 diabetes.

Lobbyists' influence over policy makers has put corporations, not citizens, at the center of every aspect of our food system, from what and how food is grown to what is manufactured, marketed, and sold. When money rules politics, it results in our current uncoordinated and conflicting food policies, which subsidize and protect and facilitate Big Food's and Big Ag's domination of our food system to the detriment of our population and our environment. Big Ag and Big Food co-opt politicians, public health groups, grassroots advocacy groups, scientists, and schools and pollute science and public opinion with vast amounts of dollars and misinformation campaigns. The consolidation and monopolization of the food industry over the last 40 years from hundreds of different processed-food companies, seed companies, and chemical and fertilizer companies into just a few dozen companies make it the largest collective industry in the world, valued at approximately $15 trillion, or about 17 percent of the entire world's economy. And it is controlled by a few dozen CEOs who determine what food is grown and how it is grown, processed, distributed, and sold. This affects every single human on the planet.

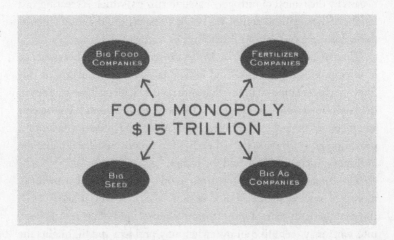

Our children's future is threatened by an achievement gap caused in large part by their inability to learn on a diet of processed foods and sugar served in schools. Fifty percent of schools serve brand-name fast food in their cafeterias and 80 percent have contracts with soda companies. Food companies target children and minorities with billions in marketing of the worst "foods."

Poverty, social injustice, and violence are perpetuated by the harmful effects of our nutritionally toxic and depleted food environment on children's intellectual development, mood, and behavior. Violent prison crime can be dramatically reduced by providing a healthy diet to prisoners. Our national security is threatened because our young adults are not fit to fight and not eligible for service, and many of our soldiers are overweight.

We are also depleting nature's capital—capital that, once destroyed, may only be able to be partially reclaimed. The threat is not only to our health and our children's future, but also to the health of the planet that sustains us. Our industrial agricultural and food system (including food waste) is the single biggest cause of climate change, exceeding all use of fossil fuels. Current farming practices may cause us to run out of soil and fresh water in this century. We are destroying our rivers, lakes, and oceans by the runoff of nitrogen-based fertilizers, which is creating vast swaths of marine dead zones. We waste 40 percent of the food we produce, costing more than $2.6 trillion a year in global impact.

There is a solution, a *food fix*. Across the globe there are governments, businesses, grassroots efforts, and individuals who are reimagining our food system, creating solutions that address the challenges we face across the landscape of our food system. This book both defines the problems and maps out the policies, business innovations, and grassroots solutions, providing ideas for what we can each do to improve our health and the health of our communities and the planet.

The imperative to transform our food system is not just medical, moral, or environmental, but economic. Dariush Mozaffarian, MD, the dean of Tufts School of Nutrition Science and Policy, injects hope into what may seem like an overwhelming problem and highlights the "waves of innovation and capital now sweeping food and allied disciplines, from agriculture to processing to restaurants and retail, and in healthcare, personalization, mobile tech, and employee wellness. Catalyzing this multi-billion-dollar revolution, and ensuring its rapid trajectory is evidence-based and mission-oriented, is an essential opportunity and challenge."

As a doctor, it is increasingly clear to me that the health of our citizens, the health of our society and our planet, depends on disruptive innovations that decentralize and democratize food production and consumption, innovations that produce real food at scale, that restore the health of soils, water, air, and the biodiversity of our planet, and that reverse climate change. I cannot cure obesity and diabetes in my office. It is cured on the farm, in the grocery store, in the restaurant, in our kitchens, schools, workplaces, and faith-based communities.

All these things and more can provide the seeds for the type of transformation needed to solve one of the central problems of our time—the quality of what we put on our fork every day. We have to take back our health one kitchen, one home, one family, one community, one farm at a time! Changes to our own diet are necessary but not sufficient to truly create the shifts needed to create a healthy, sustainable, just world.

The policies and businesses that drive our current system must change to support a reimagined food system from field to fork and beyond. If we were to identify one big lever to pull to improve global health, create economic abundance, reduce social injustice and mental illness, restore environmental health, and reverse climate change, it would be transforming our entire food system. That is the most important work of our time—work that must begin now.

PART I

THE HEALTH AND ECONOMIC IMPACT OF OUR FOOD SYSTEM

*People are fed by the food industry, which pays no attention to health,
and are healed by the health industry, which pays no attention to food.*
— WENDELL BERRY

The True Cost of Food— The Health, Economic, Environmental, and Climate Impact of Our Food System

Ninety-five trillion dollars—$95,000,000,000,000—is an almost unimaginable number. Yet this is an estimate of the burden that will be put on our economy by chronic disease over the next 35 years in both direct health care costs and lost productivity and disability. To put it in perspective, that is almost five times our nation's gross domestic product of $20 trillion a year. According to the World Bank, in 2017, the entire world's GDP was just $80 trillion.

For that amount of money, we could...

- Provide free education
- Provide free health care
- Eradicate poverty
- End food insecurity and hunger
- Solve social injustice, income, and health disparities
- End unemployment
- Rebuild our infrastructure and transportation systems
- Shift to renewable energy
- Draw down carbon emissions and reverse climate change
- Transform our industrial agricultural system, which is destructive to humans, animals, and the environment, into a sustainable, regenerative system that reverses climate change, preserves our freshwater

resources, increases biodiversity, protects pollinators, and produces health-promoting whole foods

That $95 trillion is the total cost of chronic illness to the United States over the next 35 years (or 91 percent of the total tax collected by the US government), in both direct health care costs and the loss of productivity due to heart disease, diabetes, cancer, mental illness, and other chronic conditions.[1] Imagine if we had a significant portion of those resources to spend on things that matter to all of us rather than preventable chronic disease. Most of those diseases are caused by our industrial diet, which means they are avoidable if we transform the food we grow, the food we produce, and the food we eat. The $95 trillion is just the start of the value to our economy if we fix all the broken parts of our food system. Clearly not all chronic disease will disappear, nor will all those who are chronically ill be able to go back to work. But if even a conservative fraction of that money, an estimated $15 trillion, is available, it would provide crucial resources to solve our most critical problems. And $15 trillion is still about four years of our total federal tax collections.

Eleven million people die every year from a bad diet. And more than a billion people in the world are overweight and sick from eating our processed, industrialized diet and not eating a healthy whole foods diet.[2] In fact, the number one factor causing these deaths is the lack of fruits and vegetables in our diet. The sad thing is that in America only 2 percent of our farmland is used to grow fruits and vegetables, despite our government's recommendations that 50 percent of our diet should be fruits and vegetables. Fifty-nine percent of our farmland is used to grow commodity crops (corn, wheat, soy) that get turned into ultra-processed foods that we know are deadly. These processed foods make up about 60 percent of our diet!

Why does this matter? For every 10 percent of your diet that comes from processed food, your risk of death goes up 14 percent.[3] That means a lot of extra deaths because we support agriculture that creates food that makes us sick and fat and harms the environment, and not the production of fruits and vegetables and whole foods that make us healthy.

The complexity of the problem prevents people from connecting the dots and taking action. And most of the true costs are not even recognized, limiting the motivation to change the system. Let's take a journey through every aspect of the food system and connect those dots.

THE COSTS OF CHRONIC DISEASE

In 2018, the Milken Institute issued two major reports. The first, *The Cost of Chronic Diseases in the US*,[4] and the second, *America's Obesity Crisis: The Health and Economic Costs of Excess Weight*,[5] map out the staggering impact of food obesity and disease caused mostly by our current food system. It's overwhelming, but here are just a few of the key facts:

- The direct health care costs for chronic health conditions was $1.1 trillion in 2016, or 5.8 percent of our US gross domestic product (GDP).
- The indirect costs, including just lost income, reduced productivity, and impact on caregivers, but not including the impact of our food system on the environment, were another $2.6 trillion. The combined direct and indirect costs are $3.7 trillion, or one in five dollars of our whole economy. Every year!
- Most of the diseases driving the costs are related to obesity and poor diet: abnormal cholesterol, osteoarthritis, type 2 diabetes, high blood pressure, stroke, cancer, Alzheimer's, and kidney failure. It's important to note that these costs do not include pre-diabetes, which affects one in two Americans and causes heart attacks, strokes, and dementia even if it never leads to full-blown type 2 diabetes.
- In ten years 83 million Americans will have three or more chronic diseases, compared to 30 million in 2015. Today 60 percent of Americans

have one chronic disease and 40 percent have two or more chronic diseases.

■ Seventy percent of Americans are either overweight or obese—that's about 228 million Americans! Forty percent are obese, up from 3.4 percent in 1962.

Now let's think about this globally. If 2.2 billion people around the world are overweight, the costs are beyond comprehension. If the burden of chronic disease will cost the American economy $95 trillion over the next 35 years, what might the global costs be?

Global per capita health care costs are one-tenth that of the United States and the global obesity rates are lower as well, but the global costs are also staggering. For argument's sake, if you assume that there are 1,000 times (over 2.2 billion worldwide) as many people overweight in the world as there are in the United States,[6] could the global costs be in the quadrillions of dollars? That's a lot of zeros.

How does this impact us? While Democrats argue to create Medicare for All and Republicans argue to reduce entitlements to bring down our $22 trillion national debt, both are missing the obvious fact. Fix the reason why we have those costs in the first place. Stop the flow of sick people into the system and the harm to our environment and climate by fixing the cause: our food system.

Yet most of our government's policies promote the growing, production, marketing, sale, and consumption of the worst diet on the planet—billions in subsidies (known as crop insurance or other supports) for commodity crops turned into processed food and food for factory-farmed animals; $75 billion a year in food stamp payments that effectively reduce hunger but are mostly for processed food and soda; unregulated food marketing of soda and junk food; confusing food labels; industry-influenced dietary guidelines; and more. Its very policies also support agricultural practices that pollute the environment and worsen climate change.

The Congressional Research Service estimates that by 2025, 48 percent of our entire mandatory federal spending will be for health programs such as Medicare and Medicaid.[7] Bill Haslam, the former governor of Tennessee, shared with me that one in three dollars of its state budget is spent on Medicaid. This does not account for all the federal programs covering health care, including the Department of Veterans Affairs, Department of Defense, Children's Health Insurance Program, and Indian Health Service, among others. All in all, our government covers 50 to 60 percent of health care costs in America. The Government Accountability Office (GAO) projects that by 2048, Medicare and Medicaid will account for $3.2 trillion in federal spending. To put that in perspective, our entire federal tax collections are only $3.8 trillion.[8] There will be almost nothing left for the government as a whole—for defense, education, transportation, or anything else. Neither cutting Medicare nor creating Medicare for All will solve this problem.

HOW TO FIX HEALTH CARE: BEYOND CUTTING ENTITLEMENTS OR MEDICARE FOR ALL

In 2013 I spoke at the World Economic Forum, and at a big gathering of the world's health care leaders from government, the pharmaceutical industry, insurers, and health care systems, I asked a simple question. It was after a distinguished panel focused on fixing health care by better health information technology, improved care coordination, reduction of medical errors, improved efficiencies, and improved payment models, all necessary but not sufficient. Their plan was akin to moving the deck chairs around on the *Titanic*.

Here was the question: Wouldn't it make more sense to address the root causes of chronic disease that are driving the costs, rather than trying to clean up after the fact? The room of 300 people went silent. It was as if I had just revealed the meaning of life. Afterward the panel moderator, the dean of Columbia University's School of Public Health, told me how profound this insight was and how all the health leaders were talking about it after. Really? I was shocked. This is so obvious, yet no one had thought of it.

The World Economic Forum estimated that between 2010 and 2030 the global health care costs for chronic disease will exceed $47 trillion[9] (probably an underestimate given the new, more robust analysis of $95 trillion over 35 years for the United States alone). They declared this the single biggest threat to global economic development. General Motors spends more on health care than on steel, and Starbucks spends more on health care than on coffee beans!

Other analyses from global management consulting firm McKinsey put the global cost of obesity at $2 trillion a year, which is roughly equivalent to the global impact from smoking, armed violence, war, and terrorism combined.[10] In addition, according to the McKinsey Global Institute report, obesity accounts for $2 trillion in lost productivity.[11] Any way you slice it, the costs of obesity and chronic disease are weighing the world down.

We think of these problems as diseases of affluence, but the fact is that the greatest burden, or about 80 percent of obesity and chronic disease, is in the developing world, in low- and middle-income countries. They face what the World Health Organization (WHO) classifies as the "double burden of obesity and malnutrition" and are completely unprepared for this epidemic. There is little health care infrastructure, few doctors and nurses to treat these problems, and even less money.

The "cheap" food that causes disease is not so cheap after all. The hope and promise of the Green Revolution—to use agricultural technology to create abundant cheap food to feed the world—turned out to have horrible unintended consequences. In fact, cheap food turns out to be very, very expensive.

Yes, chronic disease is costly. And kills millions. But that is only a small part of the total cost driven by our food system. Add to these costs the real cost of our food system on the environment, economy, climate, social justice issues, poverty, education, national security, and so on, and this number grows dramatically. Let's explore some of the costs.

THE COSTS WE PAY FOR FARMWORKERS AND FOOD WORKERS

Farmworkers and food industry workers are underpaid and exploited. They face high risks of injury and harm from agricultural chemicals. Most aren't protected by minimum wage or overtime pay requirements. (However, New York State recently passed the Farm Laborers Fair Labor Practices Act.[12]) Many farmworkers live below the poverty line and have no health care, instead depending on emergency rooms and Medicaid. The truth is that the food system disproportionately affects the poor, immigrants, and people of color who actually work in the food system.

The average restaurant worker makes only about $10 an hour.[13] That's why we pay their salary through billions in tips and another $16.5 billion in food stamps. Their dependence on food stamps limits their food choices at the checkout counter, and healthy options are often not affordable enough or government approved.

For those who work on a farm—there are 1 million farmworkers in our country—they have one of the most dangerous jobs in America. They die at seven times the rate of other workers.[14] The Environmental Protection Agency (EPA) estimates that 10,000 to 20,000 farmworkers are harmed by acute pesticide poisoning every year, which doesn't account for the long-term effects of being exposed to toxins day after day and year after year.[15] The herbicides and pesticides that farmers use on their crops are neurotoxins, carcinogens, and hormone disruptors. Many of those used in the United States are banned in other countries. The government agencies (the Food and Drug Administration, or FDA, and EPA) that should be regulating these chemicals for human safety are not doing their job.

THE LOSS OF BIODIVERSITY IN NATURAL AND AGRICULTURAL SYSTEMS: WHY IT MATTERS

While these chemical inputs damage human health, they also disrupt natural ecosystems, deplete the diversity of life in the soil, threaten the loss of most of the plant and animal species we have consumed for millennia, and severely affect pollinators, like honeybees and butterflies, we depend on for agricultural crops.[16] (Chapter 16 explains these consequences in depth.) But the loss of biodiversity, the result of industrial agriculture, is a much bigger problem that threatens global food security. Not only are we threatening insects essential for agricultural production but we are also losing varieties of plant foods and animals at an alarming rate.

According to the UN's Food and Agriculture Organization (FAO), more than 90 percent of plant varieties and half of livestock varieties have been lost to farmers (and the world).[17] Most of our food comes from just twelve plant varieties and five animal species, threatening our food security. Thirty percent of livestock breeds are facing extinction, and six breeds become extinct each month. Just three crops (wheat, corn, rice) account for 60 percent of our food. This occurred because of the centralization of seed production (farmers can't even collect, store, or breed their own plants) by corporations such as Monsanto (now Bayer) as part of the "improvement" of agriculture promoted globally through the Green Revolution and the industrialization of agriculture. Most farmers no longer grow local, resilient, genetically diverse and nutrient-dense varieties. They use only genetically uniform (or GMO) high-yield varieties that require intensive use of fertilizers, pesticides, and herbicides—further destroying the organic matter and biodiversity of the soil that results in less nutrient-dense plants and increased need for irrigation and fertilizer. In all ecosystems, complexity is health; simplicity makes systems vulnerable. Think of monocrop corn (meaning it's the only crop grown on a farm) compared to a rain forest. One plant dies in a rain forest, no problem. One plant dies on a monocrop corn or soy megafarm—no food.

How do we even measure the costs to human health and the threats to our pollinators and the loss of biodiversity? No more bees, no more pollination, no more plants, no more animals—no more humans.

BEYOND JUST THE HEALTH CARE AND SICKNESS COSTS

Before we get too deep into all the additional costs and harm of our food system, the good news is there are solutions that can solve all these problems. In other words, a *food fix*! It is a complex set of related strategies for citizens, businesses, philanthropists, and governments to fix our food system that can occur on a global level. It will not be easy, but it is necessary for our survival as a species, for the economic and political stability of national governments, and for the health of the planet.

The costs of the food system are not borne by the companies that cause these problems. Nor are they paid for at the grocery store or restaurant. They are paid for by all of us indirectly through the loss of our social capital (human happiness, health, productivity, etc.), our natural capital (health of our soil, air, water, climate, oceans, biodiversity, etc.), our economic capital (our ability to address economic disparities and social, environmental, educational, and health care problems), threats to national security, and more.

The silver lining in *Food Fix* is the potential for "the fix" to be an enormous driver of economic growth and innovation. Billions of dollars in investment are flooding into the food and agriculture sectors, creating new businesses, jobs, and national and global economic growth for innovations in farming, food manufacturing, retail, restaurants, health care, and wellness that improve the health of people and the planet. And the side effect will be significant economic growth and jobs from entire new industries and trillions in cost savings by addressing chronic disease; restoring ecosystems that include soil, water, and biodiversity; and reversing climate change. The countries that get this right will not only help humans and the earth, but leap ahead in the twenty-first-century economy for jobs and economic growth.

In *Food Fix* we will unpack how all these factors contribute to suffering and lack in the world. We will learn how we as citizens, businesses, philanthropists, and governments can begin to restore the health of our people, our communities, our economies, and the environment.

There is a Jewish concept called *tikkun olam*, which roughly translates to "repair of the world." That is what our work must be, and the hope of this book.

THE INVISIBLE COSTS OF OUR FOOD SYSTEM

All of us pay the invisible costs. The true costs are not paid for by the food system that generates the costs. We must have a true accounting for this cascade of unintended consequences of our food system, including climate change; depletion of fresh water, forests, and soil; damage to our oceans; loss of biodiversity; pollution; and chronic disease and its economic burden.

Understanding these complicated and diverse effects of human activity and how they destroy our human, natural, social, and economic capital is not an easy task. Yet it is essential to our survival. Shifting our thinking from seeing health care, disease, social justice, poverty, environment, climate, education, economics, and national security as separate problems—in other words, connecting the dots, thinking of the interdependencies and the systems nature of this problem—is critical to solving it. It will require collaboration and action by governments, businesses, nonprofits, and citizens to solve. But the first step is to understand these connections.

There is no way I can create a comprehensive catalogue of all these impacts and all the solutions (and there are many) in this book, but giving examples and mapping out the big picture I hope will stimulate a new wave of thinking and actions to solve this problem. Sometimes I feel like I am standing on a beach watching a tsunami approach while everyone around me is sunbathing and playing in the water, oblivious to the implications of what is about to happen.

ACCOUNTING FOR SUSTAINABILITY AND CONSEQUENCES OF OUR FOOD SYSTEM

The true cost of food is not on the price tag. If the true price of food were built into the price we pay, or if Big Ag and Big Food had to pay for the harm caused by the food they produce—the pollution, the loss of biodiversity, the loss of soil and cropland, the depletion of our water resources, chronic disease, the loss of intellectual capital due to harm to our children's brains from ultraprocessed food, farmworker and food worker injustices, the threat to national security, and other damaging outcomes—then your grass-fed steak and organic, regeneratively grown produce and food would be much cheaper than industrial food. Sometimes it takes litigation to hold these companies accountable. For example, over a 30-year period General Electric dumped 1.3 million pounds of polychlorinated biphenyls (PCBs) into the Hudson River. Eventually they were held to account and were forced to pay more than $1.7 billion to clean it up. All the costs of food need to be quantified and measured. What gets measured gets managed.

A movement is underway to truly account for the real costs—to humans, to the environment, and to the economies of our current industrial food system. It is called *true cost accounting*. Some costs are easy to measure, like direct health care costs. Some are harder to measure, such as the damage to climate and environment, or social justice impacts. But many groups are working hard to assess all these factors and map out an honest view of the consequences of how we grow food, what we grow, and how it affects those who grow it and eat it, as well as the impact on governments and economies. Changes in our food policy to account for these costs and leveraging taxes and incentives can have a profound impact on and improve the overall health of humanity and the planet.[18]

In their report *The True Cost of American Food,* the Sustainable Food Trust details exactly how seemingly unrelated silos in health care, policy, environment, climate, agriculture, and the food industry are all connected. The UN Environment's TEEBAgriFood (the Economics of

Ecosystems and Biodiversity for Agriculture and Food) group and their recent report *Measuring What Matters in Agriculture and Food Systems* also help define the problems and solutions. We need to analyze all the impacts of our food system, good or bad, and their costs or savings to create a new economic model that reflects the true cost of food and build the business case for a sustainable, regenerative food system.

A TALE OF TWO FOODS: AN INCONVENIENT AND INVISIBLE TRUTH

Let's take a journey with your average hamburger or steak and a can of soda. It's a powerful mental exercise to track the entire path of the food we eat. We don't typically think of the life cycle of anything we eat; we happily chomp along without much thought to how our choices affect all the things we care about. It's easier just to enjoy and stay oblivious. But we cannot afford to be unconscious anymore. The stakes are too high.

The story starts in Iowa or maybe Brazil. And it winds its way through the food chain to your plate. If the corn that fed the factory-farmed cattle came from Brazil, the only added baggage is that you helped cut down ancient rain forests, which are essential to suck up carbon from the atmosphere and keep our planet cool. The two main products of soy are soy oil (the building block of processed food) and soy meal, used for chicken, pig, pet, farmed fish and dairy cow, and processed human food like plant-based burgers. Corn and soy mono-crop megafarms and CAFOs (confined animal feeding operations) or factory farms in Iowa and Brazil all create the same problems. Here's how:

THE MONOPOLY OF THE SEEDS

First the GMO seeds are sold to farmers by Big Ag seed monopolies. Four big companies, Bayer (which recently purchased Monsanto), Chem-China and its subsidiary Syngenta, Corteva, and BASF, formed by giant mergers over the last few years, control most of the seeds in the world, including 60 percent of the vegetable seeds. These companies burden farmers with less choice and higher prices, making them dependent on their seeds and their chemicals. These companies produce the seeds but also the pesticides and herbicides that are used on the crops. The consolidation and centralization of seed production means that we have less food biodiversity and resiliency, which threatens our food security. It also means the loss of autonomy to save and collect seeds for farmers, especially for the 2.5 billion small farm holders across the globe. They have to buy their seeds only from the seed monopolies.

Only 1 percent of corn grown in America is sweet corn actually consumed by humans. The rest is *dent* corn, used for food oils, animal feed (for cattle), ethanol, high-fructose corn syrup (HFCS; for your sugary soda), biodegradable plastic, alcohol, food starch, and food additives (for your hamburger bun). Soy is increasingly used for biodiesel, which will drive the price up. Soy and corn monocrops account for 53 percent of all farmland. Much of that food goes to feed animals on CAFOs or factory farms, which in many places in the developed world are now the main way we produce animals for human consumption. It varies globally, but in the United States only 27 percent of cropland is used to grow food for humans, while 67 percent is used to grow food for factory-farmed animals.[19] According to the UN FAO, worldwide, 70 percent of total agricultural land is suitable only for grazing animals (and not suitable for growing crops) and, as we will see in Part 5, is a key part of the solution for climate change.

THE DESTRUCTION OF SOIL AND RAIN FORESTS: CLIMATE CHANGE AND DESERTS

The problem is not only that portions of the crops are grown for feedlot animals (including the cattle for your burger) and HFCS for your soda. How those crops are grown also creates massive destruction. The crops are grown through intensive industrial farming that leads to massive soil erosion and loss of soil carbon, worsening climate change. In Iowa, we lose 1 pound of topsoil for every pound of corn grown. The cost of soil erosion from industrial agriculture is $44 billion a year. We lose almost 2 billion tons of topsoil a year.[20] That's about 200,000 tons every hour. We have lost a third of all our topsoil—which took billions of years to create—in the last 150 years. The UN projects that in 60 years we may completely "mine" all our topsoil, making it almost impossible to grow food. Soil gone. No food. No people. That's sixty more harvests. What will your grandchildren eat?

Soil erosion and the loss of carbon in soil lead to the massive global problem of desertification, the decline of farm- or rangeland into deserts. Twelve million hectares of land, an area the size of Nicaragua or North Korea, are lost every year to desert. The land we lose every year could produce 20 million tons of grain.[21]

And this is not just in developed countries. There is a big demand for palm oil (even used in "health" foods), which comes from cleared rain forests in Southeast Asia. This drives soil erosion, river and air pollution, and climate change. It destroys habitats for wildlife and threatens extinction of animals such as orangutans.

There is a difference between dirt and soil. Dirt is lifeless and dead and cannot hold water or carbon. Dirt contains very few microorganisms, fungi, or worms, all of which are needed to extract nutrients from the soil to feed the plants. So dirt requires massive inputs of fertilizer, pesticides, herbicides, and water just to grow our food. This further ruins soil. In the United States we use more than 1 billion pounds of pesticides a year, and globally we use 5.4 billion pounds of pesticides and over 200 million pounds of fertilizers, both of which destroy soil life.[22] Healthy soil, on the other hand, is alive, teeming with microbes. Just 2 square centimeters of soil have more life and microbial diversity than anything else in the universe. Soil can hold hundreds of thousands of gallons of water per acre, protecting against droughts and floods. Soil is the biggest carbon sink on the planet. Think of it as the rain forest of the prairies; it can sequester more carbon and do more to reverse climate change than all the rain forests in the world. Restoring all our dirt on the planet to soil could completely draw down carbon in the environment to preindustrial levels. Healthy soil reduces or eliminates the need for pesticides, herbicides, and fertilizers. Healthy soil extracts nutrients from the earth, making them available to plants and humans. Over the last 100 years mineral levels in our food have dropped dramatically.[23] Soil feeds plants by making micronutrients and macronutrients available to the plants; dirt doesn't—it requires chemical inputs to grow plants.

THIS IS NOT SUSTAINABLE

All the aspects of our food system make it the number one cause of climate change, exceeding that of the energy sector, mostly because of deforestation, CO_2 emissions and methane from factory farms, nitrous oxide, CO_2, and methane from the overuse of fossil-fuel-based fertilizer, food transport and storage, and food waste. In fact, the process of producing fertilizer creates one hundred times more methane than reported by the fertilizer industry.[24] One-third to one-half of all greenhouse gas emissions come from industrial agriculture, which releases 600 million tons of CO_2 equivalent into the air every year.[25]

In addition to the direct harms of our current system is the lost opportunity to provide the economic and ecosystem benefits of innovations in agriculture, including regenerative agriculture, forests on farms, silvopasture (raising animals among orchards to increase soil fertility and reduce need for water and fertilizer), etc. The benefits of these innovations in agriculture (see Part 5) have been estimated to be twice as big as the harms from our current agricultural model.

The media, governments, and even the Paris climate agreement focus almost entirely on the energy sector, not agriculture. The Paris Agreement didn't even mention that the food system itself is a bigger cause of climate change than the energy sector. Our agricultural system is both the greatest cause of and at risk of being the most affected by climate change. The inconvenient truth is that our climate is heating up. The invisible truth is that our food system is the biggest cause.

THE LOSS OF THE WORLD'S FRESH WATER

Now back to the GMO corn used to feed the beef cattle. We have to irrigate these crops because soil that has been depleted can't hold water (which of course leads to the increased number of floods and droughts we have seen in recent years). Seventy percent of the human use of the world's fresh water is for agriculture.[26] Significant portions of it are used for growing food for animals rather than humans or for ethanol. The thing is, these animals are supposed to eat grass, graze on rangelands, and drink rainwater or eat grass grown with rainwater, not eat corn irrigated by fresh water from precious aquifers and rivers.

Water is a limited resource. Only 5 percent of water on the planet is fresh water. Lake Baikal in Russia contains 1 percent. We are depleting our ancient aquifers faster than rainfall can replenish them. The biggest one in America, the Ogallala Aquifer in the Midwest, is being depleted by more than a trillion gallons more a year than can be refilled by rain.[27] Irrigation of crops is the main cause. Dirt can't hold water. Soil can. If we switched to range (grass)-fed regenerative livestock production, we would restore soils, draw down carbon (reversing climate change), and store massive amounts of water, which can prevent floods and droughts. No water, no food, no humans. The solution is soil, not oil. According to a 2019 UN report, $300 billion invested in regenerative agriculture would be enough to restore 900 hectares of the 2 billion hectares (5 million acres) of degraded land in the world, build soil, and slow down climate change enough to give us more than 20 years to innovate climate-change solutions.[28] That is the total global military spending in just 60 days, or less than one-tenth the annual cost of obesity and diabetes in the United States.

FERTILIZERS: DESTROYING LAKES AND OCEANS

The nitrogen fertilizer, pesticides, and herbicides used to grow the plants that in part feed the beef cattle that becomes your burger all come from fossil fuels—and one-fifth of fossil fuels are used for agriculture and our food system.[29] That's more than all transportation from cars, planes, and ships combined. There are 10 million tons of fertilizer used just to grow corn in America. There are 200 million tons of fertilizer used across the world every year.[30]

The nitrogen fertilizer runs off these megafarms into rivers and down to lakes. Recently Lake Erie in Cleveland was suffocated by algal blooms, killing the fish and creating a big dead zone in the lake and toxic drinking water for Toledo, Ohio. Lake Erie is dying partly because of your hamburger or feedlot steak. Toledo alone spent $1 billion just to address the polluted water for its residents.[31]

The nitrogen-rich fertilizer also dumps into rivers that run to the ocean. When the runoff from Midwest industrial farms hits the Gulf of Mexico, it creates an 8,000-square-mile dead zone—that's the size of New Jersey. In the Gulf of Mexico alone, it kills 212,000 metric tons of seafood a year.[32] That's a boatload of sushi and gumbo! There are almost 400 similar dead zones around the world, collectively the size of Europe. We produce massive amounts of soy and corn used to make factory-farmed meat, ethanol, biofuels, cooking oils, and ultraprocessed food, and the "side effect" is destroying one of the healthiest protein sources in the world—seafood. The cost of nitrogen pollution is estimated at $210 billion a year.[33] And there are other unintended consequences. The nitrogen runoff ends up in our tap water, resulting in increased cancer rates and birth defects, preterm labor, and low birth weights.[34]

Raising animals through managed grazing and regenerative agriculture will protect our waterways and save millions of tons of fish. (More on this in Part 5.) We will also produce meat that is healthier for humans and the planet and more humane for the animals and farmworkers.

It's not just big soy and corn operations that cause the problem, but giant beef, hog, and chicken factory farms that dump massive amounts of waste (full of more nitrogen) into giant lagoons that run off into rivers and lakes too. Remember Hurricane Florence in North Carolina, which swamped these operations? More than fifty hog lagoons overflowed and flooded local waterways.[35] Guess what happened to all that waste.

Depressed yet?

It gets worse. I am not going through this to depress you—but to help you connect the dots so we can solve this problem as a whole, not piecemeal. Telling Americans to eat less and exercise more only blames the victim. The food industry produces that addictive burger and soda that override willpower, driving your body to gain weight.[36] Toxic foods like that create an astounding amount of secondary consequences for humans, the environment, and the economy.

THE TRUE COST OF YOUR FOOD: JUST A FEW MORE UNINTENDED CONSEQUENCES

I hope you are getting the picture of all the additional costs—the ones you don't pay at the grocery store or restaurant. What if the real cost of food and our food system was actually built into the price? What if farmers who provide ecosystem services (building soil, improving water use, and biodiversity) were paid for those services, while Big Ag, seed, chemical, and fertilizer companies that use up ecosystem services (depleting organic matter in the soil, overuse and pollution of freshwater resources, destruction of biodiversity such as pollinator species, and the contribution to climate change) were charged for their impact and ecosystem destruction? Maybe the factory-farmed burger should cost $1,000 a pound. Maybe the can of soda would be $100. Maybe the cost of grass-fed steak would be only $3 a pound. On Amazon, Smartwater (made by Coca-Cola) is 9 cents an ounce. Pepsi is 2 cents an ounce (in a 2-liter bottle). When water is more than four times the cost of soda, we have a problem.

Here are some of the rest of the costs hidden in your feedlot steak or burger (or pretty much any food grown in our industrial agricultural system):[37]

- Pesticide poisoning and related illnesses cost $1 billion a year.
- Other pesticide costs including death of birds and insect pollinators (bees and butterflies), loss of biodiversity, crop loss, and groundwater contamination are about $7 billion a year.

- Cleanup of manure from CAFOs costs about $4 billion a year. There are millions of these animals, and they produce more than 300 million tons of manure a year, which is held in open pits or manure lagoons and contaminates land, water, and air. This cost doesn't account for all the illnesses, like asthma, in nearby communities from aerosolized toxins caused by this pollution.
- Declining property values around CAFOs are $26 billion a year. Who wants to live near a stinky, polluted hog, chicken, or beef operation?
- Taxpayer subsidies for these factory farms from our Farm Bill are about $13 billion a year.
- Fast-food employees make so little money to serve up your burger (and fries and soda) that they need food stamps to buy their own food. That costs us about $7 billion a year.
- Increasing CO_2 in the atmosphere acidifies the oceans, killing phytoplankton, which produce 50 percent of the oxygen we breathe. Cost? What is the price of losing 50 percent of our oxygen?
- Antibiotic use in animal feed to promote growth and prevent infection from overcrowding is a big contributor to antibiotic resistance in humans, which kills 700,000 people a year and costs trillions globally every year. The antibiotics also end up in manure and slurries that are spread on fields (including organic crops) and destroy the soil microbiology.

This is not a complete list. But you get the point. The global cost is not in the billions or even trillions but in the *quadrillions*. Much of it is hard to measure. How do you measure the loss of biodiversity or the destruction of coral reefs, or the decimation of phytoplankton, which produce so much of the oxygen we breathe? Who is paying that cost? You are. I am. We are. The planet is. Natural habitats and oceans are. Even the historical diversity of seeds used to grow our food is suffering. We are losing our nutritional heritage due to seed monopolies. And the list goes on. If you get that feedlot burger (or any food), you may not finish it but may toss the remains in the trash, contributing to the massive problem of food waste. Another $2 trillion in costs!

FOOD WASTE: WHAT A WASTE!

Food waste is enormous. Up to 40 percent of our food is wasted in the field, in transport, in the retail environment, in restaurants, by food service companies, or in our homes and sent to landfills.[38] Think of all the resources that go into growing, transporting, distributing, and buying the food: seeds, water, energy, land, fertilizer, labor, and financial capital wasted. Mind-boggling. We have more than enough food to feed all the humans in the world and more (up to 10.5 billion people) with our existing food supply. Yet 800 million go to bed hungry and 2 billion are malnourished. The waste of all that food, the additional farmland and farming practices used to grow it, the need for deforestation to grow more food because so much is wasted, and the rotting of that food in landfills, producing toxic methane that heats up our climate, make food waste the third-biggest emitter of greenhouse gases on the planet, after the United States and China. (More on this in Chapter 17.)

But there are solutions. Some cities such as San Francisco mandate composting. France made it illegal for supermarkets to throw out food and instead requires them to send it to food banks, compost companies, or farms for animal feed. Nonprofits such as Feeding the 5000 have had forty global events feeding 5,000 people entirely from food waste. Even top chefs like Dan Barber showcase gourmet meals made entirely of food scraps—for example, carrot peels, ends of celery, and stems of mushrooms.

These solutions are just the beginning, but solving this problem will reduce hunger, reduce the need for croplands and deforestation, and reduce CO_2 in the environment by 70.53 gigatons, making it the third-most important solution for drawing down carbon and reversing climate change, according to Project Drawdown.

THE UNEXPECTED CONSEQUENCES OF CLIMATE CHANGE FOR PUBLIC HEALTH

The 2018 Report of the Lancet *Countdown on Health and Climate Change: Shaping the Health of Nations for Centuries to Come*[39] documents the human health impacts of climate change. Climate refugees are real, displaced by natural disasters and extreme weather events. The UN projections estimate that by 2050 there will be 200 million to 1 billion climate refugees.[40] That was the entire population of the world in 1820. To put it in perspective, the Syrian refugee crisis, which was in part due to climate change and drought, amounted to just 1 million refugees.

Vulnerable populations around the world are exposed to weather extremes, increased infectious disease, and threats to their food security. In 2017, 712 extreme weather events resulted in $326 billion in economic losses, triple the economic losses from just a year earlier.[41] Heat waves resulted in 153 billion hours of labor lost because it was too hot to work. Higher temperatures increase disease—cholera, malaria, and dengue fever, among others. The heat also worsens health and increases the demand for limited health care services for those with heart disease, type 2 diabetes, and lung diseases. Agriculture is also in turn affected by climate change and increasing temperatures, with downward trends in yields in thirty countries threatening food security. This is clearly not all about our food system, as other factors drive climate change, but since our food system is the single biggest contributor, if we fix it, it would be the single biggest solution. In 2019 the Intergovernmental Panel on Climate Change (IPCC) issued a landmark report entitled *Climate Change and Land, an IPCC Special Report on Climate Change, Desertification, Land Degradation, Sustainable Land Management, Food Security, and Greenhouse Gas Fluxes in Terrestrial Ecosystems.*[42] This report lays out the imperative of reimagining our agricultural system as a key solution to climate change and food and political security.

In Chapter 17 we will take a deeper dive into climate change and how our food system and innovative agricultural solutions can help us solve this unprecedented crisis, which is worse than we think.

We also have a co-opted government. When I asked Ann Veneman, the former secretary of agriculture under George W. Bush, why we couldn't have science guide our policies for food and agriculture, or why we don't stop the marketing of junk food to kids, or have more transparent food labels, or stop subsidies for commodities turned into processed food, or create subsidies for fruit and vegetables, she told me that it was the food and agriculture industry's influence on Congress and the administration.

The Farm Bill, which controls most of our food and agricultural policies, is heavily influenced by lobbyists. Over 600 companies spent $500 million to influence the 2014 Farm Bill to get what they wanted.[43] Almost 73 percent of the members of the Senate Committee on Agriculture, Nutrition and Forestry and 90 percent of the House Agricultural Committee receive donations from Monsanto (Bayer) and Syngenta. If you add in all the other food and agriculture companies, 100 percent of the members would have received donations.[44]

SODA AND SUGAR-SWEETENED BEVERAGES: THE WEIGHT OF CORN

The soda and sugar-sweetened beverage story is pretty much the same as that for your burger or steak—damage to the environment, huge costs to society, and massive economic consequences from drinking the high-fructose corn syrup that sweetens your soda, energy drinks, teas, and coffees. But there is one big difference. Feedlot meat isn't great for you. But eating it doesn't kill people except through the downstream effects we just reviewed. Sugar does! Especially high-fructose corn syrup, which is used for sugar-sweetened beverages. These kill 186,000 people a year from heart disease, diabetes, and cancer caused by drinking sugar-sweetened beverages.[45] The risk goes up with every additional soda.[46]

A recent study found that your risk of death from heart disease was

31 percent higher if you consumed two sugar-sweetened beverages a day.[47] Every extra drink caused the risk to go up by another 10 percent. I was recently shopping at a convenience store in Utah and at the checkout counter was a very overweight woman buying two 2-liter bottles of soda while she sucked on the straw of her 40-ounce Big Gulp Mountain Dew. I wish this was an aberration, but it is a common practice in America.

The other big problem with the soda industry is that as taxpayers we pay for 31 billion servings of soda to the poor through SNAP (Supplemental Nutrition Assistance Program), or food stamps. That is $7 billion a year, the biggest line item in SNAP, which accounts for almost 10 percent of the "food" purchased by SNAP recipients. You can do the math yourself. If a 2-liter bottle of Coke is $1.79 at Target, that's 22 cents per 8-ounce serving, and that's 31 billion servings. Soda is one of the very few things that has been proven to cause obesity.[48]

THE REAL PRICE OF CORN

We actually pay four times for our corn.

First, we subsidize the growing of corn to the tune of about $250 million a year. About 8 percent of that corn is used to make high-fructose corn syrup. The rest is used for feed for factory-farmed animals, ethanol, cooking oil, alcohol, industrial products, and processed-food additives.

Second, we pay for the environmental consequences of modern corn production. Modern chemical-intensive till farming causes compaction and loss of topsoil. This causes an increase in greenhouse gases because industrial monocrop, chemical agriculture depletes organic matter in soils. Then we pay for all the damage from the nitrogen runoff to waterways and oceans, the harm from the pesticides and herbicides, and the depletion of our water resources.

Third, through SNAP we pay for a lot of the junk food and sugar-sweetened beverages made from corn syrup—that's about $75 billion a year. In fact, money earned from SNAP makes up about 20 percent of

Coca-Cola's annual revenue in the United States. That doesn't include any revenue from noncarbonated sugar drinks like Powerade or Vitaminwater. That makes Coca-Cola a billion-dollar welfare recipient.

And fourth, we pay for all the health care costs of obesity and chronic diseases (caused mostly by diet), or about $3.7 trillion a year.[49] Sadly, there are other costs to our children. We are overfed but undernourished. Obesity, food insecurity, and malnutrition occur in the same people. In the United States, 7 percent of our children are stunted, which causes permanent developmental, neurological, and long-term economic impacts for them and for society.

So, what should that can of soda cost? A lot more than 22 cents for an 8-ounce serving! Maybe it should be $100 a can or more.

Turns out that your fast-food burger and soda are far more expensive than a grass-fed steak and a glass of water when the true cost is taken into account.

And we pay for it all through our government supports for industrial agriculture, including the euphemistically named crop insurance, which mostly go to large, multimillion-dollar industrial farms, and most of those dollars end up in the pockets of the chemical, seed, and fertilizer companies that supply those farms. Taxpayers fund the SNAP program. Weirdly, the USDA won't disclose where those dollars are used, saying it is protecting the privacy of big retailers like Walmart and Kroger. A South Dakota newspaper decided this data should be public under the Freedom of Information Act (FOIA) and has filed a lawsuit to make the data public. The case has gone to the Supreme Court.[50] Shouldn't the government protect citizens, not corporations? What are they hiding?

We indirectly support the food industry's marketing of junk food to children, the poor, and minorities by allowing it to deduct $190 billion a year in advertising costs,[51] while absolving it of the responsibility to pay for the chronic disease caused by that food. Taxpayers pay for all the sickness caused by eating this food, through Medicare, Medicaid, and all the other medical coverage the US government provides for more than 50 percent of the population.

This simply isn't just, ethical, moral, or right. It must be fixed. We need full transparency and honesty about the costs of our current food system on each one of us and on our communities, society, economy, and environment.

FOOD FIX: THE TRUE COST OF FOOD

There is not one simple solution to the challenges of farming, diet, public health, the economy, the environment, the climate, workers' rights, education, national security, social justice, health, income inequities, health disparities, and more. But they are all connected in one way or another by one thing.

Food.

We need to think about these issues as one interconnected, intersecting set of challenges that we can and must address if we are to reverse the crises we now face and avert the disasters just over the horizon: rising global temperatures, loss of all our topsoil, depletion of our freshwater resources, loss of the earth's biodiversity, increasing desertification, hunger, malnutrition, and obesity, the burden of chronic disease, and the instability of governments and economies, to mention just a few. Many of these problems started as unintended consequences of good intentions and policies:

- Food stamps (SNAP) started as a way to address hunger and malnutrition but now drive obesity and disease for 46 million Americans. While it effectively addresses food insecurity, SNAP is not leveraged to improve the nutrition or health of its recipients.
- Agricultural policies historically protected farmers from weather and price fluctuations and supported increased crop production, but now these same policies and agricultural practices are the number one cause of climate change, deplete global water resources, and drive environmental destruction and the production of cheap ingredients that are mostly turned into processed disease-promoting food-like substances.

- Fertilizers were created to increase crop yields and help farmers around the world produce more food.
- The discovery of vitamins, the Great Depression, and World War II focused the nation on producing inexpensive and vitamin-rich shelf-stable starchy calories. The food system we have is not an accident but is mostly the result of good intentions and conscious goals that were mostly met. Though 800 million around the world still suffer from hunger and many more from food insecurity, the efforts of the mid-twentieth century food system were very successful. According to Tufts University's Dariush Mozafarrian, "the unintended consequences were the focus on a few staple commodities, the hyper-processing of foods, which led to the erosion of land, soil, water resources, and climate, and the failure to increase protective minimally processed foods, all leading to the chronic disease and sustainability crises we see today."
- This juggernaut is linked to things seemingly unrelated: the $22 trillion US national debt, chronic disease and obesity, destruction of our environment by pollution, climate change, poverty, social injustice, loss of our children's ability to learn and develop, political instability, and the destruction of our communities. Food connects them all. How we grow it, process it, produce it, distribute it, consume it, and waste it affects almost everything that matters in our world today.

Yet this is a fixable problem. Taking a step back, looking at the problem holistically, as one system out of balance, will help us reimagine the world we want, the world we can create by addressing the overall dysfunctions in our food system. We can solve these problems. Solutions exist. They will call on multiple sectors and stakeholders—from citizens and consumers, businesses and farmers, and policy makers in every level of government, including city and state, to nonprofits, philanthropists, and scientists—coming together in global agreement and efforts to transform our food system.

Think of it as the Paris Accord, where 195 countries came together to create voluntary agreements to address climate change, but this will be an accord for food, or for the UN Sustainable Development Goals for our food system (which in part already address these issues). Imagine if opposing groups come together to fight a common problem, like the various kingdoms in *Game of Thrones* who come together to fight the army of the dead, because the survival of them all depends on it. Imagine if aliens came to threaten our planet; we would form a global effort to fight back. This is what we urgently need right now. This affects every single one of us. And it is the defining problem of our time.

Throughout each part of this book, I will share some of these solutions. Some are well-formed programs that already exist. Some are proposed solutions by experts. Some are easy to implement, others more difficult. They are meant to highlight what is needed and what is possible, rather than be a comprehensive set of solutions. Citizens, farmers, businesses, investors, nonprofits, and governments all must play their part. This is a starting point for a deeper exploration as a society, a road map for the change that is needed to address these challenges together. These ideas are meant to inspire, educate, and motivate individuals, businesses, and government policy makers to innovate and think differently about these issues—to see the linkages, the need for systems thinking, the need for thoughtful integrated solutions.

In 2018, Dariush Mozaffarian, MD, dean of Tufts School of Nutrition Science and Policy, and I met with Representative Tim Ryan of Ohio and suggested that all of our government's various policies on health, nutrition, agriculture, and food were not integrated, often working at odds with one another, and overseen by eight different agencies, without any awareness of their effectiveness, influence on public health, or economic impact. That led to a request by Congress for the Government Accountability Office, the government's independent assessors of the effectiveness and cost of government policies, to examine these issues in detail and report on recommended actions to fix them. We each can make a difference.

We need new ideas, strategies, policies, and business innovations to fix these problems and bring diverse groups together to solve them. It is possible. Solutions exist. They are achievable, and we need the push from the grass roots and from the top down to shift public opinion, to create a movement that forces legislatures and policy makers to take notice and take action. We can use the power of our forks and our collective behaviors to move in the right direction. Throughout *Food Fix* we will explore the specific ways in which citizens, businesses, and policy makers can solve the biggest problem we face today—our broken food system and all its consequences.

I hope you will join the **FoodRx Campaign,** take personal action, and urge our policy makers to fix our food system so we can improve the health of millions of Americans, our economy, and our environment. To learn more and join the movement, go to www.FoodRxCampaign.org.

CHAPTER 2

THE GLOBAL EPIDEMIC OF CHRONIC DISEASE: THE ROLE OF OUR FOOD SYSTEM

The chronic diseases that are sweeping across the globe and weighing down global economies can't be cured by better medication or medical care. Food is the biggest cause of chronic disease and the economic burden it places on families, societies, and nations. While the cost of health care is only going to balloon as we move into the future, we don't need to wait 35 years to see the damaging effects of our food system.

In 2019 *The Lancet* published an analysis of dietary risk factors in 195 countries based on the Global Burden of Disease Study, the most comprehensive study of the effects of diet on health ever conducted, covering a 27-year period.[1] Despite the limitations of the study, the bottom line was this: A diet without enough healthy foods (fruits and vegetables, nuts and seeds, whole grains, etc.) and with too many bad foods (processed foods, refined grains, sugar-sweetened beverages, trans fats, etc.) accounted for 11 million deaths and 255 million years of disability and life years lost. Most striking was the finding that the lack of protective foods (whole real unprocessed foods) was as or more important in determining risk of death than the overconsumption of processed foods. This is a big deal.

We are facing an unprecedented threat from biological weapons of mass destruction—the food produced by our food system that drives disease, suffering, environmental destruction, and climate change.

Imagine if an infectious disease like Ebola or Zika or AIDS or cholera killed 11 million people a year. We would have a global effort to find a cure, to address the public health factors—and governments, scientists, philanthropists, and businesses would be aligned to fight these threats. Yet there is silence when it comes to our global response to the most common kinds of preventable deaths.

I was recently at the Milken Global Conference listening to a panel of the leading thinkers and actors in health care—the head of the National Institutes of Health, the CEO of the Bill and Melinda Gates Foundation, the head of the Center for Medicare and Medicaid Services, and the CEO of Kaiser health systems. They spoke of important things—eradicating polio, malaria, and AIDS, gene editing to cure rare genetic disorders, improving the interoperability of medical records, data sharing, and improving medical payments systems to pay for value. All great advances. But no one talked about the elephant in the room: the tsunami of disease, death, and costs driven by our poor diet, not to mention the effects of our food system on the environment, climate, and even social justice. It dwarfs every other problem.

The reason this problem is pretty much ignored or attacked piecemeal is that this epidemic has come on fast and furiously over the last 40 years and blindsided society and governments. And better medication or medical care can't solve these chronic diseases. The solution? Our forks.

Yes, it is true. There is no denying it now. The food we eat (or the food we don't eat) is the single biggest cause of death worldwide, exceeding tobacco and every other known risk factor. Historically, infections, poor sanitation, or what we call communicable disease caused most deaths. Now more than 70 percent of deaths worldwide are from what we call "noncommunicable disease," conditions like heart disease, obesity, type 2 diabetes, cancer, and dementia. However, as we'll see in Part 4, there is a problem with the term *noncommunicable*. It implies that these conditions—such as heart disease, cancer, diabetes, dementia, and depression, among others—just appear randomly, or that they are the result of poor judgment. However, these diseases are highly contagious and driven by the structural environment—

government policies, poverty, and a pervasive and increasingly toxic global food system and environment that create conditions ripe for poor diet and chronic disease, often referred to as the social determinants of health.

We often blame the victim for these diseases. No one blames someone for getting malaria or tuberculosis. But for chronic disease we put the blame on individuals, on personal responsibility. It turns out that it is our social environment—what Paul Farmer from Partners in Health has called structural violence—the social, economic, and political conditions that drive disease. If we live in a world where our food system mainly produces disease-causing foods, where a food carnival makes it almost impossible to make the right choice, where our government supports the production and sale of these foods, where these foods are biologically addictive, then personal choice is a fiction.

The science is clear: Noncommunicable diseases, it turns out, are very communicable. You are more likely to be overweight if your friends are overweight than if your family is overweight.[2] Depending on your neighborhood, your life expectancy may be 20 to 30 years shorter than that of folks from another county, city, or state. Simply moving an overweight diabetic from a low socioeconomic neighborhood to a slightly better one leads to weight loss and improvement in diabetes, without any other intervention.[3]

This is far more than an issue of personal choice and behavior. The food we have available to eat (ultraprocessed food) and the food we don't eat (fruits and vegetables and whole foods) are determined by the food system itself—what we grow and produce and how we market and distribute it, and what we don't.

According to the lead author of the *Lancet* study, "There is an urgent and compelling need for changes in the various sectors of the food production cycle, such as growing, processing, packaging, and marketing. Our research finds the need for a comprehensive food system intervention to promote the production, distribution, and consumption of healthy foods across nations." Basically, our whole food production system from the field to the fork focuses on producing foods that make us sick and fat and cause us to die early, rather than on foods that make us healthy, prevent disease, and help us live a long, productive life. Sadly, both the intended and unintended consequences of our global food system provide too much of the bad stuff and not enough good stuff. It is killing us.

THE PERILS AND PROMISE OF FOOD

I recently saw a picture of a beach scene from the 1970s and another from Woodstock. I could not find a single image of anyone overweight, never mind obese, in a sea of humans. What has happened to us reminds me of the story of the frog in boiling water. If you put a frog in boiling water, it will jump right out. If you put a frog in tepid water and slowly heat it up, the frog will just boil to death. That is us today as we head into the middle of the twenty-first century.

Over the past 40 years, since the government's first dietary guidelines encouraged us to cut the fat and increase the carbs (a deadly idea), and since the expansion of extractive, industrial agriculture, which has produced hundreds of thousands of food-like substances from a very few raw materials (wheat, soy, and corn), we are now a nation where being an optimal weight is an anomaly. We have created the worst diet in the world and are exporting it to every country on the planet.

When I graduated medical school, there was not a single state with an obesity rate over 20 percent. Now there is not a single state with an obesity rate under 20 percent, and within the last few years we have seen many states surpass an adult obesity rate of 40 percent and most others are closing in on 40 percent.[4] Obesity, now officially considered a disease, and its downstream diseases (heart disease, cancer, type 2 diabetes, dementia, arthritis, and others) are literally weighing down our species, our communities, our environment, and our economy, depleting human, social, economic, and natural capital in ways both visible and invisible.

Approximately 60 percent of our calories in the United States come from ultraprocessed foods, with the poor, minorities, the young, and the less educated consuming the most.[5] This leads not only to obesity and disease, but also to micronutrient deficiencies and malnutrition. More than 90 percent of Americans are deficient in one or more nutrients at the level that creates vitamin deficiencies such as scurvy, rickets, and others.[6] The paradox is that we provide our population with too many calories and not enough nutrients. We are overfed and undernourished. Surprisingly, the most obese adults and children are the most malnourished.[7] And globally this problem is even worse.

What is the root cause of this tsunami of chronic disease that affects more than one in two Americans and increasingly our global population? The reasons are complex, but it is a combination of physical inactivity, smoking, excess alcohol consumption, and diet. But our diet and our food system are by far the biggest contributors to the structural factors that have led to this epidemic of chronic disease. The shift in our food quality, our food and health policies, our agricultural practices, and business "innovations" in product development and marketing in the more than $15 trillion food industry (food[8] and agriculture[9]) have created a disease-creating food system and economy. This shift grew from both the unintended consequences of policies and practices thought to be innovative and "better for you" such as the promotion of margarine and shortening—which has likely killed millions since the development of Crisco in 1911—and the deliberate practices and policies driven by an amoral food system hungry for profit and market (or stomach) share.

But we can change this trajectory—first in our own homes, then in our country, and finally globally.

THE PROBLEM OF ULTRAPROCESSED FOODS

Despite the fact that we produce more than enough food for our global population, we still have more than 800 million people who go to bed hungry and 2 billion who have nutrient deficiencies that result in stunting, impaired cognitive development, risk for infectious disease, and chronic diseases, among other risks. At the same time, 2.1 billion go to bed every night overweight. As we will see in Part 5, the world food system produces an average of 2,870 calories per day for the 7.5 billion humans on the planet. The average calorie need per person is 2,550. Globally, we produce 320 calories more than we need per person per day. We currently produce enough food for 10.5 billion people.[10] But even in the United States food insecurity affects 12 percent of the population, or about 15 million people, including 6.5 million children.[11] And the 46 million Americans on food assistance, or SNAP, half of whom are children, are at risk for hunger and food insecurity.[12] I am embarrassed to live in the richest country in the world, where one in four children are food insecure.

How is it possible that we create so much food but so many people are still undernourished? Food security is defined as access to affordable nutritious food, but when SNAP was developed, "nutritious" meant vitamin-fortified starchy calories. The calories are abundant, but the nutrition is not, technically leaving nearly everyone on the planet food insecure because of lack of access to whole fresh nutrient-dense foods.

It may be surprising that the most food insecure are also the most obese, have twice the risk for type 2 diabetes, and are also malnourished because much of the food we produce is calorie-rich, nutrient-poor processed food and sugary beverages.[13] Calorie for calorie, these foods cost less than nutritionally rich fruits and vegetables or whole foods. If you have $1, you can purchase either 1,200 kcal of cookies or potato chips or 250 kcal of carrots.[14] And if you are poor and live in a food desert, good luck finding a carrot. The cost of processed food per calorie is low. The cost per nutrient is high, very high, often because there are almost none! Ultraprocessed foods and the food system that produces them are at the root of the chronic diseases that account for 80 percent of the deaths from noncommunicable disease worldwide (heart disease, diabetes, cancer, etc.).[15]

A recent study of more than 44,000 people published in *JAMA Internal Medicine* found that for every 10 percent increase in the intake of ultraprocessed food, the risk of death increases by 14 percent.[16] If 60 percent of our calories come from processed foods, the math adds up to a lot of unnecessary, food-caused, preventable deaths.

Just as the wrong foods can cause disease and death, the right foods can dramatically reduce disease and death. Mounting research proves that food is medicine and demonstrates how whole foods, especially an increase in vegetables and fruit, can prevent or reverse chronic disease.[17] At Geisinger Health Systems, providing food-insecure poorly controlled type 2 diabetics with a year's worth of whole foods reduced health care costs by 80 percent and dramatically improved their health outcomes.[18]

According to Dr. Dariush Mozaffarian, "The idea of food as medicine is not only an idea whose time has come. It's an idea that's absolutely essential to our health care system."

The truth is that our agricultural system doesn't produce enough for everyone to eat even the minimum requirement of fruits and vegetables, which may be even more important to prevent disease than reducing industrial processed foods (although that is still critically important). We have all heard we should eat five to nine servings of fruits and vegetables a day (one serving is a half cup).[19] This is a bare minimum, with some research suggesting we should be consuming 15 servings (about 8 cups) a day for optimal health. The government's dietary guidelines advise us to make 50 percent of our plate fruits and vegetables. Globally about 78 percent of the world's population does not eat the minimum of five servings of fruits and vegetables a day.[20] We tell people to eat more fruits and vegetables, but we don't grow them. How does this make any sense?

Even worse, ultraprocessed foods (corn, soy, wheat) are turned into sugars, refined oils, and starch that are the building blocks of processed food, which is made into every size, color, and shape of extruded food-like substance but is essentially the same garbage. These foods hurt us twice. First, they damage the environment by depleting soil, water, and oil resources and are the largest source of greenhouse gases. Second, they are the greatest cause of human suffering, disability, disease, and death.[21] We produce far too many calories for the world's population and not enough of the real nutrients, found in whole foods, needed to create health.

Refocusing our agricultural system along with our national and global food policies on production of foods that support human health and the restoration of natural capital (soil health, water quality and availability, drawdown of carbon, limits on fossil fuel, etc.) would go a long way toward reducing the economic, social, and human burden of chronic disease and improving the health of our soil, water, and climate.

A DECLINE IN LIFE EXPECTANCY

The data is clear. Those who consume the most of those ultraprocessed foods, the staple building blocks of industrial food, which are processed into white flour, high-fructose corn syrup, and refined soybean oil, are the sickest. They have higher body weight, more dangerous belly fat, and worse cholesterol and blood sugar.[22] And they die sooner.

For the first time in human history, our life expectancy in the United States is on the decline for three years in a row. Over 4 million years of human evolution, life expectancy increased. At the turn of the twentieth century, it went from twenty-one to thirty-one years old. The number doesn't reflect that nearly half the population died in childhood, making the average low. But from 1900 to 2000, life expectancy increased about 41 years, from thirty-one to seventy-two years old. In America we have more than doubled life expectancy through public health measures including sanitation, a dependable food supply, and vaccinations. Some minor gains were made by advances in medical care other than vaccinations, but that is a relatively small amount. But our current food system is eroding these advances.

Children born today are expected to live shorter, sicker lives than their parents. The average child born today will live five fewer years than their parents, and if they are poor or socially disadvantaged, they will live 10 to 20 fewer years than their parents. One in three children born today will have type 2 diabetes in their lifetime. These trends have been increasing year over year. Now for three years in a row, we have seen life expectancy go down. Some of this decline may be due to the opioid epidemic, drug overdoses, suicide, and mental health disorders. Opioid deaths have risen to 70,000 a year. While important to address, that number pales in comparison to the almost 700,000 deaths a year from lifestyle (aka diet)-related cardiovascular disease alone. There has been talk of declaring a national emergency to stem the deaths from opioid overdose. Perhaps we should have a similar initiative to address deaths from poor diet.

The maps of life expectancy tell a clear story. When overlaid upon the maps of obesity and type 2 diabetes, most prevalent in the South, there is almost a complete correlation between the states with the highest obesity and diabetes rates and those with the lowest life expectancy. Death rates from heart disease, diabetes, chronic liver disease (caused by sugar and starch), stroke, and Alzheimer's are on the rise.[23] The disparities in life expectancy in this country are driven by disparities in education, income, and socioeconomic status affecting the poor and minorities that result in obesity and metabolic disease caused by poor diet.[24]

There has also been a rise in allergic, autoimmune, and inflammatory conditions linked to poor diet.[25] Mental health has also declined, with increasing rates of depression, suicide, behavior problems, ADHD, and neurodevelopmental disorders in children, much of which has been linked to poor diet,[26] while good mental health has been linked to a healthy diet.[27]

FOOD FIX: EAT FOR THE HEALTH OF HUMANS AND THE PLANET

What is the best diet for humans, our society, and the planet? What we eat is important not only to us, but also to almost everything that matters. It would seem we should have a simple answer to this question, but there is vast disagreement from a variety of experts. I have spent the last 40 years studying nutrition, grappling with the changes in recommendations and diets, and treating more than 10,000 patients with food as medicine.

Sadly, the public is at the mercy of these constantly changing debates. Eggs were bad, then they were good, and now they are bad again. Fat was bad, now it's good, but controversy exists about whether to cut saturated fat or increase refined plant-based oils. Some science shows that meat is bad and increases the risk of heart disease, cancer, and death; other science reports that meat is benign, even healthy and necessary for optimal nutrition. (Chapter 17 will help clear up some of the confusion.)

On the one side is the regenerative agriculture movement, which suggests that animals are part of the natural biological cycle necessary to create sustainable ecosystems, that animals must be integrated into farms to regenerate soil, enabling it to store massive amounts of carbon and water. These practices can reduce the need for factory-farmed meat and its overuse of antibiotics, pesticides, herbicides, and farming practices that deplete the soil and can be done at scale more profitably than feedlots. With 40 percent of agricultural lands suited only for grazing, this seems like a good idea. Even if you wanted to grow vegetables or grains on them, you can't. According to Nicolette Hahn Niman, a vegetarian regenerative rancher, the problem is not the *cow*, but the *how*. Feedlot beef, hogs, and chickens—or regenerative farms that include animals as an essential part of ecosystem restoration? (We'll dive into this in Part 5.)

Others suggest that eating meat will destroy our health and that cattle are the equivalent of the atomic bomb in terms of the destructive capacity for the climate and inhumane treatment of animals. That a meatless diet is the only way to save our health and the planet. That animal products should not be part of a healthy diet. That vegan and vegetarian diets prevent disease and prolong life. Compared to our standard processed diet, plant-based diets are better. This does not automatically mean that diets of whole foods including sustainable, regeneratively raised animal foods are bad. Data on both vegetarian and meat-based diets are primarily studies of large populations. Some studies show no difference between omnivorous diets and vegetarian or vegan diets. Some show that vegetarian diets are healthier. Some show that diets with animal protein and fat are healthier than diets high in cereal grains. No wonder people (including doctors and even many scientists) are confused. (Chapter 9 will help clear up some of this confusion.) However, the totality of the scientific evidence makes it very clear that a whole foods, unprocessed diet is better for you and the planet. With one caveat: Factory farming of animals is bad for you, for them, and for the planet. Regeneratively raised animals can not only prevent the environmental and climate harm of factory-farmed animals but actually restore ecosystems and reverse climate change.

These simple arguments often ignore the complexity and nuances beyond the sound bites.

The types of studies we need haven't been done. We have to rely on basic science, smaller clinical trials, and the totality of all the data. A large, long-term randomized controlled study of a whole-foods-based regenerative diet that includes animals or one that is vegan has not been done and is very difficult to do. It would take decades, billions of dollars, and hundreds of thousands of study participants who strictly follow a specified eating protocol. Can you see why this hasn't and can't be done? Just to study a few hundred people over a few months while strictly controlling their diets can cost tens of millions of dollars and still may not be able to predict long-term outcomes.

Yes, factory-farmed meat is bad for us and the planet. No one is for it (except Big Ag). Regenerative grass-fed meat can restore ecosystems, improving soils while sucking carbon from the atmosphere and increasing water storage in soils. It also increases biodiversity of the soil, which is critical for human survival, and can be employed on lands unsuitable for other agriculture.

The simple "plants are good, meat is bad" argument is nuanced. What plants? What meat? Industrial soy, no. Vegetables from a regenerative farm, yes. Factory-farmed steak, no. Regeneratively raised steak, yes. A recent independent life-cycle analysis by the sustainability experts at Quantis of regeneratively raised beef versus GMO soy burger (Impossible Burger) showed that you would have to eat one regeneratively raised beef burger to offset the net carbon emissions of one Impossible

Burger.[28] The soy burger is far better than feedlot beef, but it adds 3.5 kilograms of CO_2 to the environment, while the regeneratively raised beef burger removes 3.5 kilograms of CO_2. Soy is the main staple of "healthy vegan" meat replacements and plant-based burgers. So, your soy burger or pea protein shake may not be so good for you or the planet after all. Since the soy from the Impossible Burger is made with GMO soy most likely sprayed with Roundup or glyphosate, it may have as much as 10 parts per billion (ppb) more glyphosate than those made from pea protein.[29] Research shows that just 0.1 ppb of glyphosate is enough to harm your gut bacteria or microbiome.[30] Just one Impossible Burger may have 110 times that much!

So what's an eater to do?

Well, let's get into the simple principles, based on the best available data we have today, combined with a spoonful of common sense, that will help prevent and reverse chronic disease, restore ecosystems, reverse climate change, and dramatically reduce the true cost of food.

What Is the Best Diet for Us and the Planet?

I have reviewed the research on nutrition and what makes up a diet that is good for you, good for the planet, and good for society. I have laid this all out in my book *Food: What the Heck Should I Eat?* And I provided a way to do it in my cookbook *Food: What the Heck Should I Cook?* To get a nuanced view of the research, an honest and nondogmatic, nonphilosophical view based on 40 years of studying nutrition and 30 years of applying it to thousands of patients, you can read the book. But here is my best attempt to summarize it.

What to Eat: Pegan Diet Rules

The diet wars are bigger than ever in history. Vegan, Paleo, keto, low-fat, high-fat, low-carb, high-carb, raw. The EAT-Lancet Commission recently published an analysis of diets that suggested that for healthy adults there is a "universal healthy diet." The recommendations include a dramatic reduction in animal products and an increase in plant-based foods. It presents a flexitarian approach adapted to each local culture and environment. It's a step forward for sure, but it is important to understand that the eat-less-meat argument is valid only in the context of current factory-farmed-meat production systems, not regenerative grass-fed and grass-finished meat. In fact, as we will see in Part 5, eating more of the right meat may be one of the key ways to reverse climate change.

Each of us must find the right diet for our genes, metabolism, age, dietary preferences, beliefs, and so on. Moral, ethical, and religious considerations are important on a personal level. I would never tell my Buddhist monk patients to eat meat. But I would guide them in the best possible way to optimize a vegan diet, showing them how to maximize protein requirements and indicating which nutritional supplements must be taken to ensure nutritional adequacy.

The best person to listen to is your own body. How does it feel? Try different approaches. More fat, less fat. More carbs, less carbs. More protein, less protein. But one principle remains: It should be whole food, real food, recognizable from field to fork. Pay attention to your energy, weight, digestion, and health conditions. Your body will tell you what it likes. But the core guidelines for a healthy diet apply to everyone: Your diet should be aspirational, not perfect. It should contribute to better health for you, a better world for humans, including food workers and farmworkers, and a better world for the environment, our climate, and our economy.

There are a few simple principles that I have jokingly called the Pegan Diet (poking fun at the extremes of the Paleo and vegan diet camps). These Pegan rules (which are not so much rules as guidelines) attempt to create flexibility within those parameters. You can't go wrong following these principles. And any unbiased scientist who has read the scientific literature on nutrition would have a hard time arguing with these guidelines.

■ **Eat mostly whole plants.** No argument from anyone here. Think *plant rich,* not necessarily *plant based.* And remember french fries, Coke, Twinkies, and Lucky Charms are all plant-based foods! More than half your plate should be covered with veggies. The deeper the color, the better. The World Health Organization (WHO) recommends five servings a day. That is the minimum. It should be fifteen servings, or 7 to 8 cups of veggies and fruit a day.

- **Go easy on fruits.** If you are fit and healthy, more fruit is fine. But if you are overweight (like 70 percent of Americans), then go easy on the fruit. I find that most of my patients feel better when they stick to low-glycemic fruits like berries and enjoy other, sweeter ones as a treat.

- **Eat more foods with healthy fats.** Start with fats in whole foods. Good fats include nuts, seeds, avocados, pasture-raised eggs, extra virgin olive oil (don't heat), avocado oil (good for cooking even at high heat), and organic virgin coconut oil, omega 3 fats from fish, and even animal and saturated fat, and 100 percent grass-fed and grass-finished or sustainably raised meat, grass-fed butter, or ghee.

- **Eat more nuts and seeds.** They have universally been shown to prevent and reverse disease.

- **Choose regeneratively raised animal products whenever possible.** They are better for you and better for the animals and help draw down carbon and reverse climate change. The data on meat is conflicting, mostly because of the challenges of nutritional science. We'll review it in Part 5. Vegetables should take center stage, and meat should be the side dish. Servings should be 4 to 6 ounces per meal (ideally also regeneratively raised or no-till organic, which is hard to find but addressed in Part 5). The "eat less meat to save the planet" meme is not so simple. In fact, more of the right meat regeneratively raised may actually be a big part of the solution to climate change (and conserving water, increasing biodiversity, and reducing agricultural pollution), according to the 2019 IPCC report on climate and agriculture mentioned earlier.

- **Eat pasture-raised eggs.** They are rich in vitamins, minerals, antioxidants, protein, and more. They are also a cheap source of high-quality and bioavailable nutrients including B_{12}, which you can't get from a vegan diet. The 2015 Dietary Guidelines determined that dietary cholesterol does not cause heart disease and eliminated recommendations to cut it out of our diet. Dietary cholesterol, the type found in foods like eggs, doesn't significantly impact your blood cholesterol levels. In fact, your blood cholesterol is actually worsened more by sugar than by fat, and some fats, like olive oil, avocados, and nuts, actually improve your cholesterol.

- **Eat sustainably raised or harvested low-mercury fish and high-omega-3 fish.** Choose low-mercury and low-toxin varieties such as sardines, herring, anchovies, mackerel, and wild-caught salmon (all of which have high omega-3 and low mercury levels). Avoid big mercury-laden fish such as tuna, swordfish, Chilean sea bass, and halibut. See www.ewg.org for a guide on safe fish consumption.

- **Eat only unprocessed or minimally processed whole grains (not whole-grain flours).** All grains can increase your blood sugar. Stick with small portions (½ to 1 cup per meal) of low-glycemic grains like black rice, quinoa, teff, buckwheat, or amaranth. They can be a source of protein, but it takes 3 cups of quinoa to provide the same amount of protein found in 4 ounces of chicken. Beware of modern wheat—it is mostly consumed as refined flour (aka sugar), which is worse for your blood sugar than table sugar. The hybridized version has higher starch content and more inflammatory types of gluten and is sprayed with the toxic herbicide glyphosate right before harvest, then preserved with calcium propionate, which has been linked to behavioral issues, headaches, and stomach inflammation. In fact, in the most rigorous type of study in children, a randomized, placebo-controlled crossover trial, calcium propionate in bread caused kids to be irritable and restless and have trouble focusing and sleeping. And it's in every processed food that contains wheat and all bread. You can eat organic wheat berries, but stay away from the rest.

- **Eat beans.** Beans can be a great source of fiber, protein, and minerals. But they cause digestive problems for some, and the lectins and phytates they contain can impair mineral absorption. Pressure cooking is the best way to get the most out of your beans with the least risk. Moderate amounts (up to 1 cup a day) are okay. But remember it takes 3 cups of beans to get the same amount of protein found in 4 to 6 ounces of meat, fish, or chicken. Just a side note on beans versus meat for protein. The oft-quoted figure that 1,800 gallons of water is required to produce 1 pound of beef while only 216 gallons is required to grow 1 pound of soybeans is based on factory-farmed meat, where large amounts of water are used to grow the corn used to feed the cattle. However, 97 percent of water used to raise grass-fed and grass-finished beef is green water (rainwater), while the growing of beans requires irrigation, or blue water from lakes, rivers, and aquifers, which uses 5.25 times more water per acre than growing grasses for grass-finished beef.[31]

- **Stay away from sugar** and anything that causes a spike in insulin production and blood sugar—flour, refined starches, and carbohydrates (which sadly make up more than half of most diets). Think of sugar in all its various forms as an occasional treat. "Don't drink your sugar calories" may be the most important diet advice you will ever get.

- **Stay away from most refined vegetable, bean, and seed oils,** such as canola, sunflower, corn, grapeseed, and especially soybean oil, which now accounts for 10 percent or more of the calories in processed foods. They are unstable, easily oxidized, processed with heat and toxic solvents, and can be inflammatory. Stick with the fats noted previously.

- **Choose the right dairy.** Dairy today is not what it used to be. It is bad for the environment (from cows raised in feedlots) and not well tolerated by most people (except Northern Europeans and the Masai people) because 75 percent of the world's population is lactose intolerant. The way we raise dairy cattle is bad for the cows, the environment, and humans. Dairy has been linked to cancer, osteoporosis, autoimmune disease, allergic disorders, digestive problems, and more. Although in my clinical practice I find that most patients do better without dairy, some studies have shown reduced risk of type 2 diabetes, heart disease, and stroke among other benefits. Find dairy from heirloom cows that contain A2 casein, which doesn't cause the same digestive or inflammatory problems as modern cow products. Try goat or sheep products instead of cow dairy; they also contain A2 casein. Some producers such as Organic Pastures raise grass-finished A2 cow milk. And always go organic and 100 percent grass-fed.

- **Stay away from pesticides, herbicides, antibiotics, food additives, hormones, and, ideally, GMO foods.** Choose foods raised or grown in regenerative ways if possible. Also, no hormones, pesticides, herbicides, antibiotics, chemicals, additives, preservatives, dyes, artificial sweeteners, or other junk ingredients.

- **Eat for you and the planet.** Remarkably, food that is good for you is also good for the environment, our depleted soil, our scarce water resources, and the biodiversity of plants, animals, and pollinators, and it helps reverse climate change. When choosing any food in any category explore where and how it was grown. Was it grown regeneratively, organically, and sustainably with no or minimal use of agricultural chemicals? While it may seem healthy to eat a "plant-based" burger, ask how the raw materials were grown. Were the soybeans doused in glyphosate and pesticides and farmed in ways destructive to the soil and in ways that overuse our scarce freshwater resources? Does it contain highly processed ingredients or novel proteins with unknown long-term effects? Choosing the right foods also helps invigorate the economy, heals chronic disease and helps end social injustice, restores the environment, and reverses climate change. It's a win-win-win-win on all sides. This way of eating allows for vast flexibility within many cultures and dietary preferences. While there may be nuances in interpretation of the data, these principles can form the foundation of a universally healthy diet. And they include sustainability principles that will restore soils, preserve water and biodiversity, draw down carbon, reverse climate change, reduce the use of pesticides, fertilizers, and herbicides, and save trillions in health care costs, among other benefits.

FOOD FIX: FOOD AS MEDICINE

Not too long ago a group of doctors and public health experts at Massachusetts General Hospital noticed something striking: Many of the patients who routinely showed up in the emergency room requiring the most medical services were also the patients who seemed to be the most nutritionally vulnerable. They were patients with heart disease, type 2 diabetes, cancer, and other largely food-related chronic diseases. For hospitals and health insurers, these are among the highest-cost, highest-need patients. Working with a local nonprofit group called Community Services, the doctors decided to launch a study to see whether providing these patients with nutritious meals would have an impact on their health care outcomes.

The researchers recruited Medicaid and Medicare patients and split them into groups that either received nutritious meals or did not receive nutritious meals. What the study found was astonishing. The patients who had nutritious meals had fewer hospital visits, ultimately resulting in a 16 percent reduction in their health care costs. And that was after deducting meal expenses. The average monthly medical costs for a patient in the nutrition group shrank to about $843—much lower than the roughly $1,413 in medical costs for each patient in the control group.[32]

Another group of public health experts in Philadelphia studied what happened when a nonprofit health group called the Metropolitan Area Neighborhood Nutrition Alliance (MANNA) delivered healthy meals to people with diabetes, heart disease, cancer, and other chronic diseases. Over twelve months, the patients in the nutritious meal group visited hospitals half as often as a control group and stayed for 37 percent less time. Ultimately, their health care costs plummeted more than 50 percent, or $12,000 a month per patient.[33] Considering that the sickest 5 percent of patients account for 50 percent of overall health care costs in the United States according to the Agency for Healthcare Quality and Research, providing meals to the sickest provides a big return on investment.[34] The problem is that insurance will pay for expensive hospital stays but not for food that could literally save billions in health care costs. This must change.

A similar effort is underway in California, where researchers are studying the health care impact of providing nutritious meals to 1,000 chronically sick patients insured by California's Medicaid program, known as Medi-Cal.[35] Studies have shown a 32 percent reduction in health care costs and a 63 percent reduction in hospitalizations.[36] Many of these programs are funded through private donations and coordinated by the national Food Is Medicine Coalition, which is a group of nonprofits that want to use nutrition to solve the health care and chronic disease crisis. The Food Is Medicine group hopes to get these medically tailored meals included in health care coverage.

These groups recognize what our federal government sadly does not: To tackle the crisis, our national food policies must be aligned with our health care policies. Instead of just treating rampant chronic diseases with medication and surgery, we have to start preventing and treating with food.

A CASE STUDY ON FOOD AS MEDICINE

At the Cleveland Clinic Center for Functional Medicine, we see daily how food can transform chronic disease and obesity. Janice, a patient there, provides a clear example of the power of eating well. She joined one of our group programs and with the support of her peers and our staff, she did the impossible. Only it's not impossible because it happens every day when food is used as medicine.

Janice lived in the environment that surrounds us all—a toxic nutritional landscape, or food swamp, compounded by confusing science, media headlines, food industry marketing, and government regulations and policies that make the right choice the hard choice and the easy choice the wrong choice.

Janice was dancing with death. At sixty-six years old she was severely obese, suffering from heart failure, type 2 diabetes, and coronary artery disease. She also had early kidney failure from diabetes, a fatty liver, kidney stones, low thyroid function, and emphysema, and was taking a boatload of medications, including insulin injections, blood thinners, cholesterol medications, blood pressure medication, diuretics, and more to "manage" her illnesses. She saw multiple specialists to care for her complex medical problems. She was on a low-calorie, low-sodium, diabetic diet, and her blood sugars and weight were still going in the wrong direction.

Janice had already had two stents put in her heart for blocked arteries and was headed toward dialysis and a heart transplant. At her heaviest she weighed 254 pounds, with a BMI (body mass index) of 43.6 (normal is less than 25 and obese is greater than 30).

She decided to join our Functioning for Life program, a ten-week group medical visit program supported by doctors, nutritionists, health coaches, and behavioral therapists. The fundamental premise of functional medicine is to address the root causes of disease. In her case, for almost all her issues, the problem was eating too much of the wrong foods and not enough of the good foods. She grew up in a household where all they ate was processed food. It was all she knew.

At her first visit her blood sugar was out of control, averaging almost 300 (optimal is less than 85, and 126 is the threshold for diabetes). Her hemoglobin A1c, a measure of the average last six weeks of blood sugar, was 11 (normal is less than 5.5). Her kidneys were failing; her blood pressure was high despite her medication. Her cholesterol was severely abnormal, at more than 350 (normal is less than 180), and her triglycerides were 306 (normal is less than 70). She had severe omega-3 fat deficiency, which can contribute to diabetes, high blood pressure, and heart disease. Her ratio of omega-6 oils from refined processed food to omega-3 fats was 15 (optimal is less than 4). And she was severely vitamin D deficient.

In the first three days of changing her diet to an anti-inflammatory, low-sugar, and low-starch diet higher in good fats and whole foods, she got off her insulin and her blood sugar improved. She was still very overweight, but her blood sugar went to normal in three days! It's not the weight; it's the food. In three months, she lost 43 pounds, got off all her medication, normalized her blood sugar, blood pressure, and cholesterol, and reversed congestive heart failure (which never happens in traditional medicine); her fatty liver went away, and her kidney functions normalized. In one year, she lost 116 pounds and went from 254 pounds to 138 pounds (see photos below). She went from unable to function most days due to fatigue, joint pain, and brain fog to feeling healthy.

Her blood sugar, kidneys, and cholesterol are all normal, and now she is not on any medication. Her diabetes is gone. Her blood sugar is in the 80s and her hemoglobin A1c is 5.5—totally normal. Her BMI went from 43 to 23! It was like a gastric bypass without the pain of surgery, vomiting, and malnutrition, and with the pleasure of eating delicious whole foods. She is thriving as an active member of her community, a great-grandmother, a grandmother, and a mother! She was retired and disabled and now is going back to work, traveling around the world teaching, and doing archaeological exploration. She saved $15,000 to $20,000 a year in medication copay costs, especially from the insulin (imagine what Medicare was paying). And that is just one person. Imaging scaling that to the 30 million diabetics in the United States. That's a savings of $450 billion a year (most are not on as much medication as she was, but close). She said to me, "I felt I was done, and now I feel like I am beginning again!"

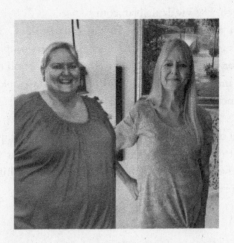

You may think this is impossible, but it is something we see every day at the UltraWellness Center, my practice in Lenox, Massachusetts, and the Center for Functional Medicine at the Cleveland Clinic, which I head. It is not a miracle. It is just good science. And this is possible when people switch from the ultraprocessed industrial diet that is killing them to real, whole foods.

FOOD FIX: SPREAD THE WORD

Follow Janice's lead: Change your eating habits for your health's sake and then take this way of eating into your world. Instead of being influenced by your family, your neighborhood, or your workplace, be the influencer.

1. Start a faith-based wellness program in your place of worship. In 2011, Pastor Rick Warren, Dr. Daniel Amen, Dr. Mehmet Oz, and I launched the Daniel Plan, a faith-based wellness program in Warren's church. In the first week 15,000 people signed up; they lost a quarter of a million pounds in the first year by supporting one another in small groups to live healthier lives. Now the program is in more than one hundred countries and thousands of churches around the world. You can learn more at www.danielplan.com.

2. Be an agent of change in your workplace. Start a lunch group, rotating who brings healthy lunches for your group. Start a wellness group for walking or being active together. Get rid of the candy, doughnuts, and sodas. They are bad for both the employer and the employees, increasing sickness, disability, and costs.

What you choose to eat every day is the single most important thing you can do to create health, spread social justice, repair the environment, and reverse climate change. It is not all-or-nothing. Do your best. One bite at a time.

FOOD FIX: HEALTH CARE INNOVATIONS

Instead of being the country with one of the worst chronic disease epidemics, we could become a model for health. While there are many ideas proposed by many groups, here are a few that could make a big impact in addressing the burden of chronic disease. Many of these have been outlined in a key paper published in *BMJ* in 2019 entitled "Role of Government Policy in Nutrition—Barriers to and Opportunities for Healthier Eating."[37]

▪ **Reimburse food as medicine.** Change medical reimbursement to pay for food as medicine through all federal and state health insurance programs such as Medicare and Medicaid for at-risk populations. The data is clear. Giving people food instead of drugs saves money. A new study providing medically tailored meals to sick patients reduced hospital and nursing home admissions and saved about $9,000 per person per year after providing free food.[38]

Pilot projects include the $25 million Produce Prescription Program in the 2018 Farm Bill to test how doctors' prescriptions of fruit and vegetables bundled with financial incentives, education, and better access can improve health outcomes and reduce the use of health care services. California provided $6 million in support of food prescriptions and medically tailored meals for chronic disease. Similar programs have found that health care costs are reduced by 55 percent and hospital and long-term-care admissions are reduced.[39]

In 2018, John Hancock turned life insurance upside down by making all their policies part of the John Hancock Vitality Program, which provides financial incentives for healthier lifestyles, including $600 a year for purchasing healthy food.[40] These types of business innovations will inspire other businesses, proving that it's possible to increase profits while promoting social good.

Geisinger's Food Farmacy provided $2,400 in food to food-insecure diabetics with education and social support and reduced costs by 80 percent while improving health care outcomes.[41] The Food Is Medicine

Coalition, an association of twenty-seven member organizations in eighteen states and Washington, DC, that provides medically tailored food to people with serious or long-term illnesses, helps advance this strategy. There is even a bipartisan Food Is Medicine Working Group in Congress today.[42] It's a start. And the return on investment is dramatic.

■ **Create a Food Savings Account,** like a Health Savings Account (HSA), where money can be stored tax free in an account that can only be used to by whole, real, health-promoting foods. It could ultimately save billions in health care costs.

■ **Fund research and change reimbursement to pay for functional medicine,** a systems approach to addressing the root cause of chronic disease. Functional medicine is how we healed Janice. Imagine scaling an approach that changes both the medicine we do and the way we do medicine:

- Addressing root causes
- Using food as medicine
- Treating the body as a system rather than a set of symptoms
- Shifting delivery of care in the community, putting patients and communities at the center of health care, not doctors and hospitals
- Using proven behavioral change strategies such as peer support models, group visits, and health coaching to change people's lifestyle.

Vida Health is a company that provides digital one-to-one or group personalized health coaching via video, text, and an app. Their research has shown dramatic improvement in health outcomes, but it is not reimbursed. Eighty percent of health is determined by our lifestyle, our social environment, and our genes. Yet we spend more than 80 percent of our health care dollars on doctors and hospitals and medical care. Not the right target if we want a healthy nation.

Cleveland Clinic has been the first major academic medical center to start a clinical and research program in functional medicine to bring new thinking to how we address the burden of chronic disease, including cardiometabolic diseases like heart disease and type 2 diabetes, autoimmune disease, and mental health issues, among others. Innovations in care delivery must also be funded: community-based programs, group models of care, and digital solutions. Initial research at Cleveland Clinic has shown that this approach increases value—that is, better outcomes are achieved at lower cost.[43] How many Janices will it take to make this available to everyone?

Virta Health developed an online program to reverse diabetes with a ketogenic diet, and within one year diabetes was reversed in 60 percent of the participants, 100 percent stopped their main diabetes medication, insulin was reduced or stopped in 90 percent, and there was an average weight loss of 12 percent, or 30 pounds, results rarely seen in medical research, where 5 percent is considered success.[44] Yet this digital program, outside the health care system, is not reimbursed.

▪ **Integrate nutrition into health care** through support for nutrition education in medical schools and by changing licensing exams to include nutrition, which would change what doctors have to study, thus forcing medical school curriculums to change. Reimburse nutrition visits for chronic disease and obesity. Integrate nutrition into electronic health records. Develop reimbursement and quality metrics, which will incentivize the integration of nutrition into medical practice. In other words, if doctors don't document nutrition status and use food as medicine, they don't get paid! Develop quality metrics and payment reform that support community-based programs to address the upstream causes of poor health. Integrate public health and health care.

FOOD FIX: BUSINESS INNOVATIONS

Innovations in food, health, medicine, and agriculture are among the hottest investment opportunities that exist today. Billions in capital are flooding into the system, often disrupting the traditional industries of food, agriculture, medicine, and health care.[45] A 2015 report mapped out a $2.3 trillion annual investment opportunity in sustainable food and agriculture. Dr. Dariush Mozaffarian suggests a number of initiatives that could facilitate the already booming investment in food, ag, and health care solutions that can solve the major problems facing our current food system. Many examples of business innovations and solutions are highlighted throughout *Food Fix*.

- **Innovation incentives:** Institute tax policy and other economic incentives across sectors (agricultural, retail, manufacturing, restaurant, health care, wellness) for development, marketing, and sales of healthier, more accessible, and more sustainable foods.

- **Opportunity zones:** Expand and support opportunity zone incentives focused on food, nutrition, and wellness investments to improve equity and reduce disparities. Opportunity zones are tax incentives to encourage those with capital gains to invest in low-income and undercapitalized communities.

- **B-corporations:** Encourage and highlight B-corporation status across these sectors to recognize and reward companies for integrating major social and environmental priorities for health, food justice, and sustainability.

- **Mission-driven investment vehicles:** Encourage and convene investment vehicles that focus on food- and nutrition-related companies centered on health, equity, and sustainability.

- **National entrepreneurship:** Develop and support a national strategy to build an ecosystem of evidence-based, mission-oriented innovation for a healthier, more equitable, and more sustainable food system.

For a quick reference guide on the Food Fixes and resources on combating chronic disease, go to www.foodfixbook.com.

CHAPTER 3

THE GLOBAL REACH OF BIG FOOD

The intentions and underpinnings of our current food system—industrial agricultural and food processing—were well intended. Diseases of hunger, starvation, and vitamin deficiencies were rampant in the early twentieth century, and while many around the world are still food inse-cure, we have taken giant steps in fixing these issues with mass produc-tion of abundant (albeit highly starchy processed) calories and vitamin fortification. But over the last 40 years the very systems that helped humanity now endanger it and our environment. The legacy methods and products of the food and agriculture system are a monstrous ship to turn and often resist threats of change and fear financial loss. However, new global problems of overconsumption, undernutrition, obesity, chronic disease, and increasingly destructive agricultural production methods driv-ing environmental degradation and climate change demand a new per-spective. The current food and agriculture monopoly sees change as a financial threat. But innovations and consumer and market pressures, espe-cially the millennials' demand for brand integrity, sustainability, and health promotion, are driving very rapid innovations in the food and ag sectors. Taking a sober look at the existing food system and the corporations behind it and their behavior is important in defining the obstacles and opportun-ities for transforming our food system.

Obesity and chronic disease are no longer just first-world problems. For a long time, I thought our Western diet was just that—a diet that was killing mostly people in the developed world with access to lots of processed foods and fast-food outlets. Turns out we created the worst diet on the planet and shipped it across the globe. As sales of processed food are going down in the United States and Europe, they are dramatically rising in Asia, Africa, and Latin America. This is not an accident. It is by design. The globalization of processed, industrial food has allowed Big Food and Big Ag to flood the world with their disease-causing products. From Mexico to Nigeria, India, China, and the South Pacific, giant food companies are transforming the local diets, uprooting the healthy traditional foods that people have eaten for centuries and replacing them with ultraprocessed Frankenfoods.

"Growth is very stagnant for global food companies in places like Western Europe and the United States and Japan because they've saturated the market," says Barry Popkin, an expert on global obesity and professor of nutrition at the University of North Carolina at Chapel Hill. "All the profit gain that every global food company sees is in low- and middle-income countries."

Not only are multinational companies pushing aggressively into developing markets, but they are also proudly explaining their strategy to investors. "Half the world's population has not had a Coke in the last 30 days," Ahmet Bozer, the president of Coca-Cola International, told a group of investors in 2014. "There's 600 million teenagers who have not had a Coke in the last week. So, the opportunity for that is huge."[1] With data showing that soda kills, that sugar is addictive, I would argue that this thinking is immoral and unethical.

Chains like McDonald's, Burger King, and KFC now have more locations in other countries than they have in the United States. Only a couple of decades ago Yum! Brands, the parent company of KFC, Pizza Hut, and Taco Bell, derived less than a third of its profits from outside the United States. Today, more than 60 percent of its profits come from outside America. As of 2019, the company had more than 1,000 Pizza Hut and KFC locations in Indonesia, 600 locations in Mexico, and more than 800 fast-food outlets in India.[2] In Ghana, where KFC has a growing presence, obesity rates have increased by 650 percent since 1980.[3] Yum! is spreading across the globe like wildfire and shows no signs of slowing down.

As top company executive Keith Siegner told investors at a conference in December 2018, the company is operating at an unprecedented scale: "We've got 46,000 restaurants. We're opening seven new restaurants a day. In the last 12 months alone, we opened—we've got 10,000 more restaurants doing delivery."[4]

This phenomenon has had a dramatic effect: Obesity rates have doubled in more than seventy countries since 1980 and tripled in children.[5] A 2014 *Lancet* study found that two-thirds of the world's obese live not in affluent countries but in low- and middle-income countries.[6] There are now more overweight people on Earth than there are people who are hungry (2.1 billion vs. 800 million), though the two aren't mutually exclusive. In many developing countries the new trend is people who are simultaneously overweight and malnourished, thanks to a steady diet of foods that are energy dense and nutrient poor. In some developing countries, it is common to find an obese mother and father raising underweight children with vitamin deficiencies.

In countries such as Vietnam, China, Indonesia, and Brazil, up to two-thirds of households suffer from this dual burden, creating what one recent report in the *International Journal of Obesity* called "a significant public health concern."[7] The Population Reference Bureau, a nonprofit that works to protect public health and the environment, studied the double burden of disease and found that it was a direct result of steering people in developing nations away from their traditional diets and physically active lifestyles.[8]

Traveling to countries where political barriers have kept out Big Food underscores the difference. I recently traveled to Cuba, where there are no chains and few Big Food brands, the result of the American trade embargo. Almost no one was overweight. Cuba's life expectancy is greater than that of the United States while spending only 1 percent of what the United States spends on health care.

BIG FOOD = BIG MANIPULATION

Food industry marketing in these emerging markets is clever and insidious. In the Western world, fast food is associated with low socioeconomic status. McDonald's, Burger King, and KFC are not exactly fancy food choices in New York or London. But in poorer countries, fast-food companies market their brands as "aspirational"—a symbol of wealth and high status. In China, KFC uses cosmopolitan young professionals to create the impression that their fried chicken and biscuits can provide a taste of high society.

In addition to slick and manipulative marketing, fast-food chains establish a foothold by catering to local tastes. In Ghana and Nigeria, for example, Domino's Pizza franchises offer a pizza topped with jollof rice—a popular West African staple made with spices, peppers, and onions. Fast-food companies use these local favorites that would otherwise be nutritious and satisfying on their own as a Trojan horse. Travel to China and you can get a dried pork and seaweed doughnut full of sugar and vegetable oils at Dunkin' Donuts. In Japan you can get a giant pizza topped with tuna at Domino's Pizza. Take a trip over to India and you can pick up a veggie burger dripping with melted paneer served alongside a mango shake at one of the more than one hundred Burger King locations across the country.

The effects of Big Food's incursions into these countries is clear. India is now known as the diabetes capital of the world, with more than 73 million people suffering from the disease.[9] One public health watchdog in India described the country as sitting on a volcano of diabetes. This is in a country where obesity was once unheard of. Only a couple of decades ago infectious diseases like malaria, pneumonia, and tuberculosis were the leading causes of death in India, but today those infections have been eclipsed by the epidemic of heart disease, which is now India's number one killer.[10] What is worse is that those infectious diseases haven't gone away. They still kill hundreds of thousands of Indians every year. It's just that now the country's health care system has to grapple with the crises of infectious and chronic diseases simultaneously.

China is close behind. Diabetes is spreading so quickly there that some experts say the country cannot build enough hospitals to keep up. The International Diabetes Federation projects that by 2030 roughly 130 million people in China will have diabetes. That's more than 1 in 10 people, whereas 30 years ago it was 1 in 150![11]

The Arab world has also been flooded with soft drinks and processed food. The Middle East and North Africa have had the second-
highest increase in diabetes globally; the number of people with the
disease is projected to soar more than 95 percent by 2035.[12] In some
Arab countries, one in three or four people have type 2 diabetes. In one
or two generations they transformed from a nomadic people without
chronic disease to a people with the highest rates of obesity and type 2
diabetes in the world.

The unintended consequences of free trade in Mexico (NAFTA)
allowed the American food industry to quickly expand there as purvey-
ors of soda and fast food.[13] Now water costs three times as much as
Coke in Mexico. In the United States one in ten American adults have
type 2 diabetes; in Mexico one in ten *children* have it. We used to call it
adult-onset diabetes because it never existed in children until recently.

The fast-food pandemic has spread to some surprising places too.
Thailand is well-known for its large population of Buddhist monks,
many of whom follow an age-old tradition of daily intermittent fasting
to protect their health and aid their meditation sessions. But in 2018,
public health experts reported that nearly half of all Buddhist monks in
Thailand are obese and at least 10 percent are diabetic. When researchers studied the monks' dietary habits, they were initially baffled. The
monks generally consume fewer calories than the average man in Bang-
kok, and they fast daily. What could be making them so fat and sick?
Then they discovered the problem: The monks tend to sip on soft
drinks throughout the day to keep up their energy levels. "When we
really do research about this, we are surprised," a Thai nutritionist told
the Australian Broadcasting Corporation. "It is the drink."[14]

In the same week that Thai health experts raised the alarm about the
outbreak of obesity among Buddhist monks, the WHO declared that
the home of the world's so-called healthiest diet, the Mediterranean,
was also being ravaged by the spread of ultraprocessed food. Mediterranean countries now have some of the highest rates of obesity in
Europe. In Italy, Spain, Greece, and Cyprus, childhood overweight and
obesity rates have surged past 40 percent. If the birthplace of the world's

healthiest diet is not safe, then no place is—the food industry is certainly making sure of that.

PLANET FAT: THE FOOD INDUSTRY'S TACTICS

In 2017 the *New York Times* published an investigative series called "Planet Fat" that exposed some of the more brazen and shocking tactics that Big Food is using to uproot traditional diets in its quest to squeeze profits out of developing countries. The series showcased how the world's largest food company, Nestlé, recruits thousands of women in some of the poorest towns in Brazil to go door-to-door selling candy and processed foods as part of its plan to expand its reach to a quarter million Brazilian households. The series profiled one young woman named Celene da Silva, a twenty-nine-year-old mother of three who sells candy in Fortaleza, where many people do not have access to grocery stores.

> As she dropped off variety packs of Chandelle pudding, Kit-Kats and Mucilon infant cereal, there was something striking about her customers: Many were visibly overweight, even small children. She gestured to a home along her route and shook her head, recalling how its patriarch, a morbidly obese man, died the previous week. "He ate a piece of cake and died in his sleep," she said. Mrs. da Silva, who herself weighs more than 200 pounds, recently discovered that she had high blood pressure, a condition she acknowledges is probably tied to her weakness for fried chicken and the Coca-Cola she drinks with every meal, breakfast included.[15]

In Colombia, where soft drinks are cheaper than water, public health advocates were threatened when they pushed for a 20 percent soda tax and produced television commercials warning the public that soft drinks could lead to diabetes. One outspoken anti-soda advocate raced through the streets of Bogotá as food industry strongmen on motorcycles chased her, warning her to keep her mouth shut. Other anti-soda advocates in Latin America accused the industry of tapping their phones and computers with spyware. News outlets that published stories and columns criticizing the soda industry in Colombia faced enormous pressure from the food industry and censorship by the government. Even health groups that tried to run ads warning about the health hazards of soda found themselves censored.[16] The food industry made the government an offer they couldn't refuse, "encouraging" them to pass a law making it illegal to talk about soda taxes in the media or advertising.

"They have threatened advocates in Colombia physically," Popkin told me. "Walking, driving by them and making threats. They have worked their power to ban marketing in a country like Colombia, where you had to take them to court to stop it. They are doing everything they can to stall."

FOOD FIX: TRANSFORM FOOD LABELS AND REIN IN JUNK-FOOD ADS

Chile Takes the Lead

Hope is on the horizon. Big Food finally met its match in Chile. More than half of all six-year-olds and three-quarters of adults in Chile are overweight or obese. The country's health care system spends roughly $800 million every year on obesity-related conditions.

In 2006, a doctor from Santiago named Guido Girardi, also a deputy in congress, was elected to the country's senate. Having seen the health crisis firsthand, Girardi vowed to take on the food industry by aggressively going after their predatory marketing practices. Girardi became president of the Chilean senate's Health Commission, and later president of the senate in 2011, and spearheaded an alliance of nutrition experts to study and gather evidence on the best ways to rein in Big Food. The alliance brought in advisers from around the world, such as Barry Popkin. What did they come up with? A groundbreaking and sweeping new law called Ley de Etiquetado Nutricional y Su Publici-dad, which roughly translates to the Food Labeling and Advertising Law. While there are challenges in its approach, the overall effort is laudable. Here are some of its major changes:[17]

1. Food companies must display big black warning logos in the shape of a stop sign on processed foods that are high in sugar, salt, saturated fat, or calories. If a food is high in one of these, then it gets a single black warning logo. Packaged foods that are high in all four of these—whether it's ice cream, potato chips, salad dressing, flavored yogurt, or Nutella—get four warning logos on their labels. However, this unduly focuses on ingredients such as calories, saturated fat, salt, and sugar, which are easy for processed food companies to manipulate (remember low-fat SnackWell cookies), rather than on overall diet quality and protective foods. It is a step in the right direction, but this type of oversimplification, though well intentioned, may in fact lead to other unintended problems, as we saw with the low-fat revolution that resulted in our current obesity crisis.

2. Strict new limitations have been instituted on food adver-tisements, especially those aimed at children younger than four-teen. The measure bans the use of cartoon characters to market junk food to kids. Tony the Tiger was removed from Frosted Flakes. Toucan Sam was pulled from boxes of Froot Loops. Candies that use trinkets to lure kids, like Kinder Surprise, were banned. This may be the most important and effective piece of the legislation.

3. There are restrictions on the sale and marketing of junk food to children. No longer can ice cream, potato chips, and choco-late chip cookies be sold in schools or advertised during cartoons or on websites that target kids. In fact, junk-food commercials are no longer allowed on television or radio between 6 a.m. and 10 p.m.

4. Food companies must incorporate messages that promote physical activity and healthy eating in the advertisements for some of their products.

All of this came on top of a whopping 18 percent tax on sugary drinks—among the highest in the world. Girardi and his alliance tried to push the sweeping new measures into law but had to overcome ferocious resistance from the food industry, which packed the halls of congress with food lobbyists determined to block it.

For a while, the food industry's lobbying efforts worked. The former Chilean president, Sebastián Piñera, a conservative businessman, vetoed the measure in 2011, offering an alternative: a health initiative financed by Big Food companies that emphasized the importance of exercise and moderation. But Girardi and his allies refused to give up. They spent weeks protesting outside Piñera's home, holding cardboard signs accusing him of turning his back on the Chilean people.

"When transnational companies put pressure on Piñera to veto the law, we mobilized," Girardi said in an interview. "I was president of the senate, and I went to the presidential palace with a big sign that said, 'President Piñera is selling out the health of the kids to McDonald's and Coca-Cola.' I was there many days with the sign, and Piñera came out and asked me to leave because it was embarrassing. I said I'm not going to leave until you discuss this law with me. So, he took away the threat of the veto and we began to have a discussion."

In 2014 Piñera was swept out of power and a new president came to power, Michelle Bachelet, a pediatrician and former health minister who was passionate about halting the chronic disease epidemic. Bachelet resisted the food industry's lobbying efforts and in June 2015 approved the new regulations. They rolled out the changes over the next three years.[18]

The Food Labeling and Advertising Law received worldwide recognition from the UN as the Best Contribution to Global Food Security (2018–19).[19]

Researchers are now studying exactly what impact the measures have had on consumers. Already there's been a sea change in behavior. "Kids are telling their parents, 'Don't buy these foods because the teacher says they're not healthy if they have the black logo,'" Popkin says. "That's norm changing." Popkin was crunching the numbers and in the process of publishing the data in a peer-reviewed journal when I spoke to him. He told me that the results of the regulations are "fourfold in impact of what we've seen from any tax or anything else in the world on sugar-sweetened beverages, let alone junk food and other things. The impact has been amazing." No wonder the US food lobby works mightily, spending millions and millions, to prevent any restrictions on food marketing or labeling by the FDA or the Federal Trade Commission.

Chile has inspired more than a half dozen countries, including many of its neighbors in Latin America. Argentinian health officials are examining what Chile did. Brazilian health authorities are looking at adopting similar measures. And Uruguay and Peru have already taken concrete steps toward slapping the black warning logos on junk foods.[20] But one of the most admirable new food-labeling systems is in Israel, where health authorities have created new laws requiring negative warning labels for junk foods and positive logos for nutritious foods like fresh produce, whole grains, and legumes. That may be the best way to get people to purchase more whole foods. Girardi says that it's important to spread these policies because consumers need to be better informed about the food choices they're making. At the same time, lawmakers, academics, and consumers need to continue building coalitions to counter the power and manipulative tactics of the food industry.

Even beyond food labeling, the radical new system in Chile that Girardi spearheaded proves that strict regulations and taxation are the levers that can force multinational food companies to change—because they will not do it voluntarily. In the United Kingdom, for example, food companies complied with new regulations forcing them to reduce the amount of sodium in their products. But they did not make those same changes to their products in the United States until the New York City Health Department under Michael Bloomberg required similar changes. It was the same with trans fats: Even though they had the technology to replace these deadly fats with healthier ingredients, many food companies refused to make the change until laws in various countries required them to do so.

It's sad to see how far Big Food has reached with its tactics for pure profit. Fortunately, many countries are recognizing the detrimental effects and taking action to protect their people. Chile's successes with labeling and the soda tax provide an example of how in our great country we most certainly can do the same. It's time we act.

For a quick reference guide on the Food Fixes and resources on improving our health globally, go to www.foodfixbook.com.

CHAPTER 4

LEVERAGING FISCAL POLICIES TO ADDRESS OBESITY AND CHRONIC DISEASE

As we've seen in the first three chapters, the obesity and chronic disease pandemic enveloping nearly every country on Earth is in many ways an economic problem. Warren Buffett called rising health care costs the "tapeworm" of business. In the last 50 years we've gone from spending 5 percent of our gross domestic product on health care to spending almost 20 percent.[1] Meanwhile, people are motivated to buy the most cost-effective foods, and in most countries, those just happen to be the foods that are most likely to make them fat. That's why fiscal policies can help us alleviate the burden of the big three killers: heart disease, obesity/diabetes, and cancer.

Tobacco taxes were enormously successful. Tobacco was once the leading cause of preventable death. But today that distinction goes to poor diets. Just as tobacco taxes drove down smoking rates, resulting in remarkable public health improvements, taxes on soda can help drive down obesity rates.

FORCING THEIR HAND

Some of the brightest minds in economics have endorsed the idea of taxes on unhealthy foods. In 2018, Larry Summers, the former Treasury secretary and president of Harvard University, joined forces with former New York City mayor Michael Bloomberg and others to launch a global group called the Task Force on Fiscal Policy for Health. Their goal: to advocate for taxes as a solution to rising health care costs and the obesity crisis.

"What I came to realize was that in terms of human betterment in the health care area, there was enormous potential," Summers told me. "In terms of the impact you could have, even with a limited number of dollars, there was probably no sector more promising than health." Looking at global health through an economic lens, he realized that countries could derive tremendous returns by investing in health, making it one of the best financial investments. "In some contexts, the returns can be as high as nine to one or even twenty to one in terms of the benefit-cost ratio," Summers says.

As an economist, Summers is a big believer in using the power of prices to influence behavior. First, people are price sensitive. Second, taxing products like tobacco and soda creates a lot of noise about those products, which itself can make people leery of buying them. "Taxes discourage things—and it's better to tax things that we want to discourage, like tobacco and foods that cause obesity, than it is to tax things we want to encourage, like working and saving," he says. "We have evidence that we do respond to prices and we do buy less of things when they become more expensive. That's the most basic principle of economics."

That's why Summers and Bloomberg created their organization to advocate for taxes as a way to improve global health. Their argument is that government has a responsibility to protect the health of its citizens. Taxing junk foods is a great way to do that because it works. Combined with incentives for healthy food or innovations in market-based and tax-code incentives, it is a proven way to boost public health outcomes and reduce health care costs. If it didn't, then the soda industry wouldn't spend hundreds of millions of dollars fighting such taxes. Every time a soda tax is proposed anywhere in the world, the beverage industry dips into its war chest. When Oakland, San Francisco, and a few other cities asked their residents to vote on soda tax initiatives in 2016, the American Beverage Association launched a ferocious campaign, spending more than $38 million. The industry wouldn't spend that kind of money if they didn't think soda taxes would take a big chunk out of their profits. Thank God that Michael Bloomberg and the Arnold Foundation dipped into their own pockets for $20 million, which allowed those taxes to pass.

"The fact that the food industry objects so strongly is confirmation that these taxes are effective and have significant and meaningful impacts—and if they didn't change the demand for their products, the food industry wouldn't care," Summers says.

One of the main criticisms against soda taxes is that they are regressive, causing a disproportionate impact on low- and middle-income families. This is the primary talking point for the soda industry. Some politicians have embraced it as well. The thing about junk-food taxes is that they are indeed regressive: The poor pay a higher share of their income on them. But the poor also suffer a larger share of the adverse health consequences. "So, the benefits, in terms of reduced health care spending, in terms of longer life expectancy, will be disproportionately felt by the poor," Summers says. "So, I'm completely comfortable with the idea that we should put a universal tax on sugary foods, recognizing that it may be regressive but that it will be offset in other ways." If those taxes on bad food are combined with incentives and price reductions on healthy foods, it will benefit everyone. When money is used to uplift poor communities with social programs, support for education, and more, as was done with the Philadelphia soda tax—which so far has provided $500 million to fund universal pre-K, public schools, and recreation centers—soda taxes gain wide acceptance and give back to those most affected. Some soda lovers have crossed over to Delaware to buy non-taxed soda, but the net decrease in consumption, and the community and health benefits and reduction in health care costs, outweigh any downsides.

However, any taxes must be paired with incentives that support cheaper prices for consumers and business incentives for research and development, marketing, and distribution of protective healing foods. This is important to offset the regressive effect of sugar-sweetened beverage and junk-food taxes and incentivize the replacement of processed foods with whole foods, not engineered Frankenfoods that bypass the limits on certain ingredients by replacing them with something worse, like we did when we replaced saturated fat with deadly trans fats (now banned).

THE PARTNERSHIP OF TAXES AND SUBSIDIES IN SAN FRANCISCO

In 2010, Laura Schmidt, a professor of health policy at the University of California, San Francisco (UCSF) medical school, was working on a program to improve health in underserved Bay Area communities. Schmidt had previously worked on alcohol addiction but switched her focus to sugar when she discovered that one of the leading causes of liver transplants in America is caused not by alcoholism, but by sugar and its consequences obesity and diabetes: nonalcoholic fatty liver disease. Schmidt knew that the way to tackle the country's sugar addiction was to use some of the same tactics that worked on alcohol, such as taxes and warning labels.

But Schmidt and her colleagues learned something surprising from the people in low-income Bay Area neighborhoods who were most likely to be affected by sugary drink policies. They didn't care too much for soda taxes. But they loved the idea of promoting tap water consumption by installing new water stations across the city. The insights taught Schmidt and her colleagues a valuable lesson. Much like SNAP reform, it is not enough to ban or discourage bad foods. We also have to create incentives or subsidies that encourage people to consume the right foods (or drinks) too.

With Schmidt's help, the city of San Francisco took aggressive action on sugary drinks. It introduced a penny-per-ounce soda tax, passed an ordinance slapping health warnings on soft drink advertisements (which ultimately was defeated by a massive beverage industry lawsuit against the city of San Francisco claiming the warnings violated free speech), and banned the use of city funds to pay for sugary drinks. But the city did something else remarkable. It would use the roughly $10 million in annual revenue brought in by the soda tax to help pay for nutritious school meals made with locally grown produce and to install water hydration stations in schools and public buildings. An additional portion of the money would be used to subsidize healthy eating vouchers for low-income San Franciscans.[2] Thanks to Schmidt and her colleagues in the public health community, San Francisco installed one hundred brand-new water stations in parks and other public locations, mainly targeting low-income neighborhoods.[3]

"We realized that if the city is going to tax soda and restrict it, put warning labels on it and stop selling it themselves, then what are people without access to clean water going to do?" she said. "How can we help them? And do we really want people buying more bottled water? Wouldn't it be better to have them drinking safe, clean tap water?

"Taxes are regressive," she added. "And so I think it's kind of ethical, if you're going to pass a tax, that you provide people with a healthy and free substitute. Don't make people pay the jacked-up prices on bottled water. That to me is the ideal soda tax: You take some of the proceeds and you roll it into providing people with clean water."

Hospitals, Schools, and Public Institutions As Soda-Free Zones

Thankfully, Schmidt did not stop there. As she was leaving a lecture on sugar and disease at UCSF one day, she walked by a food court at the medical center and noticed one obese person after another guzzling soda. The imagery struck her. Here she was, a public health expert warning people about the dangers of sugar, promoting water consumption, and yet her own institution was profiting from the sale of sugary drinks to sick patients and their families. "I thought to myself, 'I feel like a total hypocrite, this is disgusting,'" she said.

Schmidt had spent years working on policies that governments could enact to promote healthy behaviors. But she realized that workplaces, private institutions, medical centers, and universities could do a lot. So, in 2015, Schmidt and her colleagues at UCSF pressed the school's chancellor to stop selling sugar-sweetened beverages on the campus. It was a seemingly herculean task. UCSF is one of the largest employers in San Francisco, with more than 24,000 workers on a sprawling campus that extends across the city. But the university found the policy surprisingly simple to execute. The school's beverage supplier simply started stocking the university cafeterias, vending machines, gift shops, conference rooms, and stores with water and zero-calorie beverages instead of soda. Even fast-food chains on the campus, like Subway and Panda Express, agreed to swap out sugar-laden beverages with healthier options. The initiative led to a 25 percent reduction in soda consumption and an improvement in weight, cholesterol, and metabolic markers of pre-diabetes.

BUT WHAT ABOUT THE NANNY STATE?

Critics of regulation often complain about government overreach. If the government slaps warning logos on our food, taxes sugary products, and restricts junk-food advertisements, then it is forcing people to live in a nanny state. But what do nannies actually do? They protect our children. Seems like a good thing.

Anytime a city or country tries to impose a soda tax, the beverage industry bombards the public with pamphlets, billboards, and commercials telling people to reject this so-called nanny state. It's an argument that my friend Dr. Aseem Malhotra, one of the most influential cardiologists in England, and a leading food industry watchdog, has thought long and hard about. I asked him to explain why the food industry's favorite talking point is fatally flawed.

"When you talk about nanny states, this is a term that's really used in my view as propaganda," Dr. Malhotra says. "It's used by people that want to keep perpetuating the status quo where they're benefiting and profiting from regulations that are so weak that they can mislead the people into buying products that ultimately cause them harm."

We have mandatory seat belt laws, mandatory vaccinations, mandatory car seats for children, and other public health measures. How is this different? When the government proposed mandatory seat belt laws decades ago, the car industry vehemently opposed the idea. Carmakers were also against mandatory airbags and fuel emissions standards. These were all "nanny state" ideas, they cried. But now that we've had these safety measures in place for a while, the public has grown accustomed to them and the car industry is doing just fine. We accept these reasonable regulations because they are good for society. They save lives and protect the environment. It's the same with smoking. Many critics of public smoking bans have now come around to the idea that less smoking is good for society.

"I think as awareness grows, then this nanny state argument will not stand up, and politicians will respond to the public," Dr. Malhotra says. "The way the public gets their information is the media. Mass media has a huge impact on public opinion. We really need to engage journalists and editors so these discussions can be heard. We can't keep this information from the public." But the major media is mostly supported by Big Food and Big Pharma ads, making it hard for them to do true muckraking journalism. We need government regulation to make junk food more expensive, to reflect its real cost.

Proposed Policy Solutions

In 2018 Dr. Malhotra proposed a bold new plan that could reverse the diabetes crisis in three years. He created it with two other highly respected public health experts: Dr. Robert Lustig, a pediatric endocrinologist at UCSF, and Professor Grant Schofield from Auckland University of Technology in New Zealand.[4] Here are some of the controversial solutions they proposed:

- Education for the public should emphasize that there is no biological need for or nutritional value in added sugar. The food industry should be forced to label added and free sugars on food products in teaspoons rather than grams, making it easier for the public to understand. If a can of soda says 39 grams, do people really understand that it has almost 10 teaspoons of sugar (approximately 4 grams of sugar is 1 teaspoon)? The labels are designed to obscure the truth and confuse consumers.

- Companies that make sugary products should be banned from sponsoring sporting events. We encourage celebrities in the entertainment industry and famous athletes to publicly dissociate themselves from sugary product endorsements. Examples of star athletes who have already done this include Indian cricketer Virat Kohli, basketball star Stephen Curry, football legend Tom Brady, and Beyoncé.
- Sugary drink taxes should extend to sugary foods as well.
- We call for a complete ban on ads for sugary drinks (including fruit juice) on TV and Internet on-demand services.
- We recommend discontinuing all government food subsidies, especially for commodity crops such as corn turned into sugar, which contributes to health detriments. These subsidies distort the market and increase the costs of nonsubsidized crops, making them unaffordable for many. No industry should be given a subsidy for hurting people.
- We need new policies to prevent all professional dietetic organizations from accepting money or endorsing companies that market processed foods. If they do, they should not be allowed to claim that their dietary advice is independent.
- We recommend splitting healthy eating and physical activity into separate and independent public health goals. We strongly recommend avoiding sedentary lifestyles through the promotion of physical activity to prevent chronic diseases for all ages and sizes. But it is important to remember that "you can't outrun a bad diet."

You have to walk four miles to burn off one 20-ounce soda. However, physical activity is often perceived as an alternative solution to obesity based on the idea of calories in, calories out. The quality of calories matters more than the quantity. Sugar and broccoli calories are not the same when you eat them. A Big Gulp with 750 calories of sugar has profoundly different effects on your metabolism than 21 cups of broccoli with 750 calories. The disproven energy balance or calorie hypothesis of weight gain ignores the metabolic complexity[5] and unnecessarily pits two independently healthy behaviors against each other on just one poor health outcome (obesity). To relieve the burden of nutrition-related disease we need to improve our diets, not physical activity. Big Food focuses on exercise, moderation, and energy balance as the solution.

FOOD FIX: TAX JUNK FOODS AND SUBSIDIZE HEALTHY ALTERNATIVES

1. Every government should institute a junk-food tax of some kind. Sugar-sweetened drinks are the logical place to start. Sugary drinks are not the sole cause of obesity. But they represent the largest source of added sugars in the modern diet, and they have a disproportionate impact on obesity, diabetes, and heart disease. The revenue that such taxes bring should be mandated to be used to pay for important public services like pre-kindergarten and after-school programs and other community benefits so it is not just used to cover budget shortfalls. Soda taxes are the low-hanging fruit for policy makers who understand that we have to do something about our out-of-control health care costs.

It's also clear that soda taxes work. We now have studies that prove it.[6] So I urge every government around the world to explore a soda tax. This can be done at the national level or in provinces, counties, states, and municipalities. The best option is a *tiered* soda tax, which taxes beverages based on the amount of sugar they contain. Under this tax plan, beverages that have the least amount of sugar are taxed at a lower rate, and those that have the most sugar are taxed at the highest rate. This is better than a *flat soda tax*, which taxes a bottle of kombucha, with 4 grams of sugar, at the same rate as a can of Pepsi, with 41 grams of sugar. Studies show that a tiered soda tax is best because it incentivizes companies to avoid the highest tax rates by reformulating their products so that they contain less sugar. Tiered soda taxes have faced less industry opposition than flat soda taxes. They prompt companies to make positive changes. And they work best for consumers. It's a win-win for both the food industry and the public.

More than thirty countries have passed a tax on sugary drinks, including Ecuador, Barbados, Belgium, Portugal, Ireland, Spain, the United Kingdom, South Africa, Hungary, and the Philippines. And the impact on reducing consumption and forcing Big Food to reduce sugar in its products has been significant. In 2017, Saudi Arabia enacted one of the strictest policies in the world, with a 50 percent tax on soft drinks and a 100 percent tax on energy drinks. The United Arab Emirates did the same thing. The CEO of Red Bull called them, complaining that sales were down 70 percent. Since they have no ability to lobby these governments, and these countries receive no tax revenue from those businesses, their protests are ignored. India imposed a 40 percent tax on sugary drinks in 2017. The Philippines passed a tax on drinks containing caloric and noncaloric sweeteners in 2017, but those made with high-fructose corn syrup are taxed at double the rate of other drinks.

Mexico is perhaps the most powerful example of why we need more soda taxes. The country holds the dubious distinction of being one of the world's largest consumers of soft drinks (the former president, Vicente Fox, was previously the head of Coca-Cola for all Latin America), so it's no surprise that it has one of the highest obesity rates. In 2014, the Mexican government enacted a 10 percent tax on sugary drinks and a 5 percent tax on junk foods. Researchers found that after just one year, sales of soft drinks plunged 12 percent while sales of bottled water climbed 4 percent (the increase in water consumption was likely much greater because the study didn't look at tap water intake).[7] The findings provided the first hard evidence that such taxes nudge people in the right direction. Later studies also revealed some encouraging trends. The greatest reductions in soda intake occurred among low-income Mexicans and in households with children. One study in the *Journal of Nutrition* found a 16.2 percent jump in water purchases among low- and middle-income households.[8] If that weren't impressive enough, a study in the journal *PLoS Medicine* estimated that over the course of a decade the tax could help to save almost 19,000 lives, prevent 200,000 new cases of diabetes, and lower Mexico's health care costs by as much as $983 million![9]

The United States doesn't have a federal soda tax. But thirty-three countries do, and more than a half dozen US cities and counties across the country have instituted them on their own—and more are expected. Berkeley was the first American city to institute a soda tax, in 2015, and it proved very successful. Researchers at the University of California–Berkeley found that soda consumption in low-income neighborhoods of the city fell by more than 20 percent and water intake jumped significantly. Philadelphia instituted a soda tax in 2017 for both sugar-sweetened and artificially sweetened drinks, and soft drink intake dropped significantly among low-income children.[10]

2. Use tax income to subsidize nutritious foods and incentives. The sad fact is that the price we pay for most foods doesn't reflect the true societal cost of those foods. Thanks to crop supports, sugar tariffs, tax breaks, and absurdly cheap corn syrup, a can of Pepsi costs less than $1 in many parts of America. Obesity, diabetes, and metabolic diseases cost taxpayers and the federal government trillions in health care spending, lost productivity, and suffering. Even the way that we grow and produce corn syrup and other ultraprocessed foods has a devastating effect on our soil, air, water, and climate. Why do we allow this? Why don't we acknowledge the true costs of foods and price them accordingly?

Dariush Mozaffarian, MD, and his colleagues at the Friedman School of Nutrition Science and Policy at Tufts have thought long and hard about this. Their proposal: Levy a flat tax of 20 or 30 percent on most packaged and processed foods, and then use that money to subsidize nutritious foods that reduce health care costs and have a less harmful impact on the environment. "Then you would use all that money to invest in and reduce the price of minimally processed healthy foods, like fruits and vegetables, nuts and seeds, plant oils [extra virgin olive oil, avocado oil, coconut oil], and fish and yogurt," Mozaffarian says. "You would turn the prices upside down. Or at least you would make them more normal. So now you couldn't buy a 36-ounce soda for 99 cents anymore." Instead of paying 75 cents for an apple or an orange, you'd pay 20 cents. A pound of wild or sustainably raised salmon wouldn't cost you $15 at Whole Foods. It would cost you just $4 or $5. Organic and grass-fed and finished beef, chicken, and eggs would be cheaper. If the animals we eat were raised regeneratively, and if the eco-system services provided by those farms and ranches were reimbursed, who knows? We may get paid to eat regenerative animal foods because they reverse climate change, preserve water resources, and increase biodiversity!

"We should use the revenue from junk-food taxes to create incentives and systems for making healthy food less expensive while helping farmers. We don't want to just make food less expensive by putting farmers out of business. But the price is just an absolutely crucial tool. We've learned from tobacco and cigarette taxes, for example, how important price is," Mozaffarian says. "The price is clearly one tool that the government needs to use to address healthier food."

Another way to influence prices is through fiscal incentives. We should not be handing out tax breaks to industry lobby groups or to companies for spending billions advertising junk food to kids (or the poor). We need to take away those tax breaks and provide companies with incentives for marketing, advertising, and developing healthy foods. This particular policy of ending tax breaks for bad behavior has been proposed in Congress. But it hasn't gotten out of committee for a vote. The Food Is Medicine Working Group needs to repackage it in a new bill that changes the price structure of junk foods and healthy foods. It wouldn't raise income taxes, and it would only affect certain foods, such as soda, potato chips, fast food, and candy. In fact, Congress could balance the taxes and subsidies so that the policy would be cost neutral. Right now, none of the consequences of our food system—the effect on chronic disease, the impact on children's health, and the unsustainable toll on the climate and environment—are reflected in the cost of food. Those things can and must be factored into what we pay at the grocery store, restaurants, and fast-food outlets.

3. Create soda-free zones. Public and private institutions across the country—and the world, for that matter—are now showing how this can be done. More than thirty medical centers and universities in the United States alone have stopped selling sugary beverages. Many have also implemented policies to make clean drinking water and healthy foods more available.

- In 2018 the Geisinger Medical Center in Pennsylvania, which provides health care to thousands of patients, eliminated sugar-sweetened beverages, removed all deep fryers, and started limiting sodium and using locally grown fruits and vegetables in its meals.

- The Indiana University Health System removed sugary beverages and deep fryers and made healthy food options less expensive. It also began marking foods red, yellow, and green to help people identify the healthiest options.

- The Hospital Healthier Food Initiative, which the Partnership for a Healthier America launched, says that at least 700 hospitals nationwide have committed to serving more nutritious patient meals, implementing stricter cafeteria standards, and selling more fruits, vegetables, water, and other healthy foods on their campuses.

- In 2010 my institution, the Cleveland Clinic, was among the first to remove sugar-laden drinks from its campus and offer people healthier food options.[11]

Many large companies have also begun to change their food environments. There are wonderful services that cater to companies that want to create healthier workplaces. SnackNation, for example, helps people replace the junk food in their homes and offices with better-for-you snacks like fresh fruits, nuts, seeds, trail mix, and low-carb protein bars.

FOOD FIX: WHAT YOU CAN DO

1. Stop drinking sugary beverages. If you've gotten this far, then my next recommendation probably goes without saying. But I'll say it anyway: Don't drink sugar. The best way to reform the food system is to make sugar-laden foods less profitable. If consumers demand healthy products, then eventually companies will have to comply. It's not just soda. Fruit juice has a health halo. But don't be fooled by its vitamins and antioxidants. Fruit juice is loaded with sugar and is just as harmful as soda. Avoid buying it, and certainly don't give it to your children. Cutting sugar-sweetened beverages from your diet is the single biggest thing you can do to improve your health.

2. Try my sugar detox challenge. In 2014 I challenged people to kick sugar and starch and other harmful food additives to the curb with my book *The Blood Sugar Solution 10-Day Detox Diet*. Six hundred people did a trial of the program and lost a total of more than 4,000 pounds in just ten days. On average their blood pressure fell 10 points and their blood sugar dropped 20 points. They also saw a 62 percent reduction in all symptoms from all diseases. This brief detox produced better results than any drug on the planet! Since I launched the detox, thousands of people have used it to improve their health and lose body fat. It is what Janice from Chapter 2 used to lose 116 pounds and reverse her diabetes, heart failure, kidney failure, fatty liver, and high blood pressure. It is also what Jennifer Lopez and Alex Rodriguez used to reboot their health.

Learn more about how to do the 10-Day detox sugar challenge at http://getfarmacy.com/10-day-reset.

3. Support ballot initiatives. I would love to see the US government institute a nationwide sugar-sweetened-beverage or junk-food tax. But the food lobby is so powerful that it's unlikely to happen anytime soon (more on this in Chapter 6). So rather than work from the top down, we have to make progress from the bottom up.

Most of the local soda taxes in America came about because citizens petitioned and voted for them and because the tax revenue is used for community benefit. At least five of the big soda taxes—in places like Oakland, San Francisco, and Berkeley, California; Boulder, Colorado; and Albany, New York—were a result of ballot referendums that grass-roots supporters spearheaded.

Past successes followed a few guiding principles. Marion Nestle, a nutrition professor at New York University and author of *Soda Politics* and *Food Politics*, summarizes the principles that worked. She recommends proposing excise taxes that increase the price of soft drinks by at least 20 percent and explicitly linking revenues to the support of health, activity, or school programs or to providing direct community benefit. When taxes passed it was because broad coalitions supported them, including health, university, and government organizations, and representatives of minority groups. Funding is required to counter the opposition of Big Food.

If every city or county in America had a soda tax, there'd be no need for a national one. So, I urge you to vote in favor of soda tax referendums where you live. If one is not on the ballot, then make it happen yourself. In many places all it takes to get a referendum on the ballot is a proposal with enough signatures behind it. Find out the necessary criteria in your town through a quick Google search or a trip to your local town hall.

For a quick reference guide on the Food Fixes and resources on taxing junk foods and incentivizing healthy choices, go to www.foodfixbook.com.

PART II

THE DIRTY POLITICS OF BIG FOOD

If I had to describe the state of America's food policies in one word, it would be this: chaos! If I got a second word, it would be: disaster.

Eight agencies oversee the government's food-related policies, and they largely work in silos. They rarely coordinate with one another to achieve a common goal, which makes their policies confused and conflicted. In many cases, they directly contradict one another.

"The biggest challenge is that everything is so fractured," says Congressman Tim Ryan from Ohio, who is passionate about fixing our food system. "So, you have people who are involved in the food movement. You have people that are involved in health care. You have people that are involved in education. You have people that are really concerned about the national debt. You've got people that are concerned about government spending. Yet none of these issues are seen as interconnected."

On top of that, most of our food and agriculture policies undermine public health, harm the environment, and increase private profits.

I'll show you how Big Food is playing a big role in this mess. Through its corporate lobbying efforts, the food industry hijacked some of our most important food programs. It profits from sickness and disease and environmental malfeasance—and then it sticks you, the taxpayer, with the bill.

Big Food companies claim to be good stewards of public health. They argue that obesity is a complex issue and that they have an important role to play in addressing it. Engaging government agencies and working on policy issues is a critical part of this effort, they say. But food companies have a much more insidious motive. The real reason they spend so much money in Washington is so they can block policies that hurt their bottom lines and promote policies that make them money. Food corporations have to answer to their shareholders. They have a fiduciary responsibility to maximize shareholder profits, and they pursue this mission zealously—regardless of whether the outcomes are harmful to society and the environment or not. The good news is that due to grassroots efforts, and the undeniability of the harm our food system causes to human health, our environment, and our climate, many Big Food and Ag companies are focused on solutions including healthy product development and regenerative agriculture.

Our nation's disjointed food policies are driving a disease-creating economy (not to mention climate change, social inequities, and a host of other bad consequences), and most people have no idea.

CHAPTER 5

HOW BIG FOOD AND BIG AG CONTROL FOOD POLICY

In February 2017, not long after Donald Trump was sworn into office, the members of the House Agriculture Committee convened a hearing on Capitol Hill to address a controversial issue: Should the government stop people from using food stamps to pay for soft drinks and other junk foods? Two months prior to the congressional hearing, the federal government released a report showing that $7 billion in food stamps are spent on sugary beverages every year.[1] That's 20 to 30 billion servings of soda a year that we give to the poor.[2] Seventy-five percent of the foods purchased with SNAP are ultraprocessed junk food: Oreo cookies, Lay's potato chips, ice cream, and more. It's no surprise that studies show that people who use SNAP have high rates of heart disease, diabetes, and death compared to the rest of the population.[3]

While Uncle Sam can't force anyone to eat fruits and veggies, the government can at least make sure that taxpayer dollars aren't used to subsidize the Frankenfoods that are driving the belt-popping rates of obesity and chronic disease.

For many nutrition experts, the central question of the hearing was a no-brainer, but due to the influence of Big Food's money in politics, making positive change is never easy.

PRIORITIZING NUTRITION QUALITY, NOT JUST QUANTITY

The government created the food stamps program, known as SNAP, or the Supplemental Nutrition Assistance Program, in 1964 to help malnourished Americans. Today the program is a crucial safety net that helps needy families put food on their tables and avoid hunger and food insecurity. And it does a great job at doing exactly that. While the health of those on SNAP is better than those who are eligible but have not signed on, the health of those on SNAP is still dismal. SNAP is the country's largest food assistance program, providing benefits to more than 40 million low-income Americans each month at a cost of tens of billions of dollars a year. SNAP beneficiaries cut across all races and age groups. Roughly 36 percent of them are white, 25 percent are African American (though they make up only 12 percent of the population), 17 percent are Hispanic, about 4 percent are Asian or Native American, and the rest are unknown.[4] Millions are veterans, seniors, or people with disabilities. Almost one in two SNAP recipients is a child.

SNAP is a vital anti-poverty, anti-hunger tool. No doubt about it. But that is why other aspects of the program desperately need reform. The most pressing food problem for low-income households is no longer a lack of calories—it's a lack of *good* calories. Thanks to federal supports for corn, soy, and grains, junk food is now cheaper than ever (with the help of taxpayer dollars), and consumers are exposed to a conveyor belt of empty, disease-producing calories. We have solved the calorie problem. But we now have to solve the problem of nutrient deficiency because processed food has many calories but very few nutrients. Many people only think about provisions for farmers when they hear about the Farm Bill, but its second and most costly component is the food stamps program. In fact, nutrition programs have historically accounted for a majority of the Farm Bill funding.

While SNAP has succeeded in providing food security to more than 40 million Americans, it has failed to protect them in any meaningful way from the ravages of obesity and diet-related diseases. In fact, the food stamps program only increases the likelihood of the most vulnerable Americans consuming an unhealthy diet. In one study, researchers at the Harvard School of Public Health examined the diets of nearly 4,000 adults who lived below the federal poverty level. They looked at differences between SNAP participants and nonparticipants. They found that SNAP recipients consumed 44 percent more fruit juice, 56 percent more potatoes, 46 percent more red meat, 39 percent fewer whole grains, and, among women, 61 percent more soft drinks. Overall, they found that SNAP participants were in dire need of nutrition interventions. "Although the diets of all low-income adults need major improvement," they reported, "SNAP participants in particular had lower-quality diets than did income-eligible nonparticipants."[5]

In another study, the researchers found that children living in SNAP households consumed high levels of empty calories, soft drinks, and processed meats.[6] The findings dovetail with studies by the Mayo Clinic as well as research carried out by the USDA itself, which administers the SNAP program.[7]

BIG FOOD TARGETS THE VULNERABLE

So why do SNAP recipients eat so poorly? Part of the reason is that grocery stores and food companies know exactly when SNAP benefits are distributed each month. They time their junk-food marketing on those days to target SNAP recipients. A 2018 study in the *American Journal of Preventive Medicine* found that shoppers in poor New York City neighborhoods were two to four times more likely to encounter soda displays and sugary drink advertisements in grocery stores during the first week of the month,[8] the same week people get their food stamps. Yet the ads for low- and zero-calorie drinks didn't spike during these periods. Meanwhile, wealthier neighborhoods (where there are few food stamp recipients) didn't see the same increase in junk-food ads during the first week of the month. The implication is clear: Big Food aims its junk-food ads at low-income Americans with a laser focus. The retailers target SNAP recipients with the worst and most profitable foods.[9]

So why do companies target SNAP recipients with junk foods instead of health foods? It's simple: Soft drinks are far more profitable than fresh produce. As my friend David Ludwig, a leading obesity expert at Harvard Medical School, explains it, "There's a massive profit margin on sugary beverages, more so than for fruits, vegetables, meats, and seafood. They get heavily advertised, put at the front of the store, and put on special sales, specifically targeting SNAP recipients."

Almost every other government food program—from school lunches to military food programs to WIC (the Special Supplemental Nutrition Program for Women, Infants, and Children) —has at least some nutrition standards. But SNAP has none. And it's created a huge economic and public health catastrophe. A 2017 study by Dariush Mozaffarian and his colleagues at Tufts followed almost half a million adults over a decade and found that SNAP participants had substantially worse health than other Americans: twice the rate of heart disease, three times greater likelihood to die from diabetes, and higher rates of metabolic diseases.[10] SNAP beneficiaries account for at least 65 percent of the adults on Medicaid and 14 percent of people on Medicare.[11] The math is simple: Providing healthy and nutritious foods to SNAP recipients would reduce chronic disease rates and sharply lower health care costs. It would benefit the millions of people who depend on SNAP and ultimately save taxpayers billions or potentially even trillions of dollars.

The federal government has a duty to set nutrition standards for the food stamps program, which it ignores. Increasing access to healthier foods and removing obvious junk foods from the program would reduce obesity and diabetes rates and dramatically lower health care costs. As David Ludwig puts it, "We've allowed SNAP, due to food industry lobbying and neglect, to become a conveyor belt of terribly unhealthful calories. With modest reforms, we can continue to address the important problem of hunger in the United States and at the same time help reduce diet-related chronic diseases that are devastating low-income communities."

POLITICAL SWAY

To give you an idea of how challenging it can be to introduce even modest reforms into public programs like SNAP, let's go back to our 2017 hearing of the House Agriculture Committee, which oversees the roughly $900 billion Farm Bill that includes SNAP. Some on the panel of food and poverty experts at the hearing argued that eliminating sugary drinks from the program was a badly needed measure that could improve the health of millions of Americans, sharply reducing health care costs in the process. Other experts who opposed them said the restrictions would stigmatize SNAP users and create too much red tape. "Confusion at the checkout aisle," they cried.[12] This is a specious argument because SNAP already limits certain purchases, such as certain energy drinks, alcohol, and hot foods. Every checkout clerk knows what's covered and what's not, plus the government publishes a list.[13]

But the most striking comments came from the lawmakers themselves. One by one, dozens of congressmen and women took turns dismissing the link between junk-food diets and obesity. Congressman Roger Marshall, an obstetrician from Kansas, said a lack of exercise was the primary factor driving obesity rates. Then Congressman David Scott from Georgia took the floor and attacked what he called the food police. Preventing SNAP recipients from using their food stamps to pay for Mountain Dew, Coke, and Oreo cookies was not only cruel, he argued, but practically a violation of their constitutional rights as well. He ignored the fact that other government programs enforce nutrition standards without violating constitutional rights, such as school lunches and the WIC program.

"Look at the complexity you're going to put into the grocery store," he barked. "Who's going to pick up that extra cost to have the food police there monitoring, and why? I think that a better way of going about solving many of these things is to look at how we educate people. You can't force them. You can't deny them their freedoms to be able to make choices without violating their pursuit of happiness." Oh yes. Coke = Happiness. Pursuit of happiness. Not sure that's what Thomas Jefferson had in mind in the Declaration of Independence.

Congressman Scott then made a series of claims even though decades of research on diet and exercise contradicted him. "Sodas, candy, sweet things—that's not what makes us obese. It is the lack of our children exercising," he insisted. "Look at the history of this country. Look at us 30 years ago, 20 years ago. What has happened? Our children, and us, we don't exercise. We don't have physical education in the schools anymore."

Scott's argument was a masterful attempt to distract attention from the real issue, America's diet, and shift the blame onto exercise. Of course, exercise is part of the obesity problem, but you can't exercise your way out of a bad diet. It sounded as if Scott's statements had been taken straight from the food industry's playbook—and that was no coincidence. Lobbying reports show that Big Food companies and their deep-pocketed trade groups routinely shower the members of the House Agriculture Committee with campaign contributions and political gifts. Guess who is a top recipient. Congressman Scott.

If lawmakers were required to wear the logos of their corporate sponsors, Scott would look like a NASCAR driver sponsored by Big Food. Since 2006, Coca-Cola has given him more than $42,000 in direct financial donations. The company was his single largest campaign contributor in 2018, followed closely by the National Confectioners Association, the biggest trade and lobbying group for the candy industry.[14] Scott took an additional $105,000 from an influential political action committee, the Blue Dog PAC, which is funded by a roster of food industry giants that includes Coke, Pepsi, the American Beverage Association, Dunkin' Brands (the parent company of Dunkin' Donuts), and the Grocery Manufacturers Association, the largest (now relaunched) food industry lobbying group.

Scott wasn't the only one at the hearing who benefited. Top contributors to Congressman Roger Marshall were sugar industry giants Archer Daniels Midland and American Crystal Sugar, one of the country's largest sugar producers.[15] The sugar industry was a top contributor to both the chair of the House Agriculture Committee, Frank Lucas, and the committee's ranking member, Collin Peterson.[16] In total, the forty-six members of Congress that make up the House Agriculture Committee took roughly $1.2 million in campaign contributions from the soda and sugar industries between 2015 and 2018.[17] While the hearing was full of theatrics, it ended with a collective shrug from Congressman Scott and the other members of the committee, who decided not to implement any junk-food restrictions on SNAP programs. Congress: bought and sold. Government of the corporations, by the corporations, and for the corporations.

The food industry is no fool. Junk-food companies are acutely aware that sugary-drink restrictions on SNAP would wipe away billions of dollars of their annual revenue. So behind closed doors, their lobbyists have worked closely with lawmakers and government officials to stop that from ever happening. Many anti-hunger groups and national food banks, like the Food Research and Action Center, or FRAC, have also used their political influence to resist efforts to ban sugary drinks from SNAP. SNAP is just one of many government food policies that suffer from a systemic problem. Instead of prioritizing public health and the interests of society, lawmakers and government agencies are often forced to do the bidding of Big Food. That explains why the $7 billion question at the heart of that 2017 hearing on SNAP and sugary drinks was decided long before the hearing even began.

FOOD FIX: PRIORITIZE NUTRITION—PUT THE "N" BACK IN SNAP

Every semester, Pamela Koch, a professor at Columbia University who researches the connections between a sustainable food system and healthy eating, gives the students in her community nutrition class a fascinating assignment. She makes them eat on a $40 budget for exactly one week, so they see what life is like for the average low-income SNAP recipient. Students have to buy all their food from SNAP-eligible locations, like supermarkets and small grocery stores. That means there's no stopping and picking up a $10 salad and a $4 bottle of kombucha from Whole Foods. Often, they can't even afford to buy lunch. "It's an eye-opening experience for them," Koch says. "Truthfully, the amount that people are given for SNAP is based on what's called the thrifty food plan, which is unrealistic in a lot of ways."

The assignment shows her students why SNAP is so vital for people who are food insecure—people who often have no idea where their next meal is coming from. It also makes it crystal clear why food insecurity and obesity go hand in hand: When you only have $40 a week for food, you have to buy cheap food that comes in large quantities: big bottles of soda, boxes of cookies, bags of potato chips, processed meats, sugary breakfast cereals, Wonder Bread, and on and on and on. Since people on SNAP are not allowed to buy hot foods, you can't go to your grocery store and buy a $5 rotisserie chicken, but you can stock up on 2-liter bottles of 7Up and frozen chicken nuggets. Is it any surprise that these toxic foods are the most popular purchases for people on SNAP?

How do we make sure that SNAP recipients have access to nutritious and affordable foods? We can't just eliminate soda and expect that the program will be fixed.

Koch and other experts say the real way to fix SNAP is to combine junk-food restrictions with incentives to buy healthy foods. A study published in *JAMA Internal Medicine* in 2016 shows how this would work. Researchers recruited adults in the Minneapolis area who were living below the federal poverty line and were not already on SNAP. Then they split them into groups and gave them debit cards with money for food—the same way SNAP benefits work. One group was not allowed to buy sugary drinks, candy, and other junk foods. Another group was told they would receive a 30 percent financial incentive to buy fruits and vegetables. In other words, their money would go much further if they spent it on fresh produce. A third group got both the junk-food restrictions and the healthy food incentives. The fourth group, which served as the control, just received the standard SNAP benefits.

After three months, the group that ate the smallest amount of junk food and the largest amount of fresh produce was the group that had both the healthy incentives and the junk-food prohibition. Even more interesting was that the incentive-only and the prohibition-only groups didn't see much of a difference in their diets. That is pretty solid evidence that the best way to reform SNAP is to eliminate the worst foods while making the best foods more affordable and accessible.[18]

FOOD FIX: OFFER INCENTIVES FOR HEALTHY FOODS

Some successful real-world experiments are finding ways to enable and encourage SNAP participants to eat healthy, whole food. The USDA makes fresh vegetables and other healthy ingredients at farmers' markets more affordable for SNAP participants through its Food Insecurity Nutrition Incentive Program. Many states are also starting to step up to the plate with their own healthy food programs for SNAP participants. In 2017, Massachusetts launched a program that gives SNAP recipients extra money for every dollar they spend on fruits and vegetables grown by local farmers. More than 35,000 SNAP recipients in Massachusetts have taken advantage of the program, including people like Rebecca Martin, a single mother with disabilities from Northampton who purchases seedlings with her extra SNAP benefits and uses them to grow fruits and vegetables in a community garden near her home. Rebecca says the program not only boosted her family's health and well-being but also helped her reverse a painful chronic condition.[19]

At the popular Birdhouse Farmers Market in Richmond, Virginia, SNAP participants can stock up on locally grown mushrooms, apples, kale, and other fresh veggies while participating in family activities like cooking demos and classes that teach them how to compost. Nearly half of the more than 225 farmers' markets in Virginia are authorized to accept SNAP benefits. Thanks to a statewide program called Virginia Fresh Match, Birdhouse is among the farmers' markets where SNAP dollars are worth double their value when they're used to buy fruits and vegetables.[20]

Across the country, in Michigan, another program has found a way to give incentives to SNAP recipients to eat healthier: For every $10 in food stamps they spend on locally grown produce, they receive a $10 coupon that enables them to buy additional fruits and vegetables of any kind. The program, called Double Up Food Bucks, was such a hit that it has spread to more than twenty-five other states, including Alabama, Arkansas, California, and North Carolina.[21]

All these programs serve a double purpose. They encourage low-income Americans to use their SNAP benefits for healthy foods instead of junk foods, and they increase business for America's small farmers, who need all the support they can get (more on this in Chapter 15). Unfortunately, healthy incentives have not been a priority for the federal government. The 2014 Farm Bill, for example, contained just $100 million in funding (out of $70 billion) for these healthy incentives programs. While that may sound like a lot, it's insignificant compared to everything else in the Farm Bill, like the billions in support to grow and insure commodity crops and animal feed. It's also a drop in the bucket compared to the billions in SNAP money that pays for soft drinks and junk foods.

Imagine if all the supports the government poured into commodity crops and soft drinks were used to ensure that every city or town in America could provide locally grown produce to low-income families at little or no cost. Thankfully a group of experts at Tufts' Friedman School of Nutrition Science and Policy did the math, and they found the following: Providing a 20 percent incentive for fruit and vegetable purchases to Medicaid and Medicare beneficiaries would *prevent at least 1.93 million cardiovascular disease events and a net savings of $40 billion in health care costs.* An even broader 20 percent incentive for nuts, fish, whole grains, and olive oil would *prevent 3.31 million cardiovascular events and a net savings of $102.4 billion in health care costs after the cost of the healthy food incentives.*[22] Not bad for a bit of fresh food.

FOOD FIX: POLICY ACTIONS FOR FIXING SNAP

We know what needs to be done to fix SNAP—and there is surprising agreement across the political aisle. In March 2018, the Bipartisan Policy Center, a respected think tank that combines the best ideas from Democrats and Republicans, issued a report entitled *Leading with Nutrition: Leveraging Federal Programs for Better Health* on ways to improve SNAP.[23] The group came up with a series of recommendations, including some that I and others have long advocated for.

- **Make diet quality a core element of SNAP.** Congress can add a diet-quality component to SNAP under the next Farm Bill or through a presidential executive order. Or the USDA could make a policy change and then check progress by tracking the nutrition content of SNAP recipients' diets and publishing studies.
- **Eliminate sugary drinks from the list of items that can be purchased with SNAP benefits.** As we've seen, virtually every major health organization—WHO, the CDC (Centers for Disease Control), the National Academy of Medicine, the USDA, and Health and Human Services—urges people to limit them. The average low-income adult consumes three servings of sugary drinks a day. Just one soda a day increases the risk of diabetes by 32 percent.[24] The USDA needs to promote healthy diets and improve the health of the poor by removing sugary drinks from the food stamps program. Right now.
- **Strengthen incentives for purchasing fruits and vegetables.** Congress should up the paltry $100 million in the last Farm Bill for healthy incentives programs. How? By diverting subsidies for crop insurance and commodities to the programs we discussed in the last section that make fruits and vegetables more affordable and accessible. These programs should be available at farmers' markets and large supermarkets and grocery stores in low-income neighborhoods. We know that combining restrictions on soda purchases along with incentives for buying fruits and veggies improves the

nutritional quality of diets much more than either measure alone.[25] And a report from the USDA found that a majority of families using the SNAP healthy incentives programs reported buying larger amounts and greater varieties of vegetables as a result of it.[26]

- **Authorize funding for the USDA to launch experimental new pilot programs.** The small pilot programs that encourage SNAP users to purchase more fruits and vegetables have been so successful that Congress should authorize more funding for innovative programs for SNAP users. According to the Bipartisan Policy Center's report, an investment of $100 million over five years would allow the USDA to pilot a range of other programs. The USDA could look at encouraging not only healthy eating but also sustainable diets and environmental change strategies and a program that delivers low-cost nutritious meals to SNAP users with disabilities and others with special needs.

- **Align SNAP and Medicaid.** Many SNAP users are also Medicaid beneficiaries. Because poor diet is responsible for so many chronic conditions and procedures that drive up Medicaid costs, these two programs need to align. How about pilot programs using SNAP funds that deliver highly nutritious meals to SNAP and Medicaid recipients suffering from malnutrition, chronic disease, or disabilities that limit their ability to prepare home-cooked meals? Studies show that these kinds of services can improve health outcomes and reduce Medicaid costs.[27] Using SNAP to prioritize nutrition for Medicaid patients is just plain common sense. It can save lives and prevent billions of dollars in unnecessary medical costs.

On a more personal level of action, I urge you to ask your elected leaders about this. These are *your* tax dollars at work. Find out where your local member of Congress stands on SNAP reform. Are your elected leaders in the pocket of Big Food? Find out on Food Policy Action's website if they vote for Big Food or for you. You can look up your member of Congress and their voting records on food and agriculture issues. Find out if they have the courage to stand up to the big moneyed interests. And if they are failing on this issue, write to them or tell them about it at your next town hall. Tell them you want your tax dollars to be better spent. Reforming SNAP will improve the health of millions of Americans, and it will help reduce the enormous strain on our health care system.

For a quick reference guide on the Food Fixes and resources on changing the government's role in promoting bad food and reforming SNAP, go to www.foodfixbook.com.

CHAPTER 6

THE POWER OF FOOD INDUSTRY LOBBYISTS

Many of Big Food's tactics, like the widespread marketing of ultrapro-cessed foods, are plain and easy to see. You cannot watch television, flip open a magazine, or drive down a highway without seeing an ad for Coca-Cola, McDonald's, or Burger King. But the dirty politics of food often play out behind closed doors in the halls of Congress, far from public view. As we saw in the SNAP hearing in the last chapter, government lobbying is arguably the food industry's most effective strategy. Armies of high-powered lobbyists have long occupied Capitol Hill to promote the interests of Big Food, pushing multibillion-dollar efforts to influence our laws, politicians, and government programs and agencies.

FOLLOW THE MONEY

The voices heard by our legislators are those of industry, not citizens. Lobbyists for Big Food, Big Ag, and Big Pharma spent $500 million on influencing the 2014 Farm Bill alone. Hundreds of millions more in the past decade were spent in lobbying across the whole government to influence food and agriculture policies.

Food industry lobbying occurs at every level of government, from city halls and state capitols to the halls of Congress, the White House, the USDA, and the FDA, and extends globally. The lobbyists' goal is to protect the food industry's profits at all costs. Much like Big Pharma, Big Oil, and other large and powerful industries, Big Food and Big Ag have what the vast majority of Americans do not: deep pockets and access to the highest levels of government. And they use those to capture the agencies and lawmakers that are supposed to regulate them.

Lobbyists and food companies accomplish this in many ways. They shower politicians with campaign contributions, a practice that studies have shown directly influences legislation, causing lawmakers to alter the wording of bills or add lucrative earmarks (banned since 2010) that favor their donors.[1] Lobbyists invite politicians to lavish receptions and give them expensive gifts, like golf outings, Super Bowl tickets, and pricey concert seats. (While there have been restrictions on the gifts that politicians can accept since 1995, lobbyists often find and exploit many loopholes.) One analysis found that in a single year, Utah lobbyists gave state lawmakers more than a quarter million dollars in gifts, including vacation trips to Florida, tickets to Utah Jazz games, and Billy Joel concert seats.[2] In some cases they gave lawmakers American Express gift cards.

Another lobbying tactic involves the use of PACs, or political action committees, and super PACs, which pool money from companies and large donors to fund candidates and political parties. They also buy ads supporting their candidates and attacking their opponents. Super PACs have fundamentally altered the landscape of money in politics. Thanks to a Supreme Court ruling in 2010—called *Citizens United v. FEC*—there are very few limits to their financial donations. This gives corporations or wealthy individuals inordinate power to influence elections.

Through super PACs, corporations and special interest groups are now free to inject unlimited amounts of money into public discourse with limited public disclosure. As Congressman Tim Ryan from Ohio described it to me, "Nobody knows where the money comes from. It's dark money. You can literally write millions of dollars' worth of campaign donations to these super PACs, and no one will ever know who you are." This applies to both Democrats and Republicans.

The lawmakers can return the favor by writing legislation and implementing policies that benefit their donors. If the owner of a large coal company donates $15 million to a super PAC, the lawmakers who

benefit from that money can ease environmental regulations that benefit the coal industry, boosting profits. Same goes for benefits to unions
from their donations. It is not transactional, or a quid pro quo, but the
intent of the donations is clear.

THE REVOLVING DOOR

Many corporate lobbyists share a similar background. They are often
former politicians and political aides who have an inside track into their
former agencies and the clubby chambers of Congress. Even worse is
the revolving-door phenomenon, where lobbyists and government
officials cycle back and forth between jobs in the industry and jobs in
the government. It is a practice that industry insiders take advantage of
to pull strings for corporations and special interests. When President
Obama was in office, he took steps to clamp down on the practice. In
2009 he signed an executive order forbidding lobbyists from working
for agencies that they had lobbied at any point in the previous two years.
It was known as the "cooling off" rule, and it became the centerpiece
of what his White House called "the most sweeping ethics reform in
history." Although the intent was good, the Obama administration also
hired many industry lobbyists.[3]

When President Trump took the reins, despite vehemently promising to "drain the swamp" on the campaign trail, his administration
ignored the cooling-off rule in some cases and in other cases simply
issued waivers that allowed lobbyists to jump straight from their firms
to the government agencies they had lobbied only days or weeks earlier. A report from the government watchdog group Public Citizen
found that at least 133 registered lobbyists were appointed to government positions in the Trump administration's first six months. At least
60 of them had been active in the two years prior to being appointed,
and 36 had lobbied agencies and issues that were directly related to their
new government roles. Some were required to sign ethics "pledges"
that turned out to be vague and largely unenforced. For instance,
Trump's FDA commissioner, Scott Gottlieb, joined the board of Pfizer

just months after stepping down from his government post. A win for Big Pharma, a liability for the average citizen.

One agency where the revolving door has had a striking impact is the USDA. The agency hired a sugar lobbyist named Kailee Tkacz to work as an adviser on its 2020 Dietary Guidelines.[4] Immediately prior to joining the agency, Tkacz was a lobbyist for the Corn Refiners Association, which represents the biggest producers of high-fructose corn syrup. Prior to that she was a lobbyist for the Snack Food Association (now SNAC International), nicknamed Washington's voice for sugar, fat, and salt because its members include such companies as Kraft and Frito-Lay. Even though Tkacz had a blatant conflict of interest that should have disqualified her, the White House permitted her appointment, saying she was "uniquely qualified to assist the Secretary of Agriculture and his senior leadership team in issuing the 2020 Dietary Guidelines for Americans."[5]

A short time later, the agency plucked three other lobbyists from the food industry to help shape policy:

- Maggie Lyons was hired to advise the head of the USDA and other senior officials on SNAP, WIC, and the school lunch program—the very issues she lobbied the agency on while working for the National Grocers Association only a few months earlier.[6]
- Brooke Appleton, a corn and wheat lobbyist who spent years lobbying the USDA on elements of the Farm Bill, was hired by the agency to advise it on elements of the 2018 Farm Bill.[7]
- Kristi Boswell had lobbied Congress on behalf of the Farm Bureau in support of legislation that would have made it easier for agribusinesses to deny health care coverage to seasonal farmworkers. Boswell was hired by the USDA to work on the same issues that she lobbied on: regulations involving seasonal farmworkers.[8]

The food industry contends that hiring lobbyists for government positions makes political sense because lobbyists often have unique insights and expertise on obscure regulatory issues. To some extent that might be true. But it's also naïve to believe that a former sugar lobbyist would advocate for sugar restrictions in the dietary guidelines. Or that a lobbyist who spent years opposing mandatory health care coverage for seasonal farmworkers would suddenly fight to protect farmworkers' rights. Not to mention that these men and women know that, once they leave their government roles, they can walk through Washington's revolving door and immediately return to their lucrative lobbying positions.

PROTECTING PROFITS IN THE SHADOWS

Louis Brandeis, the Supreme Court justice, famously said that sunlight was the greatest disinfectant. Publicity, he argued, can be a powerful remedy for social injustice. Though he wrote those words more than a century ago, they remain as true today as they were then—and they are the reason food industry lobbyists are so careful to do the bulk of their work out of the public eye. In 2017, more than 11,500 lobbyists registered with the federal government. That's 21 lobbyists for every single member of Congress. Some of the biggest corporations, like Walmart, have as many as 100 lobbyists working for them at any given time.[9] But even that is just the tip of the iceberg. Studies show that thousands of unregistered lobbyists—so-called shadow lobbyists—work off the books thanks to obscure loopholes and lax enforcement. James Thurber, a professor at American University who studies the issue, has found that the true number of lobbyists working in Washington is around 100,000.[10] This estimate may be debatable, nonetheless it is a big number. That is enough lobbyists to fill two Yankee Stadiums or enough to have 187 lobbyists for every member of Congress. The amount spent on lobbying is staggering, about $3.4 billion a year in 2018.[11]

It should not surprise you to learn that many of the biggest names in the food industry deploy sophisticated lobbying operations to protect their profits. According to the Center for Responsive Politics, a non-profit that tracks special interest spending, the food companies and trade groups that lobby the government the most are Coke, Pepsi, Monsanto, the American Beverage Association, Nestlé, General Mills, McDonald's, Kellogg's, the candy and dairy industries, and the Grocery Manufacturers Association (GMA), who collectively spend literally hundreds of millions of dollars to influence lawmakers.

Although the Big Food companies claim to be good stewards of public health, the real reason they spend so much money in Washington is so they can block policies that hurt their bottom lines and promote policies that make them money. Food corporations have to answer to their shareholders. Unfortunately, because their products are frequently toxic, it just so happens that more often than not they end up taking a position that undermines public health. An analysis of their lobbying tactics found that 97 percent of the time the soda industry took positions antagonistic to public health, opposing limits to marketing junk food to kids or for better child nutrition.[12]

What exactly is Big Food lobbying against? Here are just a few examples.

Protections from Dangerous Chemicals

In 2009, the American Beverage Association filed eighty different lobbying reports related to twenty-four bills in Congress. Among the legislation it sought to influence was the Ban Poisonous Additives (BPA) Act of 2009, which would have ended the use of bisphenol-A (commonly known as BPA) in children's food and drink containers. BPA, a synthetic hormone that imitates estrogen in the body, has been linked to cancer, obesity, and heart disease.[13] Why would anyone want to keep these chemicals in children's food and beverage containers? It's simple: For many in the food industry, including soft drink companies, profit trumps public health and replacing BPA costs money. The American Beverage Association filed more than a dozen lobbying reports documenting its efforts to scuttle the BPA Act. They were ultimately successful. The bill failed, never making it out of committee for a vote.[14] While some states have banned the use of BPA, the FDA still declares it safe.

Fast-Food Lawsuits

Tobacco companies have been sued for giving people lung cancer. Oil companies have been sued for polluting the environment. Fast-food companies do not want to be sued for making people fat, sick, and diabetic. For more than a decade, they have spent millions trying to get politicians to pass laws shielding them from obesity-related lawsuits. As of 2018, at least twenty-six states have passed these so-called Commonsense Consumption measures, which are better known as "cheeseburger laws."[15]

Federal lawmakers have tried to enact them too. The biggest proponent of these measures was Ric Keller, a Republican congressman from Florida who sponsored two separate bills protecting fast-food makers from obesity-related lawsuits.[16] The Personal Responsibility in Food Consumption Act passed in the House but not in the Senate. Why would Keller sponsor these ridiculous bills? It could be the fact that he took hundreds of thousands of dollars in donations from a PAC representing McDonald's, Wendy's, and Burger King. He also took roughly $60,000 from Darden Restaurants, the parent company of Olive Garden, as well as $50,000 from the National Beer Wholesalers Association and more than $30,000 from the National Restaurant Association, which represents Taco Bell, Dunkin' Donuts, and Domino's Pizza. While fast-food lawsuits might strike some as frivolous, there is a reason Big Food companies are so desperate to stop them. As Michele Simon, a public health lawyer and food industry expert, argued in her book *Appetite for Profit*, the food industry is terrified of forced disclosure: "What scares food companies even more than costly jury verdicts is the prospect of the discovery process—when lawyers are allowed access to the defendant's documents and other inside information—unearthing damning information about dishonest industry practices. This in turn, can open the door to a plethora of new government regulation. An avalanche of damning documents discovered through litigation against the tobacco industry revealed so much information that an entire research group at the University of California is currently dedicated to its study. The food industry has learned from tobacco that litigation is a powerful public interest tool."[17] The buried information includes acknowledgment of the addictive nature of processed food, the specific and deliberate targeting of children, minorities, and the poor, and the strategic manipulation of science and scientists to influence policy and public opinion, among other revealing information.

GMO Label Transparency

When it comes to your health, nothing is more important than what you put in your mouth. As I always say: Food isn't just calories; it's information. That's why the more we know about our food—what's in it, where it's from, and how it was grown or raised—the better. But the food industry would rather keep you in the dark. The most damaging result of Big Food's battle against transparency was a bill passed in 2016 that limited your right to know whether GMOs lurk in your food. This is an issue that should be concerning to everyone. Genetically modified crops were sold to us with great promise: The technology was supposed to make crops immune to weed killers and pests, leading to an abundance of foods that would solve the problem of world hunger. We were told that genetically engineered crops would require fewer pesticides and herbicides and produce higher yields. But none of that has turned out to be true.

Studies have found that genetically modifying crops has little or no benefit to crop yields. At the same time, genetically engineered crops are undoubtedly bad for the environment (see Chapter 15). They've fueled the spread of herbicide-resistant superweeds on more than 60 million acres of American farmland, leading farmers to increase their use of toxic weed killers like Monsanto's Roundup, the most widely used pesticide in the world and a known carcinogen.[18] These toxins leach into the ground, contaminate rivers and streams, and taint our food supply. Genetically modified plants are the most pesticide- and herbicide-laden crops—and shockingly, an estimated three-quarters of the food in our supermarkets contain them.

At least sixty-four countries have laws mandating GMO labeling, including the twenty-eight nations of the European Union and most other developed countries including China and Russia, not generally known for consumer protections or transparency.[19]

For a while, the United States was headed in that direction as well. In 2014, Vermont became the first state to pass a law mandating labels on GMO foods. Then Maine and Connecticut followed suit. The measures were so popular that GMO-labeling initiatives were added to statewide ballots across the country, supported by grassroots advocates. Then Big Food got involved and quashed the movement.

The industry complained that labeling GMO foods would increase their production costs, leading to higher prices for consumers. It didn't matter that independent studies refuted this claim.[20] Big Food turned to its allies in Congress and spearheaded a bill overturning state laws requiring GMO labeling, commonly referred to by opponents as the DARK Act, for Denying Americans the Right to Know.

Big Food poured a shocking amount of money into this bill, underscoring just how terrifying it found GMO labeling. An analysis by the Environmental Working Group found that food companies spent more than $50 million lobbying for the legislation in the first half of 2015 alone.[21] That is money they could have easily spent on better labeling and better ingredients in their products!

It's no surprise that some of the biggest spenders were companies that depend heavily on high-fructose corn syrup, vegetable oils, and other GMO ingredients. Six companies—Coke, Pepsi, Kraft, Kellogg's, Land O'Lakes, and General Mills—spent at least $12.6 million lobbying against GMO labeling laws. Meanwhile the GMA hired thirty-two lobbyists and spent more than $10 million lobbying against the measures. Ultimately, the Environmental Working Group analysis found that the food and biotech industries together spent a combined $143 million lobbying against GMO labeling between 2013 and 2015. They also launched a widespread public campaign to influence public opinion—paying for billboards, radio and television commercials, social media ads, flyers, and other materials to mislead Americans into thinking that GMO labels would hurt their pocketbooks.

The industry's exorbitant campaign did not fool the public. One *New York Times* survey found that three-quarters of Americans expressed concern about GMO ingredients in their food and 93 percent favored labeling them.[22] But the industry used its political clout to subvert the will of the people. The DARK Act nullified labeling laws in Vermont and other states. Instead of mandating clear GMO identifiers on all packages containing them, it made labeling voluntary. It also gave food companies convenient options. They were told they could slap a barcode on packages that consumers could scan to find out if an item contains GMOs or an 800 number that consumers could call. While the food industry portrayed this as a compromise, it put an enormous burden on consumers. How many shoppers are going to walk through the supermarket scanning every single item they pick up, or making phone calls to find out if the dozens of groceries in their shopping carts contain GMOs? And what about poor and elderly people in rural areas who may not have access to the digital technology required?

The DARK Act deprives Americans of what should be easily accessible information about their food. But the law isn't written in stone. With enough pressure on politicians and the Big Food companies they're beholden to, Americans who want truth and transparency on food labels can overturn it.

DARK MONEY PROPAGANDA THROUGH FAKE GRASSROOTS EFFORTS

An earlier battle over GMO labeling illustrates one of the most insidious ways that Big Food controls public opinion, through benevolently named front groups that pretend to promote the interests of citizens and the science.

Long before the DARK Act was signed into law, food activists like Chris and Leah McManus, a couple of organic-loving vegans from northwest Washington, were doing their part to push for strong GMO labeling laws. Early one Friday morning in the summer of 2012, Chris and Leah walked into the Washington State Capitol building in Olympia with a petition for a statewide referendum. They wanted to launch a state law requiring that all genetically modified foods carry a clear and easy-to-read GMO label.

The couple had a groundswell of grassroots support: About 350,000 people across the state had signed their petition. Supporters of the referendum, called Initiative 522, included some of Washington's most recognizable icons, like the fishmongers who toss freshly caught salmon and halibut at Seattle's famous Pike Place Fish Market, who were worried about genetically modified farmed salmon escaping and interbreeding with wild salmon.

Initiative 522 also attracted the attention of the Grocery Manufacturers Association. Most people have never heard of the GMA, the food industry's largest and oldest lobbying group, but they most certainly know its 300 or so member companies. They include food industry titans like General Mills, Hershey's, Kellogg's, Procter & Gamble, Welch's, Coca-Cola, PepsiCo, H.J. Heinz, and Kraft. The GMA is a major player in DC.

In fact, a senior executive at one of the largest food companies in the world told me that the GMA has aggressively obstructed regulation and legislation that can improve the food system. That is why Nestlé, Unilever, Danone, and Mars quit the GMA and started the Sustainable Food Policy Alliance to improve the food system. What they do remains to be seen, but it was a big statement for them to leave GMA and a step in the right direction resulting from consumer demand for different food and different polices.

Between 2005 and 2016, the GMA spent roughly $50 million lobbying the federal government. At the top of the group's agenda in 2012 was GMO labeling. In a speech that year to the American Soybean Association, Pamela Bailey, the GMA's president at the time, called it "the single-highest priority for GMA this year."[23] The food industry hated the idea of a labeling requirement. Almost every processed-food maker would have to slap GMO labels on most of their products. General Mills would have to put it on packages of Cinnamon Toast Crunch and Honey Nut Cheerios. Coke and Pepsi would have to put it on their soft drinks. Kellogg's would be forced to put it on their frozen waffles, Pop-Tarts, and cornflakes. Even Welch's fruit juice would have to carry a GMO label.

The GMA was prepared to stop the Washington State initiative at all costs. The board members hatched a plan to fund an aggressive "No on 522" campaign to discredit the GMO labeling measure, using television, print, radio, and Internet ads to call it unscientific, costly, and confusing. The resulting ads were blatantly misleading, claiming that "farmers, food producers and scientists" were against the labeling initiative, making it appear to the public that there was grassroots opposition to GMO labeling. This tactic is known as astroturfing, and it has a long and notorious history. Perfected by tobacco companies, astroturfing involves creating *fake grassroots* campaigns against policies and regulations to dupe the public.

There was one problem for the GMA, though: Because it was trying to influence the outcome of an election ballot initiative, it was required under campaign finance laws to disclose that it was funding the "No on 522" campaign. But it's hard to convince Americans that farmers are raising their pitchforks against GMO labeling when your ad has a disclaimer that it was paid for by Coke and Pepsi.

The GMA and its member companies knew this tactic could backfire because they had already used it to discredit a similar labeling initiative in California earlier that year: Prop 37, the California Right to Know Genetically Engineered Food Act, spending more than $30 million on a misinformation campaign. Though Prop 37 narrowly failed at the polls, the ensuing media coverage cast the food companies and their tactics in a harsh light, and heavy pushback from consumers and health advocates soon followed, including threats of boycotts.[24] At a board meeting in January 2013, Pamela Bailey lamented to the board that although their astroturf campaign in California was successful, it carried the costs of heavy criticism and shrinking consumer confidence in all the brands that were involved. That was something they had to avoid in future battles.[25]

Louis Finkel, a GMA staff member, said they would need to develop a covert strategy that shielded the companies from the kind of pushback they got after the mudslinging in California. He suggested a "multiple use fund"—a war chest—that the individual corporations could pour their money into. The reason for the fund was twofold. First, it would provide a long-term pot of money that the GMA could draw from to attack the patchwork of state measures. And second, the companies could use it to skirt campaign finance laws.

Altogether the GMA member companies spent more than $15 million on "No on 522":

- Pepsi dumped almost $3 million into the war chest.
- Coke and Nestlé each poured $1.7 million into it.
- General Mills contributed a million dollars, as did Conagra Brands, and so on.

Only this time, because the GMA was acting as a front for the companies, the companies were able to bankroll the "No on 522" campaign without disclosing their direct roles in it. In a particularly brazen sign of the con they pulled, the GMA coached its member companies on what to say if any journalists asked them whether they were paying for the campaign. Internal documents show that the companies were instructed to simply tell reporters "No"—a flagrant lie. The GMA warned the companies not to say much more than that because "it will lead the press and or NGO groups right where we don't want them to go— meaning, 'are you assessing your members, or do you have a "secret" fund of some kind?' "[26]

In mid-2013, as the campaign blanketed the Washington State airwaves with attacks on the labeling measure, the GMA's plan seemed to be working flawlessly. Except for one major problem: It was illegal. The state's attorney general, Bob Ferguson, noticed that the campaign was identical to Big Food tactics employed in other states. As Washington voters prepared to cast their ballots, Ferguson filed a restraining order in October 2013, demanding that the GMA publicly disclose who was funding the campaign.

In November, the initiative narrowly failed, with 51 percent of voters opposing it and 49 percent supporting it—the same slim margin that took down the California proposition. Big Food and its deep pockets once again made the difference, and in the process helped to set a new record for money spent against a Washington State initiative.

When Ferguson and his office dug deeper and began to uncover the extent of Big Food's deception, they filed a lawsuit against the GMA alleging gross campaign finance violations in an attempt to mislead the public. In a case that featured some dramatic and tense moments, the GMA employed a strategy that could best be summed up as deny, deny, deny. Finkel and Bailey both testified that their intentions were not to hide the sources of the money, that shielding the member companies from public scrutiny was not their goal, and that they had no intention of violating the law. Unfortunately for them, the judge presiding over the case didn't see it that way. In her decision, Judge Anne Hirsch lashed out at Bailey and Finkel for their behavior and said it was simply not believable that they believed all along that their scheme was legal. "The totality of the record establishes under a preponderance of the evidence," the judge wrote, "that GMA intentionally violated Washington State public campaign finance laws."[27]

And, boy, did they pay for it. Judge Hirsch slapped the GMA with a record-setting penalty, ordering the group to pay an astounding $18 million for knowingly breaking the law to conceal the identities of the corporations behind its astroturf campaign. It was the largest campaign-finance penalty in American history, and several million more than the $14.6 million penalty that the attorney general had requested. On top of that, the GMA was ordered to pay the state's legal fees too.[28] The penalty was later reduced by an appeals court to $6 million, but the Washington attorney general said in 2018 that he would fight that decision. It was a good day for the law and for integrity, and a bad day for Big Food and its playbook of dirty tricks. "It's one of my happiest days as attorney general," Ferguson told reporters. "GMA's conduct was just so egregious."[29]

Still, what's a few million in fines compared to hundreds of billions in profit? They lost the lawsuit but won the battle anyway. There are no GMO labels in Washington State.

> While this book was on its way to press, news came out that the GMA is changing its name and its mission in 2020 as a result of the many food companies that have left the group. Its new name will be the Consumer Brands Association. Only time will tell if they really do change their mission.

FOOD FIX: FIGHT THE FOOD LOBBYISTS WITH REAL GRASSROOTS EFFORTS AND LOBBY REFORM

Synthetic hormones in food and beverage containers. Obesogenic chemicals in fast food. Roundup in your morning oatmeal. These may seem like health hazards to you and me, but to Big Food they are business as usual. These practices are big moneymakers, which is why the food industry is willing to spend billions lobbying against regulations designed to rein them in.

We often think of ourselves as being at the mercy of big corporations. But the reality is that they answer to us, not the other way around. When we disapprove of their practices, we can force them to change by voting with our dollars. We need to support and invest in companies that are socially, environmentally, and nutritionally responsible. And we should effectively boycott companies that are doing the opposite. Companies can only sell what consumers will buy.

Think this kind of public pressure won't work? Plenty of grassroots efforts have spurred food industry changes. Though we've seen a few examples of how Big Food has overcome attempts at GMO labeling laws, they are a great example of how public sentiment can be as important as legislation. Some big companies saw the writing on the wall when Vermont's law was on the verge of taking effect in 2016 and decided to accommodate consumers instead of fighting them. Several big companies, led by Campbell Soup Company, announced that they would start disclosing GMO ingredients on all their packages nationwide—not just in Vermont. Ben & Jerry's said it would switch to using only non-GMO ingredients, and companies like General Mills said they would seek Non-GMO Project certifications on some of their products. Many of these companies received widespread praise from non-GMO activists and applause from consumers. Walk into any big supermarket and you will now see that a lot of companies use GMO labels that go above and beyond what the law requires. Even better, more and more companies are deciding to avoid GMOs entirely. They recognize not only that it's better for their products and the environment, but that it's also a smart business move.

Other giant food corporations are also evolving in response to grassroots consumer campaigns. Take a look at the dairy industry. Sales of cows' milk have been plunging for years over concerns about hormones, antibiotics, animal welfare, and the environmental impact of dairy farms. Plant-based beverages like almond, coconut, and cashew milk have quickly become a billion-dollar industry as consumers reach for more ethical and sustainable alternatives. But almond milk may not be a great alternative to regeneratively raised dairy cows. The large almond orchards are draining the aquifers in the San Joaquin Valley in California and require large amounts of nitrogen fertilizer (problems addressed in Part 5). While some in the dairy industry have attacked plant-based milks, others have recognized the demand for them and capitalized on the trend. In 2016, Danone, one of the world's largest dairy companies, announced a deal to buy the WhiteWave Foods company—the makers of Silk nut milks, Vega protein, and other popular plant-based dairy substitutes—for about $12 billion. The acquisition allowed Danone to build up its plant-based portfolio.[30]

Meanwhile Cargill, Tyson, and a host of other global beef and poultry producers have invested millions in companies that are bringing animal-free "clean meat" products to market, like Memphis Meats and Beyond Meat. Nestlé acquired Sweet Earth Foods, the makers of Harmless Ham and Benevolent Bacon, and Unilever and Walmart are pushing further into the so-called meatless meat market. These products aren't aimed at vegans. They're aimed at meat eaters who are concerned that their hamburgers and chicken wings come with a hefty carbon footprint and a big dose of hormones and antibiotics. The market for alternative meat grew to almost $5 billion in 2018 alone.[31] But plant-based meat alternatives like Beyond Meat and Impossible Foods are not the perfect solution. They are highly processed foods whose raw materials are grown through extractive, not regenerative, agriculture.[32]

Let's all work together to send a message to Big Food.

FOOD FIX: WHAT YOU CAN DO

1. **Donate to campaigns with integrity.** We need to get money out of politics by reversing *Citizens United*, the Supreme Court decision that allows corporations to give near unlimited financial contributions to candidates and parties through super PACs in anonymous ways, often called dark money.[33] Just 132 Americans have given 60 percent of the money to super PACs. This is 0.00042 percent of the population that is driving the candidates they choose and who will likely get elected. Just 11 donors have given $1 billion (or one-fifth of all donations) to super PACs since they were established in 2010.[34] Most of the rest of the funding for candidates comes from 0.05 percent of Americans. (For more information, Harvard professor Lawrence Lessig has mapped out this problem in great detail in his book *America, Compromised*.)

This system allows very few, very rich Americans to influence government and policy. The antidote is for more Americans to vote for candidates willing to act with integrity and change the policies needed to fix our broken system. And for more Americans to donate small amounts of money. If each of us gave $10, we would raise more than $3 billion for elections. It matters.

2. Buy non-GMO foods.

- **Shop at non-GMO retailers.** One of my favorites is Thrive Market, an online retailer that sells natural, organic foods and products at discounted prices. I have personally invested in Thrive to support affordable access to whole foods through online purchases. Thrive is the largest seller of exclusively non-GMO foods. Compared to other retailers, their products are affordable, often at 25 to 50 percent off the retail price. Plus, when you sign up for a Thrive membership, the company donates a free membership to a family in need. In 2016, after a large advocacy campaign, a USDA pilot program explored the opportunity to use food stamps to shop at Thrive Market and other online food providers. Check them out at www.thrivemarket.com.

- **Look for the Non-GMO Project verified seal.** The Non-GMO Project is a nonprofit that tests and verifies products to ensure they don't contain GMOs. It also audits companies and requires that they adhere to rigorous standards to avoid GMO contamination. Support companies that are doing the right thing by choosing products that have the Non-GMO Project seal on their labels. I recommend going to their website, nongmoproject .org, to search their database of retailers in your region. As of 2019 they had more than 14,200 registered retailers across the country!

- **Look for the USDA organic seal.** The USDA oversees the National Organic Program, which certifies organic products and makes sure they are free of GMOs. Organic producers who receive the seal are prohibited from using GMO seeds or giving their animals GMO feed. Their farms are inspected every year, and they are not allowed to use chemical fertilizers, synthetic substances, and irradiation. Nor are they allowed to use artificial colors, preservatives, or flavoring. Buying products that carry the USDA organic seal is one of the best ways to steer clear of GMOs while sending a message to Big Food to change its practices. Look for the seal when you buy fresh produce, meat, and other foods.

3. Use refillable containers. One way to avoid BPA and protect the environment at the same time is to minimize your use of plastic containers. Choose reusable glass and stainless steel containers instead. Plastic containers are bad for your health and bad for the environment. They are made with BPA, BPS (bisphenol-S), and other synthetic chemicals that can leach into your food. Some of these containers can be recycled, but often they end up in landfills or they work their way into rivers, streams, and parks.

Thanks to public awareness campaigns, companies are beginning to address the problem. In 2019, two dozen of the world's biggest brands announced that they're going to start offering their products in reusable glass and stainless steel containers. Through the project, called Loop, companies like Unilever, Quaker Oats, Tropicana, Procter & Gamble, and others will be using this more sustainable and BPA-free packaging for many of their bestselling products. The way it works is that the products will be delivered to consumers in a reusable tote. When the containers are empty, you put them back in the tote, and a UPS driver will pick them up—at no extra cost.

These kinds of innovative strategies are exactly what we need from big brands. In the meantime, try to minimize your use of plastics. Use glass food-storage containers, reusable glass or metal water bottles, and other containers that are better for your health and the environment.[35]

4. Buy locally sourced meat. So how do you avoid meat that originated in countries where tainted meat is a problem? The easiest thing to do is to shop at stores that go beyond the lax federal requirements. Whole Foods, for example, requires country-of-origin labels on all its meat products. One grocery chain, New Seasons Market, even identifies the state or region where the meat originated, along with the name of the farm it came from.[36] I also recommend using the following sources to buy locally raised meat.

- **Eatwild** maintains a directory of US, Canadian, and international farms and ranches that you can use to find grass-fed, pastured meat and dairy products in your area: www.eatwild.com.

- **LocalHarvest** is probably the leading website when it comes to finding local food. Use their database to find meat, fruits, vegetables, dairy, and other foods that were grown or raised in your local area: www.localharvest.org.
- **Firsthand Foods** is a wholesale meat business that provides locally sourced beef, pork, lamb, and other meats to consumers. They work with a network of small-scale, pasture-based livestock producers that follows strict standards. Check out their website, firsthandfoods.com, and sign up for a monthly delivery of fresh, pasture-raised products.
- **American Grassfed Association** has a directory of 100 percent grass-finished meat producers: www.americangrassfed.org/aga-membership/producer-members/.

5. Engage your representatives to shift nutrition and agriculture policies to ones that promote health and regenerative, sustainable agriculture. And support strict new rules on lobbying and corporate responsibility. We have to better regulate corporate lobbyists. Since there is no money to be made in lobbying for health and nutrition, we must use politics and vote for major changes. When I went to Congress to lobby for incorporating lifestyle medicine into the Affordable Care Act, senators, congressmen, and others asked us what lobby group we were from. We said none. We are representing patients and the science. They were perplexed. It costs me thousands in airfare and hotels, but I felt a different voice needed to be heard.

FOOD FIX: SHUT THE REVOLVING DOOR AND ENFORCE LOBBYING RESTRICTIONS

The federal government can start by making the lobbying system more transparent. The more we know, the more we can change. Right now, lobbyists are held to weak disclosure laws. They're required to file quarterly reports listing their clients, their compensation, and the agencies or branches of government that they're targeting. The nonpartisan Center for Responsive Politics does an excellent job of tracking this information and making it available to the public online. But the disclosure system doesn't go far enough. All it tells us is that corporations spend a ton of money lobbying the government, which we already knew.

The public deserves to know, in a timely manner, exactly who in the government is being lobbied and why. Some research groups like the Brookings Institution have proposed a better system that would involve the federal government creating an online portal where every piece of legislation is posted before it is voted on or signed into law. There, under each bill, lobbyists would be required to state who their clients are, which members of Congress or agencies they lobbied, and their positions on that bill or its amendments. This site could also serve as a forum for the public to weigh in on proposed legislation. The Library of Congress had a website where it made legislation available online, called the THOMAS system (http://thomas.loc.gov), that has become Congress.gov. Now we just need to update this system to make it more democratic and useful for the public.[37]

Government can and should be a tremendous force for good, not for powerful special interest groups and their well-connected lobbyists. That's why the revolving door between industry and the government should be closed and locked for good. For starters:

- Elected and appointed government officials should be banned from becoming lobbyists when they leave office, or at least face an extensive "cooling-off" period of five years or longer.
- At the same time, people who worked as corporate lobbyists should be restricted from taking jobs in the federal government. If you worked as a lobbyist for the sugar industry or McDonald's, you should not be allowed to take a job at the USDA as an adviser on the Dietary Guidelines. If you worked for the FDA, you should be banned from taking a corporate job in the fast-food or pharmaceutical industry lobbying the very agency you just left. The FDA commissioner example mentioned earlier is only the most recent and egregious.

- A windfall tax could be imposed on excessive lobbying to clamp down on any one corporation's or union's ability to spend unlimited sums of money lobbying against the greater good of society. While highly controversial, Elizabeth Warren has proposed a tax of 35 percent on lobbying expenditures between half a million and one million dollars, 60 percent between $1 and $5 million, and 75 percent on expenditures over $5 million.
- Enforcing the restrictions and closing loopholes that permit personal gifts to public officials.

While changing the lobbying laws and regulations may seem far out of our realm of influence, we can vote with our dollars on the local level and pressure our senators and congressmen to support reform at the national level. Let's speak up and put an end to the politics of bad food.

For a quick reference guide on the Food Fixes and resources on reforming lobbying, go to www.foodfixbook.com.

THE US GOVERNMENT: SUBSIDIZING DISEASE, POVERTY, ENVIRONMENTAL DESTRUCTION, AND CLIMATE CHANGE

By now, we've seen many ways in which junk-food companies prioritize their profits over the health of their customers. But what should disturb you is the extent to which Uncle Sam is complicit in Big Food's destructive mission. We've seen how Big Food lobbyists have hijacked Congress, the White House, and almost every government agency involved in regulating food. The result? Government policies that promote the production, sale, and marketing of ultraprocessed foods that fuel diabesity (the epidemic of obesity and type 2 diabetes), chronic disease, and environmental damage. The government doesn't just turn a blind eye to this; it also lends a helping hand.

The Food and Drug Administration (FDA) bows down to the companies it's supposed to regulate, allowing them to churn out Frankenfoods even when they're found to contain nasty chemicals like glyphosate, BPA, and hydrogenated oils. Food labels are designed to confuse consumers and protect industry.

The Federal Trade Commission (FTC) gives Big Food permission to prey on children, paving the way for the food industry to market billions of dollars' worth of junk foods that cause weight gain, diabetes, and fatty liver in kids.

Meanwhile the Centers for Disease Control (CDC) takes millions of dollars in funding from the soft drink industry to launch obesity campaigns that ignore nutrition while focusing exclusively on physical activity.

But no agency has been more critical to Big Food and its mission than the US Department of Agriculture (USDA). To understand this, look no further than the one piece of legislation that is the single most important component of our food system: the Farm Bill.[1] Drafted by Congress and implemented by the USDA, the Farm Bill designates funding for SNAP and other government food programs, as we've already seen, but it also doles out billions in subsidies and crop insurance for farmers. These subsidies have been in place in some form or another since the Great Depression, when the government began providing aid to farmers to ensure that the country had a steady food supply. Fast-forward almost a century later, and the Farm Bill that passed in 2014 authorized nearly a trillion dollars in spending—$956 billion to be exact—through 2024. Those expenditures were largely reauthorized by Congress in the 2018 Farm Bill and then signed into law by President Trump.

The Farm Bill determines which crops farmers choose to grow. It influences the cost of groceries and the foods we eat. Whether you realize it or not, the Farm Bill plays a direct role in agriculture and your diet. And it has enormous health consequences for the entire nation.

Before we get into how farm subsidies shape what American farmers grow, let's take a look at another important task of the USDA (along with the Department of Health and Human Services): establishing the country's Dietary Guidelines.

DIETARY GUIDELINES: THE FOOD INDUSTRY'S UNDUE INFLUENCE

The US Dietary Guidelines, which are revised every five years, are intended to synthesize the latest nutrition science into simple guidelines that then form the foundation of all government food programs and are followed by almost all health care institutions and public health and professional societies such as the Academy of Nutrition and Dietetics. Since the very first Dietary Guidelines for Americans were drafted in the late 1970s, lobbyists representing different industries have been heavily involved in the process. For example, the guidelines committee wanted to advise Americans to cut back on their meat consumption. But meat industry lobbyists, unhappy about this, pressured the guidelines committee to soften their language. So instead of issuing recommendations to reduce meat consumption, the guidelines committee reached something of a compromise, recommending that Americans cut back on "saturated fat" (coded language for red meat). The advice to cut back on eggs was changed to a recommendation to cut back on cholesterol. And instead of urging Americans to limit sugar because of its emerging link to heart disease, the guidelines mentioned that Americans might want to go easy on sugar for a less urgent reason: dental cavities.

The first guidelines were based on poor epidemiological research from the 1960s that blamed fat and exonerated sugar for heart disease. Mark Hegsted, a Harvard physician, was the lead author on a 1967 *New England Journal of Medicine* paper that blamed fat and gave sugar a pass for heart disease. He headed up George McGovern's Senate commission on the first Dietary Guidelines for Americans in 1977. Turns out the sugar lobby paid him the equivalent of $50,000 in today's dollars to write that article giving sugar a pass, even though studies showed that inflammation, abnormal cholesterol, and other heart disease biomarkers were driven by sugar and starch.[2] The original guidelines evolved for the worse, piling on the low-fat bandwagon and culminating in the 1992 Food Guide Pyramid advising us to eat six to eleven servings of bread, rice, cereal, and pasta a day and to eat fat only sparingly. This led to the worst public health disaster in the history of humankind, driving a global epidemic of obesity and type 2 diabetes. Finally, in 2015, after decades of overwhelming evidence that fat was not the enemy, the US Dietary Guidelines removed any limits on dietary fat, declaring that eating fat didn't cause weight gain or heart disease. To get the full story you can read my book *Eat Fat, Get Thin*. In 2005 George W. Bush made the guidelines fully political when the final guidelines had to be approved by politicians, not scientists. The last advisory group recommended including sustainability in the guidelines. The factory-farmed meat industry didn't like it and the policy makers removed environmental considerations from the final guidelines.

Through the efforts of the Nutrition Coalition, a nonprofit advocacy group, in 2015 Congress mandated that the National Academy of Sciences (NAS) review the process by which the Dietary Guidelines are developed. The NAS found that many members of the advisory committee had consistently published work in favor of low-animal-fat vegetarian diets. Coincidentally, several members had consulting agreements with or were funded by the food industry and they ignored huge swaths of science on meat and low-carb diets.

The NAS recommendations were helpful and hopeful, but under the Trump administration things have taken a turn for the worse. The process has turned more political and less scientific. In fact, for the first time the Department of Health and Human Services and the USDA, which oversee the guidelines, have limited the research that can be reviewed to establish the guidelines. They permit review only of internal government studies vetted by agency officials and they prohibit review of any data before 2000 (when most of the relevant research was done), any outside reviews or research, and any data on ultraprocessed food, feedlot meat, sodium, or environmental impacts of the food system. The Trump administration's limits on what science can be reviewed are in direct contradiction to the NAS recommendations. Thirteen of the twenty new members of the 2020 Dietary Guidelines advisory committee have strong ties to the food industry, including the National Potato Council and the trade association of the snack food industry. Bottom line: The committee will likely ignore data that implicates Big Food or Big Ag in any of our health or environmental crises.

FOOD POLICIES AT ODDS WITH ONE ANOTHER

Today, though the Dietary Guidelines have moved in a healthier direction, even the USDA's best advice is contradicted by its actions. While the Dietary Guidelines encourage Americans to fill half their plates with fruits and vegetables to prevent obesity, the agency stacks the deck against consumers by making junk foods cheaper and easier to buy than nutritious foods. Government subsidies enable lower prices for processed food by encouraging growing of food surpluses, while not supporting farming of fruits and vegetables, even though the same agency tells us to eat five to nine servings of fruits and vegetables a day.

According to data collected by the federal government, the foods that make up the top sources of calories in the American diet are grain- and sugar-based snacks such as cakes, cookies, doughnuts, and cereal. Not far behind them are bread, sugary drinks, chicken dishes, pizza, pasta, and "dairy-based desserts" (in other words, ice cream). (See the chart "Top Sources of Calories in the US Diet" on the following page.) All of these are the products of just a handful of crops and farm foods— corn, soybeans, wheat, rice, sorghum, milk, and meat—that Uncle Sam heavily subsidizes.

Between 1995 and 2013, the Farm Bill doled out more than $170 billion to farmers and large agribusinesses to finance the production of these foods. Farmers were motivated not only to produce these foods, but also to overproduce them. The law of supply and demand no longer applied. This helped to drive down the commodity prices, ensuring that fast food, soft drinks, and other junk food were cheap and plentiful. During this period, the price of sugary drinks sweetened with high-fructose corn syrup fell nearly 25 percent, and American children increased their consumption of soft drinks by 130 calories a day. At the same time, the cost of fruits and vegetables rose almost 40 percent.[3]

Top Sources of Calories in the US Diet	
Cakes, cookies, doughnuts, granola	138 kcal
Breads	129
Chicken dishes	121
Soda, energy, sports drinks	114
Pizza	98
Alcohol	82
Pasta	81
Tortillas, burritos, tacos	80
Beef dishes	64
Dairy desserts	62
Chips	56
Burgers	53

Source: USDA Dietary Guidelines

PROCESSED CORN AND SOY HIDDEN IN EVERYTHING

You might notice that some of the most heavily subsidized foods, like corn and soybeans, are plants that are not inherently unhealthy. But the vast majority of these crops are not consumed whole. Only 1 percent of American-grown corn is sold and eaten whole as corn on the cob. Much of the rest is either fed to factory-farmed livestock to fatten them up before slaughter or converted into biofuels. As for what does hit your plate, America's heavily subsidized bounty of corn and soy may start out as whole foods, but by the time you eat them, they've been manufactured into ultraprocessed oils and sweeteners and food additives.

Corn is processed into cornstarch and high-fructose corn syrup, which are some of the most prevalent additives in the food supply, found in everything from applesauce to breakfast cereals to baby food, baked goods, bread, ketchup, frozen dinners, soft drinks, and yogurt. Soybeans are broken down into refined soybean oil (also the foundation of processed foods) and meal that is fed to livestock and pets. Soybean oil, until very recently, was then further processed into partially hydrogenated cooking oils, also known as trans fats, which cause heart attacks and strokes. Refined soybean oil alone accounts for roughly 65 percent of all the oil Americans consume,[4] which represents a thousandfold increase since 1900. Most of that is hidden in processed or fried foods. Wheat and other grains are ground into flour and refined carbs, which are worse for your body than table sugar (even whole wheat bread has a higher glycemic index than table sugar).

So how does all this impact the American diet? Marion Nestle, a professor of nutrition, food studies, and public health at New York University, did the calculations. She found that if you designed your meals to match the way the government funnels its subsidies, "You'd get a lecture from your doctor.

"More than three-quarters of your plate would be taken up by a massive corn fritter (80 percent of benefits go to corn, grains, and soy oil). You'd have a Dixie cup of milk (dairy gets 3 percent), a hamburger the size of a half dollar (livestock: 2 percent), two peas (fruits and vegetables: 0.45 percent), and an after-dinner cigarette (tobacco: 2 percent). Oh, and a really big linen napkin (cotton: 13 percent) to dab your lips."[5]

According to Dr. Nestle, on the next page is what the USDA's My Plate advice would look like if it reflected what the USDA supports with subsidies.

Big Ag grows 500 more calories per person per day than it did 25 years ago, most of it made up of corn and soy in the form of ultraprocessed food. That's because farmers get paid to grow extra food even when it's not needed. Uncle Sam also provides them with billions in crop insurance, so there's no risk of losing money if they have a bad

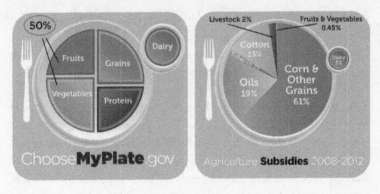

CREDIT: CONGRESSWOMAN CHELLIE PINGREE

Data from the USDA

season, and they are incentivized to grow crops on marginal land they know will fail. A lot of the crop insurance helps farmers pay for the seeds and nitrogen fertilizer used to grow on marginal land. Koch Fertilizer, run by the Koch brothers, big political donors, provides much of the fertilizer and receives big benefits from current agricultural policies. Even worse: If those farmers want to diversify and grow tomatoes and broccoli on their farms, they lose all their government support.

These government supports are essential to protect farmers (many are one bad season away from bankruptcy), but they could be better directed to help these farmers convert to regenerative agriculture, which in the end would produce better food that is more profitable for them and better for their land, the environment, and the climate.

As a result of farm subsidies, taxpayers are footing the bill for the chronic disease epidemic while simultaneously underwriting the production (and consumption via SNAP) of the very foods that are causing it. With the money used to subsidize corn and soy junk-food ingredients, the government could buy almost 52 billion Twinkies—enough to circle the Earth 132 times when placed end to end or meet the caloric needs of the entire US population for twelve days. Not coincidentally, the Twinkie offers an illustration of the degree to which government subsidies favor junk-food production. "Of the 37 ingredients in a Twinkie, taxpayers subsidize at least 17, including corn syrup, high fructose corn syrup, vegetable shortening, and corn starch."[6]

In 2016, researchers at the CDC published a study that examined the direct impact that these subsidies have on America's health. They followed more than 10,000 adults and split them into groups according to the proportion of foods they ate that were derived from the most heavily subsidized commodities. They found that people who had the highest intake of federally subsidized foods had a nearly 40 percent greater likelihood of being obese. They were also significantly more likely to have metabolic disease—with higher levels of belly fat, blood sugar, cholesterol, and C-reactive protein, a sign of inflammation. The CDC researchers concluded their paper with a thinly veiled rebuke of the USDA and its contradictory policies and nutrition advice. "Nutritional guidelines are focused on the population's needs for healthier foods, but to date food and agricultural policies that influence food production and availability have not yet done the same."[7] (Of course, the CDC has its own conflicting issues.)

FRUITS AND VEGETABLES: TOO FEW AND TOO EXPENSIVE

In contrast to huge subsidies on the crops that will end up in junk food, the percentage of federal subsidies that are actually allocated for nutritious foods is trivial. Apples are the only fruit or vegetable that receives significant subsidies (other than corn), and the amount allocated for apples between 1995 and 2010 was just $689 million—less than 1 percent of total government subsidies. Even those subsidies aren't likely to enhance nutrition; much like corn, a lot of the apples grown in America are not eaten as whole foods. They are processed into less nutritious foods like apple juice and applesauce, which are often sweetened with high-fructose corn syrup.

Uncle Sam gives farmers very little incentive to grow fruits, nuts, and vegetables. In fact, the government has long discouraged it. Many versions of the Farm Bill referred to these foods as "specialty crops"[8] and stipulated that farmers who took subsidies for commodity crops were barred from growing fruits and vegetables—if they did, they faced stiff penalties.[9] Only about 2 percent of land is used to grow fruits and vegetables, while 59 percent is used to grow commodity crops.[10]

The way the subsidy program is structured to favor large agribusinesses is no accident. Archer Daniels Midland, Bayer (which recently purchased Monsanto), Cargill, DuPont, Tyson, Syngenta, and other Big Food and Big Ag corporations have the lobbying power to mold the Farm Bill to their liking. As Marion Nestle at NYU points out:

> If you examine how its incentives line up, you quickly see that it strongly favors the industrial agriculture of the Midwest and South over that of the Northeast and West; methods requiring chemical fertilizers, pesticides and herbicides over those that are organic and sustainable; and commodity crops for animal feed, vegetable oils, and ethanol rather than "specialty" crops—translation: fruits and vegetables—for human consumption.
>
> This makes food hugely competitive and forces the manufacturers of processed foods and drinks to do everything possible to encourage sales of their products. The result is a food environment that encourages overeating of highly caloric, highly processed foods, but discourages consumption of healthier, relatively unprocessed foods.[11]

FOOD FIX: THE NEED FOR A NATIONAL FOOD POLICY

Since the food and agriculture industry is the biggest business in America and affects every single American, it is surprising that we actually don't have a national food policy. Our federal government has multiple agencies governing various aspects of food and agriculture, all acting independently, mostly without coordination, supporting a food and agricultural system that creates disease and endless human suffering and is bankrupting our economy while devastating the environment and driving climate change. We need a comprehensive reform of food policy in America (and globally) at the national and local levels. We need a food czar to head this initiative.

Countries like Brazil and Norway have taken the lead on creating national food policies. Their dietary guidelines recommend eating whole foods and their federal governments levy taxes on soft drinks and other junk food and provide assistance to farmers who grow nutritious foods. Brazil's national food policy, implemented in 2004, has already helped to reduce poverty and child mortality rates while boosting business for farmers.[12]

What would such a policy look like in America? The Union of Concerned Scientists did the research and concluded that a national food policy would ensure the following goals:

- That all Americans have access to healthy food;
- That farm policies are designed to support public health and environmental objectives;
- That our food supply is free of toxic bacteria, chemicals, and drugs;
- That the production and marketing of food are done transparently;
- That the food industry pays a fair wage to people it employs (see Part 4);
- That the food system's carbon footprint is reduced and the amount of carbon sequestered on farmland is increased (see Part 5).

So how would this actually work in practice? For starters, the government has to reform its subsidies system. Farmers need incentives to grow more nutritious foods using regenerative practices. The government needs to restructure the Farm Bill so that subsidies are used to increase the production of "specialty crops" such as fruits, vegetables, and nuts and shifted away from corn, soy, wheat, animal feed, and biofuels (which paradoxically require lots of fossil fuels to grow). The process of creating nitrogen fertilizer is energy intensive and releases a lot of CO_2 and methane, and when synthetic nitrogen is applied as fertilizer to fields, it emits N_2O, another potent greenhouse gas. Subsidies should also support farmers to transition to organically or regeneratively grown crops, grass-fed and grass-finished pasture-raised livestock, and organically produced milk. These subsidies can help farmers buy new seeds, develop new crops, and purchase new farm equipment that will help them transition to more regenerative practices. (We'll learn more about regenerative agriculture in Part 5.)

Beyond subsidies, the federal government feeds millions of people in schools, hospitals, and prisons, as well as military and government workers. It can promote healthy eating and create markets for farmers by requiring that schools, prisons, and military bases use a percentage of their budgets to buy locally sourced food from nearby farms and at the very least healthy whole foods that promote health rather than disease. As Congressman Ryan explained it, "How do we get military bases healthy? How do we get processed food out of the bases and more healthy food in? We get the bases to buy local, support the local farmers and the local area. A lot of times you'll have a military base and surrounding it will be a lot of farmland." The same goes for schools, prisons, hospitals, and other government-funded institutions.

Local and state governments can do the same. For example, Ohio State University is a public institution with nearly 70,000 students. The state of Ohio could require that the university spend 1 percent of its food budget sourcing ingredients from local farms in central Ohio. After a couple of years, that percentage could increase to 2 percent, then 4 percent, and so on. The goal would be to use public money to help small farmers transition to healthier crops while creating and opening markets for them. That is how you lay the foundation so that government agencies share a common goal. Across the country, a small but growing number of programs are making healthy food more accessible for poor families by giving them incentives to buy their food from local farmers. Innovative companies such as Azoti link local farmers and producers to big food service corporations and institutions, shortening the food supply chain and providing consumers with high-quality local and organic food.

A national food policy would transform our broken food system into one that aligns public health objectives with economic and environmental goals. It would make healthful choices the default option for Americans while slashing health care costs and helping farmers, protecting the environment, and reversing climate change.

CHANGE IS COMING

In 2018, a bipartisan group of lawmakers started the Food Is Medicine Working Group in the House of Representatives. It includes both Republican and Democratic members of Congress, like initial members Jim McGovern, a senior Democrat from Massachusetts, and Representative Lynn Jenkins, a Republican from Kansas. The group's mission is to sort out the chaos in nutrition policies to better the nation's health. McGovern outlined a number of legislative issues that the group intends to pursue:

- Incentivizing the purchase of fruits and vegetables;
- Strengthening the nutrition and education components of SNAP;
- Making hospital meals more nutritious to ensure that the sickest and most vulnerable Americans are provided nutrient-dense meals;
- Funding programs that allow doctors to prescribe fruits and vegetables to their patients instead of drugs.

"There really are areas where Democrats and Republicans can come together on this issue of 'food is medicine,'" McGovern said in 2018, before the next Farm Bill was approved.[13]

For a quick reference guide on the Food Fixes and resources on reforming our national food policies, go to www.foodfixbook.com.

CHAPTER 8

THE FOOD INDUSTRY PREYS ON CHILDREN AND SCHOOLS

Kids today are fatter than ever. Obesity rates in children have tripled since the 1970s and now one in three is overweight or obese.[1] In fact, one in four teenagers now has type 2 diabetes or pre-diabetes[2]—a condition we used to call "adult onset diabetes"; it was something I never saw in a young person during my medical school training 30 years ago. If a child is overweight, his or her life expectancy may be reduced by 10 to 20 years.[3]

A major reason for childhood and teenage obesity is the food offered in schools. School meals are often loaded with sugar, salt, processed carbs, and industrial fats. Many schools in America don't even pretend to offer healthy meals: They let fast-food chains sell pizza and cheeseburgers on school grounds and allow them to slap their logos on cafeterias and gymnasiums.

Kids spend more time at school than any other place outside their homes. The Institute of Medicine calls schools "the heart of health" because they should be a focal point in the effort to help children lead healthy lives. More than 30 million children eat school meals every day, and for many kids from working-class families, these meals make up the bulk of their daily calories. School meals are critical in the battle against childhood obesity and should be held to the highest standards.

Public health officials have long tried to make school meals more nutritious. But an enormous (and familiar) obstacle stands in the way: the food industry. In 2010, President Obama signed into law the Healthy, Hunger-Free Kids Act, a signature piece of legislation that

Michelle Obama championed as part of her effort to make a dent in child obesity rates. The law mandated that 100,000 public schools provide healthier foods to their students. It did this by granting the USDA the power to create new nutrition standards for school lunches for the first time in decades.

The law accomplished some good: It essentially banned much of the obvious junk foods from school vending machines, like soft drinks, cookies, M&M'S, gummy bears, and sugar-laden sports drinks such as Gatorade. It created standards for school meals that prioritized whole grains over heavily processed carbs, lowered sodium, and required at least a minimal amount of vegetables per meal. But that's about all the legislation got right. Sadly, it was fatally flawed from its inception because food industry lobbyists were intimately involved in shaping it.[4] And the Trump administration rolled back those improvements, giving way to the food industry lobby and harming our children in the process.[5]

SCHOOL LUNCH GUIDELINES: PROFIT BEFORE SCIENCE AND HEALTH

More than 111 food companies, trade groups, and industry organizations registered to lobby on the bill.[6] They were led by the misleadingly named School Nutrition Association (SNA), a leading industry-funded lobbying organization. About half of the SNA's $10 million budget comes from big food companies, among them Kraft, Coke, Conagra, and Domino's Pizza.[7] The SNA watered down their criteria for what could qualify as nutritious and pushed for a clause that allowed schools to opt out of the standards. The school lunch lobby fought to ensure that tomato paste would count as a vegetable, making pizza legally a vegetable, and that starchy potatoes—code word for french fries— would be favored in the standards. The two most commonly eaten vegetables in America are officially potatoes and tomatoes—eaten as french fries, ketchup, and pizza. Minnesota Democratic senator Amy Klobuchar lobbied hard for this because the nation's largest pizza provider to schools, Schwan's, is in her native state.[8]

By the time the nutrition standards were finalized, the foods allowed to be sold in schools included toaster waffles with syrup, tater tots, Uno pepperoni pizza, chicken nuggets, funnel cakes, chocolate muffins, and sugar-soaked Slush Puppie beverages.[9]

With assistance from the food industry, the USDA also created a Trojan horse policy it called Smart Snacks in School. The idea was to hold snack foods to higher nutrition standards. But ultimately it allowed branded junk foods to sneak into schools. While it sounded like a good idea in theory, the nutrition criteria for the Smart Snacks program provided an easy workaround for the industry, which reformulated their products into slightly different junk foods.

Potato chip makers created "reduced fat" versions of their chips that met the Smart Snacks criteria. Cookie companies created "whole grain" cookies and crackers (essentially junk food with a few flakes of whole grain sprinkled in). And instead of offering sugary soda, soft drink makers met the Smart Snacks criteria by offering "100% fruit juice," which you know by now typically contains just as much sugar as soda. To meet the Smart Snacks standards, PepsiCo offered schools reduced-fat Nacho Cheese and Cool Ranch Doritos, Flamin' Hot Cheetos, and Oatmeal Raisin Quaker Breakfast Cookies. Pepperidge Farm introduced lower-fat chocolate, vanilla, and "wholegrain" Goldfish crackers. General Mills created reduced-fat strawberry-yogurt-flavored Chex and a line of Fruit Roll-Ups.

All these junk foods carry the same brand names, logos, and characters as their traditional versions—and all of them were allowed into schools with the USDA's blessing. What's bizarre and contradictory is the mandate to lower fat in school lunches but allow increased starch and sugar while the US Dietary Guidelines recommend removing any limits on total fat and reducing starch and sugar. No wonder we are all confused. At the USDA, it seems like the right hand doesn't know what the left hand is doing.

In perhaps the most flagrant example of all, in 2018 the largest public school system in Texas — the Houston Independent School District — entered into a four-year deal with Domino's to market its Smart Slice pizza in Houston schools. Even though they look and taste like any ordinary pizza, the company claimed its Smart Slice pies were healthful because they contained less fat and sodium than regular pies. The crust is 51 percent whole wheat (just sneaking in under the standards for "whole grain"), and they have low-fat cheese and low-fat pepperoni. Hardly healthy, but enough to meet the government's anemic standards for "healthy." Domino's gave the Houston school district $8 million in exchange for the right to sell these branded pizzas — served in Domino's–emblazoned cardboard boxes and sleeves — in school cafeterias. The company claims it sells its Smart Slice branded pizza in more than 6,000 school districts in forty-seven states.[10] But I guess that's okay because pizza is a vegetable.

In twisting what originated as high-minded legislation to improve the quality of school food, the USDA created a monster. Its weak nutrition standards, crafted by an army of corporate food lobbyists, paved the way for "copycat" snacks to become a vehicle for Big Food to market its most popular candy, potato chips, and fast foods in schools across the country.

Kids today spend at least six hours a day at school, where they eat breakfast, lunch, and multiple snacks. Removing thinly disguised Frankenfoods from their school menus would have a huge impact on their health.

BIG FOOD DELIBERATELY TARGETS OUR CHILDREN

The government also allows unregulated food marketing in schools. Studies show that 70 percent of elementary and middle school students in America see ads for fast food, candy, and soft drinks in their schools — and those ads have a direct impact, leading children to consume more junk-food-laden diets.[11] The implicit message is that teachers and schools endorse the products; otherwise, why would they be allowed in schools? Food companies pimp their junk via direct advertising in classrooms, such as advertiser-sponsored video and audio programming; indirect advertising by corporate-sponsored educational materials; product sales contracts for soda and snack foods; ads in gyms and on school buses, book covers, and bathroom stalls; and "educational TV" such as Channel One. Channel One was available in 12,000 schools and provided ten minutes of current events with two minutes of commercials that go for $200,000 each and reach 40 percent of America's teenagers.[12] We don't let tobacco makers market their products in schools; why do we let processed-food companies, given that those foods kill more people than cigarettes?[13] (Fortunately, in 2018, Channel One aired its last broadcast, although subscribers still had access to the video library.)

Junk-food companies engage in this type of predatory marketing because it's hugely profitable. An Institute of Medicine (IOM) study, *Food Marketing to Children and Youth: Threat or Opportunity*,[14] which analyzed 123 peer-reviewed research papers, outlines in frightening detail the methods and practices used by the food industry to target youth through conventional TV, billboards, advertising, and stealth marketing. They pay the best and brightest advertising executives to develop commercials specifically designed to entice children, and they've even been known to employ brain-imaging studies to elicit the desired neural responses from the marketing. This deliberate use of brain science to manipulate our children is Orwellian but also effective. This marketing, according to the IOM, deliberately targets children who are too young to distinguish ads from the truth and encourages them to eat high-calorie, low-nutrient (but highly profitable) junk food and to demand these foods from their parents. Kids under age three demand food brands even before they can read (and sometimes even before they can walk).[15] These companies hire research firms to learn how to influence preschoolers. Shouldn't we protect our children?

Every year, companies such as Coke and McDonald's spend $1.8 billion marketing their products to children as young as two years old.[16] The average child between two and fourteen years of age sees ten to eleven of these ads per day. That's roughly 4,000 ads every year! As you might imagine, the majority of these ads aren't for apple slices and sweet potato fries. They're for Cocoa Puffs, Gatorade, and McDonald's Happy Meals that star SpongeBob SquarePants and the Minions.

Most adults can see a television ad for McDonald's and pay it little mind. But according to the American Psychological Association (APA), children under the age of eight don't instinctively recognize the difference between TV commercials and the programs they're watching, which makes them particularly vulnerable to persuasive messaging. The food industry understands this, and it is why they spend $11 billion just on television ads marketing junk food to our kids every year.[17] And that's just on television. Now kids consume most of their media online.

The IOM report was published in 2006, before the arrival of Facebook, Instagram, Twitter, Snapchat, or other smartphone apps. Now the problem of stealth marketing is much worse. The average kid now spends forty-four and a half hours a week in front of screens and is subject to intense and manipulative stealth marketing.[18] Stealth marketing is harder to track and includes embedded advertising in movies and television, toys, games, educational materials, songs, and movies; character licensing and celebrity endorsements; and less visible "stealth" campaigns involving word of mouth, cell phone text messages, and the Internet and social media. A new subversive and powerful model for marketing junk food to children is "advergames,"[19] "free" social media games and apps that integrate junk food into games for little children. These games are marketing not broccoli but obesogenic foods.[20] They drive kids to eat more junk and more food overall. Online marketing is more pervasive, insidious, and effective. In 2002 McDonald's alone spent $635 million on marketing, most of it targeted at children.[21] On their website McDonald's explains, "Unfortunately, McDonald's does not give out this kind of commercial information [how much it spends on advertising], as it could be an advantage to our competitors."

"Advertising directed at children this young is by its very nature exploitative," the APA says. Much like tobacco companies, food companies target children because they know that the way to hook them is to reach them early, when they're most impressionable. Studies show that children have an uncanny ability to remember the food ads they've seen. Exposure to just a single thirty-second fast-food commercial is enough to instill brand and product preferences in a child,[22] and repeated exposure can set the stage for that child to become a lifelong customer.[23] Fast food and the marketing behind it can lead to detrimental changes in the adolescent brain associated with dysfunctional eating and impulsive behaviors.[24] It can also thwart parents' efforts to instill healthy eating habits in their kids. Teaching your kids to appreciate real food is a herculean task when they're besieged with ads for Frosted Flakes and Pizza Hut.

Fast-food ads don't just play with a child's psyche, but also have a direct impact on their weight and long-term health. The more fast-food ads kids see, the fatter they become. Scientists have repeatedly shown in large studies that even slight increases in the amount of time kids spend viewing junk-food ads can increase their odds of becoming obese by 20 percent.[25] Teenagers are twice as likely to become obese if they see at least one junk-food ad daily.[26] One large study of thousands of teens found that 40 percent of them felt "pressured" to consume unhealthy diets by fast-food and soft drink ads. The more familiar they were with these ads, the more junk food they ate, and that was linked to a higher bodyweight regardless of their age or gender.[27]

Make no mistake: Chuck E. Cheese and Ronald McDonald are manipulating children just as Joe Camel did for decades. Only now, the consequences are more devastating. The obesity rate in kids shows no signs of slowing down. In some states, like Tennessee, almost 50 percent of children are either overweight or obese. The CDC has even begun to document a new category of severely obese kids that it calls Class 3 obesity.[28]

Even in kids who are not obese, doctors are discovering horrifying metabolic conditions driven by their junk-food diets. Ten percent of children in the United States have fatty liver disease, a condition that was unheard of 20 years ago and that is now quickly becoming the number one cause of liver transplants nationwide.[29] Liver centers across the country now have teenage patients on their transplant waiting lists—all because their livers can't keep up with the heavily processed food they're consuming.

GOVERNMENT: ON TASK OR FOOD INDUSTRY SERVANT?

With obesity rates soaring and children under siege from a barrage of sophisticated ads and marketing, a coalition of public health groups, medical experts, and children's health advocates came together to demand that the government take action on food marketing to children. In 2009, Congress ordered the FTC to work with the FDA, CDC, and USDA to recommend standards for food marketing (one of the few times these agencies collaborated). Two years later, the agencies, collectively known as the Interagency Working Group, issued a report that proposed a set of nutrition standards for foods that could be marketed to children. The proposed standards called for the food industry to market foods that were reasonably nutritious—like fruits, vegetables, whole grains, and low-fat dairy products—or products that minimized things like salt, saturated fat, sugar, and sodium.

But the standards were completely voluntary. The food industry was under no obligation to abide by them at all. Still, the mere proposition of nutrition standards sent the industry into a frenzy. Food companies realized that under the voluntary guidelines, which were fairly lax, they would not be able to market their most profitable soft drinks, breakfast cereals, and junk foods to small children. General Mills, Kellogg's, Pepsi, and an array of other corporate food giants got together and formed a lobbying group to block the nutrition standards. Calling themselves the Sensible Food Policy Coalition, the group plowed almost $7 million into their lobbying efforts. Another corporation that joined the fight against the standards was Viacom, which owns Nickelodeon, the kids' network whose cartoon characters—such as SpongeBob and

Dora the Explorer—star in many ads for junk foods targeting kids. The company poured millions of dollars into the effort.[30]

Together the companies pressured the government to drop the voluntary restrictions, saying they were unfair and would harm their business. Their lobbying coalition even released a dubious report claiming that the voluntary standards would cause $28 billion in lost sales and revenue and ultimately spur the loss of 74,000 jobs.[31] As extreme and predictable as it was, the pushback worked. The then head of the FTC, David Vladeck, issued public statements reassuring companies that the proposed standards were toothless and that the FTC had no plans to regulate them. "The proposal doesn't ban any marketing or any foods at all," he told them. "Companies can continue to market and sell the same products they do now. The proposal simply recommends that the products companies choose to market directly to kids—as opposed to the products marketed to their parents—meet the nutrition principles outlined in the report."[32] Good luck with that!

Through its intense lobbying efforts, Big Food effectively killed the already anemic marketing guidelines. As a gesture, the industry formed its own organization, the Children's Food and Beverage Advertising Initiative, through which each company set their own nutrition criteria and pledged to market only healthy foods during kids' programming, like Saturday morning cartoons. But the criteria were so absurd they were laughable. Under Kellogg's standards, the company could still advertise Froot Loops and Frosted Flakes to kids. It could also advertise Yogos, a candy whose primary ingredients are sugar and trans fats.[33]

ONLINE TARGETING OF CHILDREN

In 2016, fifty-six of the biggest food companies placed 509 million banner ads and impressions on CartoonNetwork.com, Nick.com, and other kids' sites. They also placed 3.4 billion ads on Facebook and YouTube alone.[34] In 2016 the World Health Organization issued a report warning that food companies were targeting kids on the Internet using powerful ads and extremely effective digital marketing tactics like heavily branded online video games, known as "advergames." The agency warned that fast-food chains were hooking kids in clever ways. One technique involved making McDonald's restaurants important locations in augmented reality games like the wildly popular Pokémon GO.[35] Pokémon's maker, which signed a sponsorship deal with McDonald's, said it had driven millions of visitors to the chain's restaurants.[36] The WHO warned that parents and public health experts needed to take aggressive steps to counter this new style of marketing.

"The food, marketing and digital industries have access to extremely fine-grained analyses of children's behavior," the agency said in its report. "Children have the right to participate in digital media; and, when they are participating, they have the right to protection of their health and privacy and not to be economically exploited."[37]

FOOD FIX: KICK JUNK FOOD OUT OF SCHOOLS

The Boston public school system was once a model of terrible food. Historically most of the 126 public schools in Boston, which serve 56,000 kids a day, didn't even have real kitchens. They used "satellite kitchens" that consisted of just a freezer and a warming oven. School meals were produced out of state and shipped to Boston schools, where they were heated up in the satellite kitchens—still wrapped in their plastic—and then served to students. In other words, kids were handed TV dinners for breakfast and lunch.[38] When Jill Shah, an entrepreneur and philanthropist whose husband founded the e-commerce website Wayfair, saw how Boston Public Schools was feeding its students, she was horrified.

Shah looked into what it would take for Boston to create full-service kitchens and was told it would cost more than the city was willing to spend: at least $1 million. Shah was undeterred. She came up with a brilliant plan that she called the "Hub and Spoke" model. Rather than ship prepackaged meals from out of state, the schools that already had full-service kitchens would prep food for nearby schools, whose kitchens would be retrofitted with special "combi-ovens" that could steam, roast, and even fry multiple types of food simultaneously without cross-contamination. Shah brought in a well-known local chef, Ken Oringer, to teach food service workers how to prepare meals that were healthier but still delicious. The cost of all this was far less than the city had anticipated: just $65,000 to get the program started, much less than the cost of creating brand-new full-service kitchens for every underprivileged school. In fact, the city ultimately ended up saving $3.41 per meal.[39]

The program, called My Way Café, began as a pilot program at four schools in East Boston in 2017. Prepackaged meals were eliminated. Schools were provided full salad bars and freshly prepared breakfast items—eggs, fruit, turkey, yogurt, and homemade granola. The food was healthier, and students were allowed to choose their own meals. That meant that for the first time they had options. The result? The students loved it. The rate of students eating school meals increased about 15 percent. As a bonus, the program created more jobs for local Boston residents. Shah's program was so successful that in 2018 the mayor of Boston, Martin Walsh, announced he was expanding it to all of Boston's public schools. "Boston is leading the way in making sure our students have access to fresh, healthy food," he proclaimed.[40]

Boston Public Schools, once a model of poor nutrition, is now a model for how every school district should feed its students. It is a travesty that public schools often don't even have real kitchens. Most have only deep fryers, microwaves, and displays for candy and junk food at the cafeteria checkout counters. But Shah's program and others like it are having a wonderful impact on children's health. They're models for how other school districts can save money, serve better food, and improve the health and well-being of their students.

FOOD FIX: TAKE BACK OUR SCHOOLS
FROM THE FOOD INDUSTRY

Parents, school boards and administrators, and school staff can help implement these changes.

1. Introduce salad bars in schools. It's been a struggle to get a variety of delicious vegetables into schools. It's time we introduce a salad bar in every school. It gives kids options, and it can be done at minimal cost. Cincinnati Public Schools managed to install a salad bar in each of its schools in under a year. Programs like Salad Bars to Schools (a partnership of Whole Foods, the United Fresh Start Foundation, the Chef Ann Foundation, and others) are working to do this at a national level. As of 2018 they've raised more than $14 million and have used that money to introduce salad bars in 5,354 schools, which serve fresh delicacies like pomegranates and roasted chickpeas.

In 2015 my friend Congressman Tim Ryan introduced legislation called the Salad Bars in Schools Expansion Act, which designates funding to bring more salad bars to school cafeterias across America. We need more bold and creative solutions like this. Congress should go even further and designate funding in the Farm Bill to bring this initiative to every public school in America.

If you're a parent reading this, don't rely on schools to feed your children all their nutritious meals. Make sure you introduce them to as many vegetables as you can at home. Serve low-glycemic fruits like berries and apples to them for breakfast. Cook and sauté vegetables for dinner at home and combine them with protein. Make salads for lunch and dinner on weekends and serve them with healthy proteins and fats. If you're looking for great ideas, refer to my cookbook *Food: What the Heck Should I Cook?*

2. Eliminate processed junk foods from school menus. Many parents and school administrators think that food needs to look and taste like junk for kids to eat it. That's why pizza, burgers, fries, and mac and cheese are standard fare in school cafeterias. But a number of schools are finding that kids will eat healthy food if it tastes good and they're provided the option.

In New York, a nonprofit group called Wellness in the Schools started a venture to develop what it called an Alternative Menu for New York City public schools. This menu features fewer processed foods, more vegetarian entrees, freshly made salads and dressings, and zero sugary drinks or flavored milks. Nothing on the menu costs the schools extra money: It's all made from the same ingredients provided to every school. How did Wellness in the Schools accomplish this? It's simple. The group hires recent culinary school graduates and embeds them in public schools for three years, where they show cafeteria workers how to make nutritious and delicious meals from scratch. By the time the culinary grads leave, the school food service workers are well versed in scratch cooking. Wellness in the Schools typically works with underprivileged schools, and for them the program is not costly at all: Most of the money that keeps the program running comes from donors.

3. Ban chocolate milk. Kids don't need to drink cows' milk at all; the data is clear that milk is not beneficial and may be harmful for kids, especially skim milk.[41] But the National Dairy Council lobby is so powerful that schools will not get funding for lunches unless milk is offered at every meal! At the very least, schools that offer milk can cut out 10 grams of sugar per serving by switching from chocolate and strawberry milk to white milk. San Francisco banned chocolate milk in all its high schools in 2017 after a yearlong pilot program found that removing the chocolate option from its elementary and middle school cafeterias hardly affected the amount of milk consumed.[42]

4. Support farm-to-school programs. Instead of relying on Big Food suppliers that ship processed ingredients from manufacturing facilities—often from far away—school lunchrooms should procure many of their core ingredients from local farms. This is often relatively inexpensive and easy to do. School administrators who want to learn how to do this can reach out to the National Farm to School Network, which helps schools procure foods from the farms in their area. I'm a big advocate of farm-to-school programs because ultimately kids win, farmers win, and local communities win. It would be wonderful if Congress designated more funding for these programs in the next Farm Bill.

5. Plant a garden at every school. School gardens connect kids to Mother Nature. They teach them about the environment and motivate them to love fruits and vegetables. They give them opportunities to nurture and enjoy plants that they might not otherwise get to experience. They give them an opportunity to be physically active outdoors in the sun. Most important, they can supply fresh produce to school cafeterias. Gardens are both a learning tool for soil, plant science, and entomology and a vehicle for healthy eating. Groups like KidsGardening, FoodCorps, and Big Green, and nonprofit foundations are working to bring more gardens to schools at the national level. But they need more support and funding.

6. Bring back basic cooking skills to schools as part of their curriculums. Home economics was once a given in almost every school in America. But cooking and nutrition classes fell by the wayside as America shifted to a junk-food diet. This is a travesty. Cooking and nutrition should be a part of every school curriculum. This so-called edible education nudges kids to eat more fruits and vegetables and empowers them to make better food choices. A number of nutrition education programs have embraced this mission, like CookShop, the Edible Schoolyard Project, Common Threads, and Recipe for Success. But now it's time to provide better funding and support so that every kid has access to them.

FOOD FIX: BAN JUNK-FOOD MARKETING THAT PREYS ON KIDS

Unfortunately, some problems only the government can fix. At local and state levels, we also need to limit the reach of fast food—enacting zoning restrictions on fast-food outlets near schools and instituting levies or taxes on fast-food outlets to support community programs for health, education, and so on. On a federal level, we need the FTC to get strict.

The First Amendment doesn't prevent us from protecting children from harmful marketing and advertising. More than fifty countries (not including the United States) regulate food marketing to children. Even here, Joe Camel is gone. If a foreign country were harming our children in the same way Big Food is currently doing, we would go to war to protect our children.

The food industry is never going to self-regulate to the point of making meaningful reforms. And we can't wait forever. The FTC could use its authority to rein in the industry's out-of-control marketing tactics, and lawmakers should enact legislation to protect the most vulnerable.

1. End junk-food advertising to children. The IOM report advises Congress to act to limit food marketing to kids, including bans of cartoon characters, celebrity endorsements, health claims on food packaging, stealth marketing, and marketing in schools, and to provide support for healthier foods. The IOM advises. Congress ignores. Why? They are funded by food lobbyists. Congress and the FTC should ban all junk-food ads from airing during children's programming, as recommended by the American Academy of Pediatrics. According to the Academy of Pediatrics, a ban on fast-food ads aimed at kids would reduce the number of overweight children and adolescents in America by an estimated 14 to 18 percent. Meanwhile, eliminating federal tax deductions for junk-food ads that target children would reduce childhood obesity by up to 7 percent.[43] Why should Big Food get a tax break for manipulating our kids into getting fat and sick?

2. End predatory digital ads. In addition to television ads, Congress needs to ban online, digital, and other forms of interactive junk-food and fast-food ads aimed at kids. In many ways these ads are even more harmful because children today spend increasing amounts of time on social media, where regulations are especially lax. In the meantime, pediatricians and family practitioners should discuss food advertising with their patients, encouraging parents to monitor children's exposure. Medical professionals could also emphasize the importance of good nutrition to help counteract the weekly blitz of junk-food advertising most kids are forced to endure.

Below are just a few of the governments that have taken aggressive regulatory steps. When will the United States join them?

- The **Quebec** government was the first to forbid predatory marketing, banning fast-food advertising to kids in electronic and print media way back in 1980. This one aggressive measure has had an impact that still resonates today. A study published in 2012 found that the advertising ban led to a 13 percent reduction in fast-food expenditures and an estimated 2 billion to 4 billion fewer calories consumed by Quebec children. It has the lowest childhood obesity rate in Canada.[44]

- Not far behind Quebec is **Sweden**. In 1991 the country instituted a ban on all toy and junk-food commercials aimed at children under the age of twelve. To this day, the law remains very popular in Sweden. Sweden has one of the lowest childhood obesity rates in Europe.[45]

- The **United Kingdom** has one of the highest rates of childhood obesity in Europe, but British public health officials have begun to take action in recent years. About a decade ago the government implemented a ban on junk-food TV ads aimed at children under the age of sixteen. The impact was so striking that some cities decided to go further. About 40 percent of children ages ten and eleven in London are overweight or obese. In 2018 the city decided to ban all junk-food ads from its public transport system. That meant no more ads for candy bars, soft drinks, and potato chips on its iconic double-decker buses or the Tube. The United Kingdom now has some of the strictest standards in the world. In 2018, its Advertising Standards Authority pulled several online ads created by Cadbury and other candy companies because they did not do enough to prevent adolescents from viewing them.[46]

3. Parents: Limit your children's screen time. If you have a child under two years of age, make sure he or she does not watch television or use technology. Studies have shown that it can be detrimental to their brains. Many Silicon Valley tech executives don't let their children use technology such as smartphones, iPads, or computers.[47] They are the ones who have designed them to be addictive. And many Big Food company executives don't let their kids use their own products (or eat or drink them themselves). For older children, the best thing you can do is tightly monitor their screen time and filter out the programs or channels with harmful ads. Look for programs you can download that are free of junk-food commercials and other predatory ads. Select programs for kids to watch on PBS, which tends to restrict junk-food ads, or Netflix so they won't be bombarded with food commercials every five minutes. Limit their amount of screen time to an hour or less each day. Strong evidence also exists that screen time is linked to attention deficit disorder in children[48] and is the second-biggest driver of obesity after sugar-sweetened beverages.[49]

We don't have to sit idly by letting Big Food prey on our children. Let's protect them at home and in school with nutritious foods and education that builds the foundation for a healthy life. And let's support organizations and leaders who want to do the same.

For a quick reference guide on the Food Fixes and resources on protecting the health of our children, go to www.foodfixbook.com.

CHAPTER 9

THE FDA IS NOT DOING ITS JOB TO PROTECT US

The average American eats a junk-food diet; about 60 percent of our calories come from ultraprocessed foods. But if you're in the minority that tries to eat healthy, you've probably struggled trying to make sense of food labels. It can be overwhelming. Some of them might as well be written in another language. You shouldn't need a nutritional biochemistry degree to decipher the ingredients label on a protein bar or a cup of yogurt. Have you ever read a food label and wondered what the heck mono- and diglycerides are? Or why carrageenan, maltodextrin, and soy lecithins are in so many processed foods?

These emulsifiers and chemical additives are a big red warning sign to drop the package and run. If you can't pronounce an ingredient, it's probably not something you want to put in your body. Unfortunately, most people don't take the time to read the ingredient lists, which are usually buried on the back of food packages and written in fine print. And the other important source of information, the "nutrition facts" panel, is more confusing. Most people don't know what a "percent daily value is," or whether the serving sizes listed under the nutrition facts are realistic (they are not).

The FDA regulates food labels, and they're a prime example of how the agency is failing the public. They are allowed to be deliberately misleading and confusing, which serves the interests of Big Food rather than those of consumers. As Jerold Mande, a nutrition expert who worked on food labels at the FDA and the USDA, explained it to me, many food companies do not want you to know what's in their products, so they deliberately make their ingredients hard to read. "A lot of companies use all capital letters and they squish them together and use a very small size, about 1/16-of-an-inch letter," he said. "The result is that you look at most food packages and it's very hard to read the ingredient list."

Companies are required to list ingredients in the order of their predominance. But that doesn't tell you how much is in the package. If sugar is the second ingredient listed on a package, that doesn't tell you if it makes up 30 percent of the food or 5 percent.

Have you ever picked up a jar of strawberry jam at the supermarket and looked at its ingredient list? A jar of Smucker's strawberry jam lists strawberries as the first ingredient, and then the second, third, and fourth ingredients are as follows: high-fructose corn syrup, corn syrup, and sugar. This tactic is very common. The reason companies often use several sweeteners in one product is so they don't have to list "sugar" as the first ingredient. As Mande explained, "What we know from some investigations is that companies often use five different sugars in their products so that they don't show up high on the list."

THE FDA ALLOWS HARMFUL INGREDIENTS IN OUR FOOD

In addition to regulating food labels, one of the FDA's top responsibilities is ensuring the safety of the food supply. Under a federal regulation passed in 1958 called the Food Additives Amendment, any substance that the food industry intentionally adds to its products is considered a food additive. All food additives are theoretically subject to premarket review and FDA approval. Food additives are only exempted from this rule if they are GRAS, which stands for *generally recognized as safe*. The GRAS system was designed to apply to ingredients that have been dietary staples for generations, like cinnamon, vanilla, baking powder, salt, pepper, olive oil, vinegar, caffeine, butter, and a variety of natural extracts and flavorings.[1] In other words, things our grandparents would recognize.

But thanks to aggressive industry lobbying, the FDA has ceded much of its regulatory power over food additives to food manufacturers. It's a blatant case of the fox guarding the henhouse. In many cases the FDA has allowed chemical industry trade groups like the Flavor and Extract Manufacturers Association to declare new food chemicals GRAS without any scientific explanation at all.[2] In 2013, a study published in *JAMA Internal Medicine* found that the GRAS review process lacked integrity because many of the GRAS committee members who make safety determinations have strong industry ties. "Between 1997 and 2012," the authors concluded, "we found that financial conflicts of interest were ubiquitous in determinations that an additive to food was GRAS. The lack of independent review in GRAS determinations raises concerns about the integrity of the process and whether it ensures the safety of the food supply."[3]

Today more than 10,000 additives are allowed in food—43 percent of them are GRAS additives and fewer than 5 percent have actually been tested for safety.[4] The average American consumes 3 to 5 pounds of these additives every year. Consumer watchdog groups have repeatedly urged the FDA to step up its oversight of these additives. In 2015, the Natural Resources Defense Council, the Center for Science in the Public Interest, the Environmental Working Group, and other organizations filed an eighty-page report with the FDA, laying out exactly how its failure to vet new chemicals violates the law. The report listed a number of additives that cause cancer. In a very strange statement, the FDA said those additives were not harmful even if they caused cancer in animals, but they were removing them anyway because of the law.[5]

Even more disturbing is that many chemicals and medications used in agriculture are banned in Europe and other countries, but they are still allowed to be used in the United States. Just a few of the many examples:

- **Potassium bromate and azodicarbonamide.** These are used in baked goods. Subway got outed for use of a yoga-mat chemical in their bread in 2014 (more on this story later in this chapter). That was azodicarbonamide. It causes cancer in animals, and in Singapore if a company uses it, they are subject to a $450,000 fine and 15 years in jail![6] Potassium bromate is added to flour to make it riser faster and look nice. It has been labeled as a potential human carcinogen by the International Agency for Research on Cancer. Petitions to ban it have been at the FDA for 20 years.

- **BHA and BHT.** BHA and BHT are used in many processed-food products as preservatives and flavor enhancers. These additives are severely restricted in Europe. BHA is actually listed by our own government as "reasonably anticipated" to be a human carcinogen.[7] But that's not a strong enough association for the FDA to protect us, or could it be the food lobby and the revolving door between the FDA and the food industry having its way?

- **Brominated vegetable oil (BVO).** If you have ever had Mountain Dew or sports drinks, you have had BVO. Bromine is a flame retardant that causes memory loss, nerve damage, and skin problems.

- **Yellow food dyes no. 5 and no. 6, and red dye no. 40.** If any of these dyes are used in Europe, the foods are slapped with a warning label that says "May have an adverse effect on activity and attention in children." Studies have clearly shown that these dyes cause hyperactivity and behavior changes in children.[8] They are everywhere— candy, icing, cereal, mustard, ketchup, breakfast bars, and other foods. Yellow dye no. 5 is known to cause allergies, hives, and asthma.

- **Farm animal drugs.** Drugs used in raising livestock, including bovine growth hormone to promote milk production and ractopamine to make animals fat, are also harmful to humans.

The FDA is asleep at the wheel, at best. At worst it is doing the bidding of the food industry. And sadly, we have seen this story before. The most striking example of this is trans fats, a man-made additive that persisted in the food supply for 50 years after it was found harmful and after it was known that it caused millions of heart attacks. Yet because trans fats were designated safe, Americans turned their backs on butter, tallow, and lard and ate margarine and shortening instead. It was only in the 1990s that well-designed studies demonstrated that even slight increases in trans fat consumption promoted heart disease, giving scientists their smoking gun. It took 50 years from the time scientists found that trans fats were harmful for the FDA to remove it from the GRAS list, and even then it was only after a lawsuit. Why? Trans fats were one of the main building blocks of processed and fast food. The food industry did what it usually does: It tried to downplay the science and fought against regulations.

But in a positive twist, the public health community banded together and worked hard to get trans fats out of the food supply. The beginning of the end for trans fats came in 2006, when New York City banned trans fats in restaurant food. The food industry aggressively opposed the measure, but other cities and states across the country—from Massachusetts and Vermont to Maryland and California, among others—soon followed suit. Then, finally, after years of dragging its feet, the FDA announced in 2015 that it was banning trans fats and removing them from the GRAS list. The FDA ultimately did the right thing. But it should have acted sooner. New York City's bold and early action on trans fats paid dividends: A study of its 2006 trans fat ban found that in just a few years it led to a nearly 7 percent citywide drop in hospital admissions for heart attacks and strokes.[9]

THE POWER OF ONE PERSON TO CHANGE BIG FOOD

By now, you may be thinking, *What can I really do about any of these problems in the food industry?* Well, in fact, you can do a lot. My friend Vani Hari proves it.

Vani Hari might be the single most influential food activist in America today. She has taken down Big Food companies and spurred more food industry reforms than any other person I know. She's forced multibillion-dollar corporations to remove unhealthy additives and disclose potentially harmful ingredients in their products. Her words and actions are so powerful that in 2015 *Time* magazine named her one of its 30 Most Influential People on the Internet. She's written two eye-opening and inspiring books, the most recent of which is *Feeding You Lies: How to Unravel the Food Industry's Playbook and Reclaim Your Health.*

Long before she became the self-proclaimed Food Babe and a household name, Hari was just your average person eating a junk-food diet like the vast majority of other people on this planet. As the daughter of Indian immigrants who came to the United States to pursue the American Dream, Hari was raised to believe that the American food system was among the best in the world. But eating the American diet made her sick and fat. She had asthma, eczema, acne, stomach problems, and severe allergies. Then she started reading about diet and realized her food was making her sick. She changed her diet to whole foods and her health problems and the excess weight disappeared.

She started sharing her experiences on a blog, *Food Babe,* and exposing the chemical and harmful ingredients in most fast and processed foods. She started with Chick-fil-A, which listed 100 ingredients in a chicken sandwich including MSG and TBHQ (a derivative of butane, an ingredient in gasoline). Chick-fil-A invited her to their headquarters and not only listened, but also made changes. In 2013, the company announced that it was removing artificial dyes, high-fructose corn syrup, and TBHQ from its products. The company also said it would begin using only antibiotic-free chickens. For Vani, it was a huge victory, and one that would turn out to be the first of many.[10]

She took on Chipotle, outing them for using trans fats and GMO ingredients while claiming to be a healthy restaurant. They were forced to be transparent and became the first national chain to remove GMO ingredients from their food after thousands signed Vani's petition.[11] Kraft was next in her sights for using artificial dyes and preservatives in their mac and cheese in the United States but not in the UK, where they are prohibited. Using her Food Babe Army to garner hundreds of thousands of signatures and camping out at their offices, she ultimately forced them to remove the chemicals.[12] Next on her list was Subway, whose slogan "Eat Fresh" was misleading. Why? They used a yoga-mat ingredient called azodicarbonamide in their bread in the United States but not in other countries, where it was banned. Hari got Subway to stop using it and also agree to source only antibiotic-free meat. Many of the biggest fast-food chains across the globe followed suit. McDonald's, Wendy's, Jack in the Box, Chick-fil-A, and White Castle, among others, all removed azodicarbonamide from their products too![13] Starbucks was called out for using a carcinogenic caramel color in their pumpkin spice latte and removed it. General Mills and Kellogg's agreed to stop using the toxic preservative BHT.

FOOD FIX: DON'T LET FOOD COMPANIES FEED YOU THEIR LIES

Big food companies are turning their supertanker ships slowly, pivoting to healthier product lines and encouraging better agricultural practices, often after being forced to do so by consumer demand. Not too long ago I met with the head of Nestlé USA and toured their factory in Cleveland. What I saw impressed me. The company is on a mission to remake their products so they have less junk in them. Nestlé has divested itself of its candy business, is removing additives and processed ingredients from many of its foods, and has quit the GMA because it opposed policies to improve the food system such as soda taxes and labeling of GMOs. Nestlé started the Sustainable Food Policy Alliance along with Unilever, Danone, and Mars. While these companies have legacy products that are bad for you and the planet, they are working to adapt to consumer demand.

From what I could see, Nestlé is trying hard to make real food. The company still has a long way to go. But the fact that the world's largest food company is moving in this direction is an encouraging sign — and it's people like Vani Hari who are responsible for helping to push the industry in a new direction.

ANTIBIOTICS IN ANIMAL FEED AND THE RISE OF SUPERBUGS

Antibiotics are a multibillion-dollar category of drugs that save many lives. But the majority of antibiotics aren't prescribed by doctors and used by sick patients — they're fed to livestock on factory farms. Antibiotics are widely used in industrial agriculture to reduce the spread of nasty infections caused by overcrowding, filth, and other cruel and unsanitary conditions in concentrated animal feeding operations, or CAFOs. The drugs are used to alleviate some of the horrible consequences of factory farming, like preventing cows' stomachs from exploding as a result of the excess gas produced by fermenting corn in their rumens, the first chamber of a cow's stomach.

For the food industry, a welcome side effect of stuffing animals with antibiotics is that it accelerates their growth. It makes them bigger and fatter with less food, so they are more profitable.[14] As a result, antibiotics have become a staple in industrial farming. But this comes at a terrible cost to societal health.

The spread of antibiotic-resistant diseases is a rapidly growing threat across the globe, contributing to the deaths of 700,000 people worldwide each year, and it's predicted that by 2050 this global epidemic will kill more people than cancer.[15] No one disputes what is driving this epidemic: It's the overuse of antibiotics. Two major factors contribute to this. One is the misuse of antibiotics in hospital settings, where the drugs are widely overprescribed, often for viral infections, for which they are useless. The other major factor is the excessive use of antibiotics in food animal production. The drugs reduce the infection rate in farm animals, but a small number of bacteria invariably survive and then mutate into drug-resistant germs.

According to the CDC, "Use of antibiotics on the farm helps to produce antibiotic-resistant germs. All animals carry bacteria in their intestines. Giving antibiotics to animals will kill most bacteria, but resistant bacteria can survive and multiply. When food animals are slaughtered and processed, these bacteria can contaminate the meat or other animal products. These bacteria can also get into the environment and may spread to fruits, vegetables or other produce that is irrigated with contaminated water."

The CDC reports that at least half a dozen multistate outbreaks of food poisoning have been linked to drug-resistant bacteria since 2011, including one that sickened 634 people in 29 states. Nearly half of those people were hospitalized. *Consumer Reports* testing found that meat from conventionally raised animals is twice as likely to contain superbugs as meat from animals that are raised without antibiotics.[16]

It's not just meat eaters who have to worry. One outbreak of E. coli that killed three people in 2006 was linked to spinach that had been contaminated by pig and cow manure from a nearby farm.[17] Experts have found that the drug-resistant bacteria that spawn from the indiscriminate use of antibiotics on farms can spread to people in many ways:

- Farmworkers can be infected while handling animals and manure and then pass superbugs to other people.
- Superbugs can be spread to crops and groundwater through the use of contaminated fertilizer.
- Manure and urine slurries containing antibiotics are often spread on fields, killing the microbiology of the soil the same way antibiotics harm our own microbiome.[18]
- Drug-resistant bacteria can even be spread throughout communities by the wind. One study of people living near farms in rural Pennsylvania found that they were nearly 40 percent more likely to contract MRSA infections than people who lived farther away.[19]

The economic price of overusing antibiotics is likely to be staggering as well. RAND Europe, a nonprofit research organization, looked at the impact of the overuse of antibiotics in agriculture on labor productivity. Hold on to your hats. Globally, between now and 2050, the cost of antibiotic resistance is estimated to climb as high as $124.5 trillion. That doesn't even include any associated health care costs, so this is likely a big underestimate.[20] The Union of Concerned Scientists estimates that in the United States alone the public health costs are $2 billion a year.[21]

With so much at stake, you might think that the FDA would take aggressive action to protect the public. The agency has the power to clamp down on the use of antibiotics in animal feed. It can tightly regulate them, forcing drug companies and factory farms to be more circumspect about using antibiotics. And the FDA could track their usage more closely, so that health authorities could prevent drug-resistant outbreaks or contain them more quickly when they occur. But in fact, the use of antibiotics in livestock has increased in the past decade. In 2009, the FDA estimated that 29 million pounds of antibiotics were used in this country.[22] Twenty-four million pounds were used to prevent disease in livestock in overcrowded conditions.[23] Today that number is estimated to be 32 million pounds.[24]

How could that be? Because the FDA allows the food industry to police itself. In 2013, the FDA announced that it wanted drug companies to change the way veterinary antibiotics are sold and labeled. It asked drug companies to remove indications for weight gain and growth promotion, and it said that antibiotics should only be fed to animals with a veterinarian's approval. That means that in theory the drugs should not be prescribed specifically to make animals bigger and fatter.

But the FDA made the plan completely *voluntary*. No regulation, no legislation. It just politely advised Big Ag not to use antibiotics, advice which was promptly ignored. Perhaps not a surprise when the deputy commissioner of the FDA from 2010 to 2016, Mike Taylor, was before that the vice president of public policy for Monsanto. Another major loophole is that the food industry can continue to indiscriminately use antibiotics and then claim they are doing so for reasons other than growth promotion. Even when the FDA placed a "ban" on using antibiotics for growth promotion on factory farms in 2017, it had little impact. The food industry continues to pump animals full of these drugs. Now it just says it is doing so to prevent disease.

FOOD FIX: REFORM AT THE FDA— PREVENTING ANTIBIOTIC OVERUSE AND SUPERBUGS

I once asked Peggy Hamburg, the former FDA commissioner, why the FDA didn't mandate clearer food labels, restrict toxic food additives, and end the use of antibiotics for growth and disease prevention in animal feed. She was honest. When the FDA tries to implement stricter regulations, she said, Congress (in the pocket of Big Food and Big Ag) threatens to shut down funding and programming at the FDA. Our own Congress has become the bully for the food industry. The other problem is the revolving door between industry and the FDA, where many key appointees at the FDA have worked for Big Food, Big Pharma, and Big Ag.

As consumers we have to push for change at the state and local levels. We can support groups like the US Public Interest Research Group (PIRG), a consumer watchdog group that has been leading the charge on this issue. The advocacy group helped California and Maryland pass laws banning their states' factory farms from routinely using medically important antibiotics. Thanks to California and Maryland leading the way on this issue, many more states are now looking to enact similar measures. Doing so will go a long way toward protecting the public from lethal superbugs.

Even the WHO has called on the agriculture industry to stop giving antibiotics to healthy animals.[25] It's important that we all support the following solutions proposed by PIRG, the WHO, and other prominent authorities and health experts.

1. Implement an outright ban on antibiotics for "disease prevention" in livestock. The use of antibiotics on factory farms must be limited to cases of animal sickness or direct disease exposure only.

2. Stop factory farms from using antibiotics that are especially valuable to human medicine, including fluoroquinolones, glycopeptides, macrolides, and third- and fourth-generation cephalo-sporins. The WHO describes these antibiotics as critically important for humans.

3. Bring in qualified veterinarians. Implement requirements that they oversee the administration of antibiotics to animals on factory farms, and that antibiotics be administered only in cases where these veterinarians have directly assessed the animals.

4. Promote and apply good practices at all steps of production and processing of foods from animal and plant sources. Ideally, transi-tioning from factory farms to regenerative agriculture and practices will solve this problem. (More on this in Part 5.)

5. Improve biosecurity on farms and prevent infections through improved hygiene and animal welfare.

6. Reduce the need for antibiotics altogether by adopting new technologies (for example, vaccines) to improve animal health and prevent disease.[26]

7. Track the misuse of antibiotics. The USDA and FDA don't effectively track the use of antibiotics in livestock production. The drug and agriculture industry refused to release any data until 2003 and now releases only limited data. In order to track and regulate the misuse of antibiotics there must be mandatory transparency.

FOOD FIX: HOW TO PROTECT YOURSELF

Thankfully, Vani Hari lays out a blueprint for how anyone can use food activism to fight for food industry reforms in her latest book, *Feeding You Lies: How to Unravel the Food Industry's Playbook and Reclaim Your Health*. The book exposes the industry's deceptive practices, its manip-ulation of nutrition science, its misinformation campaigns, and its label and marketing trickery. It's an empowering book that I encourage you to check out. She maps out an action plan as someone who has taken on Big Food and won. It will not just open your eyes and educate you; it will also give you the tools to follow in Vani's footsteps.

1. **Buy your meat from a trusted local farm.** Or look for meat and dairy products that have the American Grassfed Association (AGA) logo. The AGA follows sustainable and transparent practices, and it treats animals humanely. The animals are raised on pasture, are allowed to forage, and are not drugged with hormones and antibiotics.

2. **Find certified grass-fed products online,** for example, on Thrive Market or Amazon. Or you can go to the American Grassfed Association website and look for certified grass-fed producers in your area: americangrassfed.org/producer-profiles/producer-members-by-state/.

3. **Look for labels on meat, poultry, dairy, and other foods that say *hormone-* and *antibiotic-free*.**

4. **Visit localharvest.org/organic-farms to find small farms in your area that do not use hormones and antibiotics.** There are almost 2 million farms in the United States, and almost 80 percent of them are small farms.

5. **Eat real whole food,** or if you have packaged food, make sure every ingredient is something you recognize or would have in your kitchen and use in cooking. No one has azodicarbonamide, mono- or diglycerides, BHT, or carrageenan in their cupboards. An egg or almond or avocado doesn't have an ingredient list or nutrition facts label.

6. **Eat at restaurants that don't use animal products raised with antibiotics.** PIRG, along with the Natural Resources Defense Council and other groups, releases an annual "Chain Reaction" report that grades restaurant chains on their antibiotics policies for the meat they buy. In 2017, the scorecard contained A grades for only two restaurant chains: Chipotle and Panera Bread. Subway was given a B+ and Chick-fil-A received a B. Meanwhile, eleven restaurant chains received the worst grade, an F. Those that flunked included Dairy Queen, Sonic, Applebee's, Domino's, Chili's, Little Caesars, Arby's, IHOP, Cracker Barrel, and Buffalo Wild Wings. I would generally advise you to avoid these restaurants anyway. But let's be honest: Millions of people patronize these establishments, and they aren't going away anytime soon. It is good to see that the annual report is already making a difference. Many companies that see their low grades released to the public are motivated to

improve them. In 2015, Subway had the worst grade, an F, which helped inspire the company to make dramatic improvements. The sandwich giant earned a higher grade after it started serving antibiotic-free chicken and pledged to eliminate antibiotics from all its meat and poultry products by 2025. Don't patronize the restaurants with bad grades—and let their corporate management know exactly why you don't eat there. Eventually, they'll change their policies.

TEAMING WITH THE US PUBLIC INTEREST RESEARCH GROUP

Although I generally recommend avoiding chain restaurants because of their ultraprocessed foods and bad fats, you can check a restaurant's grade in regard to antibiotic-free meat. Find the restaurant scorecard on PIRG's website: uspirg.org/blogs/blog/usp/grades-are-antibiotics-more-top -us-restaurants-receive-passing-grades-year.

Join the fight by going to their website and signing up to support the campaign, called Save Our Antibiotics: uspirg.org/sites/pirg/files /programs/antibiotics/overuse.html.

Vani Hari is proof that one person can start a revolution. And if many of us join her, we'll be able to turn around these problems in our food system—for everybody's good. With enough pressure from citizens and companies that choose to make better decisions about their ingredients, eventually the FDA will have to step up.

FOOD FIX: FDA POLICIES FOR PEOPLE, NOT CORPORATIONS

The FDA has a vital job to do. It's supposed to keep our food supply safe and regulate food. But right now it gets a grade of D+, just barely passing. I propose a handful of relatively simple fixes that could vastly improve the FDA's handling of our food system. Americans should demand these changes, putting pressure on Congress to make these reforms a reality. The FDA needs to improve in three key areas. It needs to create stronger safety standards for the use of antibiotics in our food, enforce stricter food-labeling standards, and mandate safety testing before products or additives are used in our food supply. Many countries have already shown the way. The FDA just needs to follow suit.

Here's what the FDA can do to make food labels easier to understand, because now you have to have a PhD in nutrition to make any sense of them. Why does it say grams of sugar instead of teaspoons, especially in a country that doesn't use the metric system? Simple. The food industry wants us confused. If the nutrition label of a 20-ounce soda said it contained 15 teaspoons of sugar, we might think twice about buying it.

1. Use the stoplight system for food labels. Similar to the GMO-labeling tactics we've discussed, in Chile and many European countries the food labels use a brilliantly simple system. A green logo means the food is good for you: Go ahead and buy it. Yellow means it's essentially neutral: Not so good for you, but not necessarily bad for you either. Proceed with caution. And a red logo is the equivalent of a great big stop sign: This food could kill you, so either put it down and back away or be doubly sure that this is what you really want to put in your body or feed to your children. Front-of-package warning labels have been used very successfully in other countries such as Chile for foods that are harmful. The industry will fight back, all guns blazing, but it is the right choice. Don't make it hard for consumers; make the right choice the easy choice.

2. List ingredients by their percentages. The United States is one of the few developed countries that uses an outdated system. As Jerold Mande explains, "Other countries actually state the percentages of those ingredients. If it's the second ingredient, is it 30 percent or is it 5 percent? You just don't know with our current labels. Other countries require the top ingredients and their percentages [to be] listed." The FDA needs to require food companies to list the percentages of sugar, oil, food coloring, and other ingredients on their labels.

3. Restrict health claims on package labels. Food companies have a right to package their products in appealing ways. They can slap pictures of mountain springs and green valleys on their labels if they like. They can come up with clever brand names to entice consumers. But the FDA should put its foot down when companies make unwarranted or misleading health claims. Americans spend billions every year on cereal, bread, yogurt, and other foods that claim to be "all natural" despite containing synthetic and genetically engineered ingredients. Many foods are labeled "whole grain" even though their first ingredient is refined flour. There are foods that claim to "strengthen your immune system"—like Ocean Spray cranberry juice—even though they are loaded with sugar. And many processed foods claim to be "lightly sweetened" (like Kellogg's Frosted Mini-Wheats) or "a good source of fiber," even though they are nothing of the sort.[27] The FDA should stop companies from slapping false claims on their labels. They should be allowed to make health claims only when they have actual evidence to back them up. The FDA allows Froot Loops to be labeled "heart-healthy" because it has no fat or cholesterol (but tons of sugar) but deems KIND bars unhealthy because they contain "fatty" nuts, even though nuts are now universally accepted to help with weight loss and prevent heart disease and diabetes.

4. Strengthen its regulation of chemical food additives. Food industry groups should not be allowed to declare new food chemicals and other additives safe without the proper scientific evidence. The FDA must enforce the current standards under the law. The safety of our food supply depends on it.

As we'll see in the next chapter, Big Food's influence on the FDA is not the only way we are being deceived. But we will expose their tactics and show you how everyday citizens can lead the way toward transformation.

For a quick reference guide on the Food Fixes and resources to improve the role of the FDA, go to www.foodfixbook.com.

PART III

INFORMATION WARFARE

Big Food and Big Ag are clearly focused on manipulating government to implement policies that strengthen their foothold in the marketplace and quash any initiatives to limit their profits. They also focus on manipulating science, public health groups, professional societies, and public opinion through even more massive efforts.

The food industry is not going to change overnight. We have to be on the lookout for some of the industry's most nefarious tactics: dubious, if not fake, science and sly partnerships.

When I was in medical school, I thought science was a beautiful, pristine field full of integrity and truth. But as I've paid closer attention, I've discovered that nutrition studies are highly corrupted by the food industry. Big Food is furiously promoting false science.

The food industry also buys loyalty from a wide range of prominent organizations we believe to be credible and independent sources of advice. Industry spends billions on corporate social responsibility programs that make strange bedfellows, but that spending achieves two important objectives for the food industry: It can generate outspoken support, and it can buy silence. But most important, it can trick and deceive you, the consumer. After all, the industry's ultimate goal is to get you to buy more of their products.

Follow along, but be warned: What you're about to read will shock you.

HOW THE FOOD (MOSTLY SODA) INDUSTRY CO-OPTS PUBLIC HEALTH AND DISTORTS NUTRITION SCIENCE

When Coca-Cola and Skittles were created, it may be true that the manufacturers didn't know just how much obesity and disease their products would cause. But this is no longer the case. Big Food companies are not innocent actors caught in the wake of their unintended consequences. They are active participants in the disability, disease, and death of billions of people. Rather than changing or reinventing their products to be less harmful, Big Food has launched an intentional, thoughtful, and meticulously designed series of efforts to silence critics; manipulate science; distort the truth; and aggressively control and influence media, politicians, public health and consumer advocacy groups, and consumers. Let's see exactly how.

In the spring of 2012, Coca-Cola was under attack.

New York City mayor Michael R. Bloomberg had just announced a controversial new plan to ban local restaurants, movie theaters, and fast-food establishments from selling large cups of sugary beverages. Chicago, Philadelphia, and other cities were debating whether to institute sugary-drink taxes to drive down their obesity rates as well. And on social media, a video called "Sugar: The Bitter Truth" was going viral, with millions of page views and more than 50,000 new viewers every month. The video showed a charismatic endocrinologist named Robert Lustig explaining in gripping detail why sugar is toxic to the liver and the body.

Americans were starting to look at their fizzy, sugar-laden beverages as the cause of their growing waistlines. Sales of full-calorie soft drinks across the United States were plummeting, reaching their lowest point in 20 years. Coca-Cola, the industry leader, was desperate to stop the bleeding. The company deployed a powerful weapon: one of its top executives, Rhona Applebaum, a tough corporate executive with a PhD in microbiology who was Coke's chief scientist. In August 2012, Applebaum drew the battle lines. She warned the sugar executives at the International Sweetener Symposium that they needed to be more aggressive in defending their products from the public health onslaught. Applebaum put up a slide that showed a list of the food industry's biggest detractors. On the slide were photographs of Kelly Brownell— dean of the Sanford School of Public Policy at Duke University and an obesity expert and outspoken advocate of soda taxes—along with the logo of the Center for Science in the Public Interest, a consumer watchdog group and major critic of the junk-food industry.[1]

Applebaum outlined how to fund "defensive and offensive science and research" to promote industry-friendly studies—a bit bizarre because science is not a weapon; it is an inquiry into truth. She warned that the industry was under attack from "detractor activism." She complained about Lustig's viral video on sugar, calling him a crusading "tube star" and pointing out that he and other public health critics were resonating with the public. These critics of the industry "basically go unchallenged," she told the crowd, lamenting that even Coke had sometimes been too complacent in the face of criticism.[2] Applebaum told the executives that Big Soda and the sugar industry were facing a do-or-die moment. To drive the point home, she put up a slide with a famous quote uttered by Benjamin Franklin during the Revolutionary War. "We must all hang together, or assuredly we shall all hang separately."

Applebaum told the executives that she had come to them with "a plea from Coca-Cola" that "we all have to work together and use science" to defeat their detractors and win over the public. She laid out a strategy that Coke had devised to "balance the debate": cultivating relationships, collaborating on research, and communicating results.

Her not-so-subtle suggestion: Forming relationships with leading public health organizations would turn junk-food foes into friends. And she said that the industry had to be proactive in communicating about the health effects of sugar while telling consumers to exercise to avoid obesity. "Address the negatives—advance the positives," she told the audience.[3]

Applebaum's resolve at the symposium was not just for show. Internal e-mails show that Applebaum courted many prominent scientists, often inviting them to Coca-Cola headquarters in Atlanta and depositing thousands of dollars into their bank accounts.[4] Applebaum funneled millions of dollars in payments and funding to more than a dozen prominent scientists at universities around the country. And these scientists then published dubious research that benefited the soft drink industry and supported its energy-balance message to the public. Energy balance is a code for eat less, exercise more, that familiar myth that weight loss is all about calories and soda can be part of a "balanced" diet.

A thousand calories of Coke versus a thousand calories of broccoli. Are they the same when you eat them in their effects on your body and metabolism? The science is clear.[5] Absolutely not.

UNDER THE TABLE

In one case, Rhona Applebaum and Coca-Cola provided millions in funding to the Pennington Biomedical Research Center, where one of the country's leading obesity researchers, Peter T. Katzmarzyk, produced a study of a dozen countries that pinned the blame for childhood obesity on sedentary behavior.

"Pennington Biomedical Research Study Shows Lack of Physical Activity Is a Major Predictor of Childhood Obesity," announced a news release published in August 2015. A footnote toward the end of the press release included an important disclaimer that few people reading it might have even noticed: "This research was funded by The Coca-Cola Company." Pennington's big study cited lack of sleep and "too much television" as additional factors that contribute to childhood obesity. But the study was perhaps most noticeable for what it did not say — it was strangely silent on the role of junk food and sugary drinks. For their services, Katzmarzyk and the other Pennington researchers received nearly $7 million in funding from Coca-Cola.[6]

In total, Coke provided more than $120 million to US universities, health organizations, and research institutions between 2010 and 2015. From 2008 to 2016 Coke funded 389 articles in 169 journals concluding that physical activity was more important than diet and that soft drinks and sugar are essentially harmless.[7] You have to walk 4 miles to burn off just one 20-ounce Coke. You can't exercise your way out of a bad diet, but these companies continue to publish data that minimizes the effect of food and inaccurately pushes exercise as the solution to our obesity and disease epidemic.[8]

Furthermore, Applebaum and Coke's influence on researchers extended beyond money. One of the top scientists they courted was Jim Hill, a professor of medicine at the University of Colorado. Hill served on NIH and CDC obesity panels. He cofounded the National Weight Control Registry, the most prominent, long-running weight-loss study in America. He was also a former president of the American Society for Nutrition (ASN), which once called him "a leader in the fight against the global obesity epidemic." It's no surprise that ASN is heavily funded by the food industry.

Beginning in about 2011, with cities and states increasingly proposing taxes on soda and other junk foods, Hill grew cozy with Coke. He published studies paid for by Coke and the American Beverage Association (formerly known as the American Soda Pop Association), and he traveled the country giving speeches and attending conferences on

Coke's dime. Some of his research findings were so counterintuitive that they were practically unbelievable. In one study published in the high-profile journal *Obesity*, Hill reported that obese people who drank diet soda lost more weight than obese people who drank only water.[9] Independent research consistently shows that diet drinks increase weight gain and type 2 diabetes.[10] In e-mails (obtained through the Freedom of Information Act, FOIA), Applebaum had been urging Hill to publish the study, saying Coke was eager to fend off negative press about the dangers of aspartame. In one e-mail Applebaum alerted Hill that *The Dr. Oz Show* was planning to run a negative segment about artificial sweeteners. Applebaum told Hill that Coke was desperate for him to publish his paper. When he finally did, in May 2014, nutrition experts were incredulous.

"How coincidental that right as diet soda sales take a significant tumble, the soda industry's main lobbying group helps fund a study that tries to claim diet sodas are superior to water," one skeptical nutritionist told a reporter at the time.[11]

Hill's deeds did not go unrewarded. Coke paid him $550,000 for "honoraria, travel, education activities, and research on weight management." The company paid for his travel to conferences and meetings in England, Mexico, and Grenada. It also picked up the tab for Hill and his wife to fly to Australia and New Zealand.[12] In 2014, the company gave Hill's university a check for $1 million to help him start an anti-obesity advocacy group called the Global Energy Balance Network (GEBN), which was Applebaum's brainchild. She not only conceived of the organization, but also helped to recruit its 120 members, many of whom Coke had financially supported. Behind the scenes, e-mails show, Applebaum orchestrated the group's message, designed its website, and edited its mission statement.[13] Hill, with Applebaum's blessing, became the group's president.

THE PROBLEM WITH CALORIES

Science definitively proves that all calories are not the same: Sugar and starch calories act completely differently than calories from fat when you eat them. In a 2018 Harvard study,[14] researchers fed two groups identical numbers of calories, but one group ate 60 percent of calories from fat with less than 20 percent from carbs while the other group had 60 percent from carbs and 10 percent from fat. In the most overweight of the participants, the low-carb, high-fat group burned 400 more calories a day without any more exercise, and while eating the exact same number of calories. Sugar slows your metabolism. Fat speeds it up.

Calories are information, instructions that affect hormones, brain chemistry, the immune system, the microbiome, gene expression, and metabolism. The energy-balance hypothesis is dead—except in the minds of those in the fast-food industry because they have a stake in pushing the idea that weight is all about calories in and calories out. But any third grader could tell you that 1,000 calories of soda and 1,000 calories of broccoli have profoundly different effects on the body.

In one internal memo that the nonprofit advocacy group US Right to Know obtained, Applebaum characterized the GEBN as a "political campaign" and said the goal was to "develop, deploy and evolve a powerful and multi-faceted strategy to counter radical organizations and their proponents." As Applebaum saw it, Big Food was at war with the public health community and science, and the GEBN would serve as the industry's war room.

"There is a growing war between the public health community and private industry over how to reduce obesity. Sides are being chosen and battle lines are being drawn. The most extreme public health experts have gained traction with the media, with many policy makers, and with an increasing proportion of the general public."[15]

Unfortunately for Applebaum, the GEBN blew up in Coca-Cola's face. In 2015, the *New York Times* and other news outlets exposed the organization as an industry-funded front group. When the news broke, Coke announced that Applebaum was suddenly "retiring" from the company and cut its financial ties to GEBN, which promptly announced it was ceasing operations because of "resource limitations."[16] Resource limitations? Really? Their "sponsor's" annual revenue in 2018 was more than $31 billion for selling sugar water.

THE BIG FOOD PLAYBOOK

Coca-Cola's involvement in spreading disinformation is not unique. Its tactics exemplify a multipronged strategy that Big Food has been using to deceive the public for decades.

Junk-food companies routinely recruit nutrition experts to do work for them, paying them enormous sums to promote unhealthy products and to criticize studies that the industry doesn't like. The food industry spends more than $12 billion a year funding nutrition studies (while the NIH spends only $1 billion), polluting and diluting independent research, and confusing policy makers, the public, and even most doctors and nutritionists. Studies funded by the food industry are eight to fifty times more likely to find a positive outcome for their products. The food industry forms deep financial partnerships with policy makers, public health groups, and academic societies.

During medical school, I believed science was an honest field. But I've discovered how much the food industry manipulates nutrition studies. And they are frequently tainted. Their results depend on the design of the study, who is doing the analysis, and who is paying for it. The sad reality is that Big Food is furiously promoting false science.

Just looking at Coca-Cola, researchers, through FOIA, obtained 87,013 pages of documents including five agreements between Coke and public institutions in the United States and Canada.[17] The "research" contracts allow Coca-Cola to review research prior to publication and maintain control over study data, whether the study gets published, and any acknowledgment of Coca-Cola's funding of the study. If they don't like the results, Coke gets to bury the findings. And they support front groups that pose as independent organizations to mislead consumers. How is that real science?

So much for the purity of science and independent researchers! Big Food's ironclad plan to fool you with junk science and bogus claims is once again reminiscent of the tobacco industry's efforts to subvert the truth in past decades. The many ways in which Big Food is borrowing the tactics of Big Tobacco were documented in a landmark 2008 paper written by Kelly Brownell, which was titled *The Perils of Ignoring History: Big Tobacco Played Dirty and Millions Died. How Similar Is Big Food?*[18] As Brownell noted, "Disputing science has been a key strategy of many industries, including tobacco. Beginning with denials that smoking causes lung cancer and progressing to attacks on studies of secondhand smoke, the industry instilled doubt. Likewise, groups and scientists funded by the food industry have disputed whether the prevalence figures for obesity are correct, whether obesity causes disease, and whether foods like soft drinks cause harm." Unbelievably, the food industry front group the Center for Consumer Freedom claims that the obesity epidemic is a hoax.[19] Guess they have never been to Disneyland, or taken a walk down Main Street America.

This coordinated industry-wide strategy aims to influence science, public health organizations, and professional societies and corrupt government policy and lawmakers. When the food industry has contributed as much as $300,000 to the PAC of the congressman who introduces the Cheeseburger Bill,[20] which will prohibit lawsuits against food companies for any injury caused by their food—and most of Congress votes for it—you don't have to wonder who is pulling the strings.

TAINTED SCIENCE

As consumers, we depend on unbiased studies to shed light on the foods we should eat and the ones we should avoid. While some food companies do carry out legitimate and informative research, many fund their own studies for self-serving purposes. Why? One reason is marketing.

Food companies use studies to make dubious health claims about their products so they can increase sales. The other reason is so they can manufacture doubt. When independent studies point to the dangers of their products, food companies respond with their own questionable studies that say otherwise—just as tobacco companies funded studies that cast doubt on the link between smoking and lung cancer. As we already saw with Coke, the soft drink industry seems to have mastered this practice better than anyone.

In February 2001, *The Lancet* published a large independent study ("independent" being the key word) that was among the first to demonstrate that:

- Sugar-sweetened beverages increase obesity rates in kids.
- A child's likelihood of being overweight increased in direct proportion to the number of soft drinks he or she consumed.
- For every can of soda a child drank each day, their odds of becoming obese rose by 60 percent.[21]

The study was a bombshell. It garnered international headlines, and more than 1,000 other scientific articles would go on to cite it. In the days and weeks that followed the study's publication, Coke's stock plummeted. Its share price declined 20 percent relative to the Dow Jones Industrial Average, a downswing that persisted for months. In total the drop represented a loss of $20 billion in the company's valuation.

How did Coke and other soft drink makers respond? In the decade that followed, they funded a slew of studies that claimed that sugary drinks were innocent. Coke, Pepsi, the American Beverage Association, Tate & Lyle (a corn syrup producer), and other sugar and soda industry groups sponsored ("sponsored" being the key word) a half dozen systematic reviews that examined whether sugary drink consumption was linked to weight gain. Every single one of these studies found *zero* association between sugary drinks and obesity.

At the same time, *independent* researchers continued to conduct their own studies, publishing eleven extensive reviews that examined whether sugary-drink consumption was a strong determinant of weight gain and obesity. Out of these eleven studies, nine of them found that the answer was a resounding yes. Many of the studies even noted that public health authorities had enough evidence to discourage people from drinking soda.

The scope of this problem is enormous. An analysis published in *JAMA* in 2017 found that compared to independent research, industry-sponsored food studies of all kinds have a 30 percent greater likelihood of reporting conclusions favorable to their sponsors. The researchers found that this level of bias was on par with studies funded by Big Pharma, which are notorious for portraying risky drugs in a favorable light.

SCIENCE OR PROPAGANDA?

In a report entitled *Nutrition Scientists on the Take from Big Food,* Michele Simon details how the food industry has corrupted the nutrition science community. In a review of 206 studies, researchers found that not a single industry study published showed a negative outcome. Another investigation found that industry-funded studies were nearly eight times more likely than independent studies to show a positive outcome.[22] Another review of 133 studies on sugar-sweetened beverages found that 82 percent of independently funded studies show harm from sugar-sweetened beverages, while 93 percent of industry-funded studies found that soda and sugar-sweetened beverages were not associated with any health problems.[23]

Yet another recent study found that industry-sponsored studies showed no harm from artificial sweeteners, but independently funded studies found significant harm.[24] Coca-Cola and PepsiCo would have us believe that they are being good corporate actors by reducing calories in their drinks. Don't believe them.

For consumers, this means that you have to be hyperaware. When you see a company touting the health benefits of their products on food labels, in an advertisement, or on a website or television show, there's a good chance that the claim came from a dubious study that was wholly bought and paid for by industry.[25] Or when you see studies casting doubt on the harmful effects of their products, don't believe those either. Take a look at the ridiculous studies that the food industry is feeding you...

Sweet Deception

In 2011 a study in the journal *Food & Nutrition Research* looked at data on more than 7,000 kids and concluded that those who ate candy were up to 26 percent less likely to be overweight or obese than kids who didn't eat candy. The candy eaters did not have increased blood pressure, cholesterol, or other metabolic risk factors. In fact, they had *lower* inflammation than the non-candy eaters.[26] The findings were almost too good to be true. "This study suggests that candy consumption did not adversely affect health risk markers in children and adolescents," the authors wrote. Who knew candy was a health food! Shocking, right? Well, not if you know who funded the research.

The authors of this study received thousands of dollars from the National Confectioners Association, a trade group that represents the makers of Skittles, Hershey's, and Butterfingers. The candy group not only paid for the study but was also involved in analyzing the data and writing the manuscript. E-mails show one of the authors, Victor Fulgoni, a former Kellogg's executive, acknowledging to his coauthors about incorporating the candy industry's feedback in their study manuscript. "You'll note I took most but not (all) their comments."

As absurd as it was, the study nonetheless generated plenty of positive media—precisely what the candy industry was looking for. "Does Candy Keep Kids from Getting Fat?" one CBS News headline declared.[27] No, it doesn't. But that hasn't stopped the candy industry from funding other studies that claim that candy consumption has no link to heart disease, obesity, or metabolic syndrome.[28]

If you think that top peer-reviewed scientific journals publish objective research, think again. One of the most respected medical journals, the *Annals of Internal Medicine*, published a study in 2017 entitled "The Scientific Basis of Guideline Recommendations on Sugar Intake: A Systematic Review."[29] At first read I was taken aback. The conclusions contradicted almost all the science I had studied on sugar for 20 years. "Guidelines [to reduce] dietary sugar do not meet criteria for trustworthy recommendations and are based on low-quality evidence." Turns out the "study" was funded by the International Life Sciences Institute (ILSI), the food and agriculture industry front group founded by a Coca-Cola executive and whose sponsors include, along with Coca-Cola, Bayer, Dow AgroSciences, DuPont, ExxonMobil, General Mills, Hershey Foods, Kellogg's, Kraft, McDonald's, Merck & Co., Monsanto, Nestlé, Novartis, PepsiCo, Pfizer, and Procter & Gamble. And the lead author was on the board of Tate & Lyle, one of the largest makers of high-fructose corn syrup.

This problem is global. In Australasia, Nestlé partnered with nutrition societies and funded dubious studies to promote its sugary powdered drink, called Milo, to millions of parents and children. Milo is a malted sugar beverage like Ovaltine with the same glycemic index as Coca-Cola. With the backing of local nutrition experts, the company marketed the ultraprocessed concoction as a nutritious breakfast meal, running ads featuring cartoons, energized schoolchildren, and famous kid-friendly pop stars. They also promoted it as a health and sports drink targeted at kids who have an "energy gap," which they claimed four out of five kids suffer from. I must have missed the class in medical school where we learned about the dreaded energy gap that must be cured with a sugary drink. Nestlé enlisted Dr. Tee Siong to "prove" that Milo was a health drink.[30] He served as science director for more than 20 years for ILSI Southeast Asia. Is it any surprise that Malaysia is Asia's fattest country?

Dr. David Ludwig, professor of nutrition at Harvard Medical School, reviewed Siong's study and found that its design was flawed. The dietary analysis used was not validated and the Milo drinkers were more active and had far less screen time, which the analysis didn't account for. Oh, and Nestlé reviewed the manuscript.

Sugarcoated Research

While these examples are from recent years, the sugar industry has been duping Americans with deceptive research for more than a half century. Sugar executives acknowledged a link between sugar consumption and chronic disease back in the 1950s and '60s. An industry trade group called the Sugar Research Foundation funded animal research as far back as the 1960s that looked at the relationship between sugar and heart disease. But documents show that when the research suggested that sugar might cause both heart problems *and* cancer—a result they found terrifying—the industry buried the data and never published their results. Around the same time, the sugar trade group paid Harvard scientists the equivalent of $50,000 in today's dollars to publish an influential review in the *New England Journal of Medicine* dismissing the idea that sugar caused heart disease. The real culprit, they claimed, was saturated fat.[31]

In fact, the two authors of that review, Fred Stare and Mark Hegsted, were the most prominent nutrition scientists at the time. Dr. Stare started the nutrition department at Harvard, the first in the country. He and the school received $29 million over his career from the food industry, including sugar industry funding for thirty studies from 1952 to 1956.[32] In 1975 he wrote a book called *Sugar in the Diet of Man*. We need say no more. His colleague, Mark Hegsted, went on to help develop the first US Dietary Guidelines under Senator George McGovern, advising us to cut the fat and not worry about sugar and carbs, setting the stage for the greatest health crisis in the history of our species. There were no conflict-of-interest disclosure requirements for researchers in the 1960s.

Today a small handful of influential researchers are still deeply involved with the sugar and corn syrup industries. One of them is James Rippe, a scientist who runs an institute that specializes in churning out studies for the food industry. The lobbying group for the high-fructose corn syrup industry, the Corn Refiners Association, paid Rippe $10 million over a four-year period for his research and even kept him on a $41,000-a-month retainer to write editorials defending corn syrup from critics.[33] And Rippe then produced a series of studies that reported the following:

- Guidelines on reducing added sugar intake are unwarranted.
- Eating added sugar doesn't promote insulin resistance (pre-diabetes or diabetes).
- Consuming even five times the upper limit of sugar recommended by the American Heart Association (AHA) doesn't increase blood pressure or screw up your cholesterol.[34]

With almost ten times as much of this "junk" research on junk food as of true independent science, the public, the media, and the policy makers stay confused.

Whole Grains: Not the Whole Truth

If you believe the federal government, whole grains are practically a superfood. But in reality, their health benefits are dubious at best because we typically refine and process them until they are barely recognizable.

Of course, the AHA gets money from cereal makers to put their seal of approval on the packages and receives hundreds of thousands of dollars for each "endorsement." Twix is a health food according to the AHA, in case you weren't aware—and so are Froot Loops, Cocoa Puffs, and French Toast Crunch, right along with the 7 teaspoons of sugar per serving. It shouldn't be called breakfast; it should be called dessert.

When you grind it into flour, whole wheat or not, it is worse than sugar. The glycemic index of sugar is 65 and that of whole wheat bread is 75, which means that the bread raises your blood sugar more than table sugar. Below the neck, there is no difference between a bowl of sugar and whole wheat bread. Well, actually, the bread is worse.

The scientifically independent group the Cochrane Database of Systematic Reviews concluded that the favorable studies on whole grains were so weak and mired in conflicts of interest that their results "should be interpreted cautiously."[35]

Actually, whole grains can be healthy, but not when sprinkled into junk food. How about Whole Grain Frosted Strawberry Pop-Tarts with 38 grams of sugar and refined flour (9.5 teaspoons of sugar) and 47 ingredients, including proven carcinogenic compounds like caramel color, anyone? Eat the actual whole grain, not an industrially processed version, which carries more harm than good with every bite.

DOES THE STUDY PASS THE SNIFF TEST?

At the end of the day much of the nutrition research that is published in major journals is legit. But the food industry is determined to dupe you with bogus studies to promote their processed junk foods. Because industry studies tend to produce sensational findings, they are often picked up by blogs and news outlets, leading to eye-catching headlines. That's why you need to be skeptical when you see the latest nutrition science headline in the news. If it doesn't pass the smell test, then it's best to forget it. Don't share it on Facebook, don't send it to friends, and certainly don't take it as fact.

Before you buy into a headline, ask yourself some important questions. First, ask who paid for the study. Does the story mention who funded it? If it's a study on breakfast cereal and weight gain, for example, did the NIH fund it or did Kellogg's pay for it? You might need to dig a little deeper. If it says it is funded by the International Life Sciences Institute, you may feel relieved. Sounds legit. But dig deeper. Google the organization. See who is behind it. Be a sleuth.

As Vani Hari says in her book *Feeding You Lies*, "You wouldn't believe a study on cigarettes that was funded by Philip Morris, and you probably shouldn't believe a study on cereal paid for by a company whose bottom line depends on Froot Loops, Apple Jacks, and Frosted Flakes."

GET TO THE SOURCE

To find a funding source for a study, look up the study on PubMed (https://www.ncbi.nlm.nih.gov/pubmed/). Simply type in the name of the lead author and the subject of the study, click on the link to the study you're researching, and look for the part of the paper that mentions its funding source. If the funder sounds like a legitimate organization, don't trust it. Google it to see what you can find.

Don't believe everything you read. "To separate the truth from the bull," Hari says, "I have the following suggestions. Scrutinize the source of the information, the source's possible agenda, and the evidence provided in the message. If possible, ask: Is the evidence science-based? Who funded the science? Does the evidence logically support the claims being made? Does it seem like relevant facts or context have been left out? Remember that commercial pressures shape the form and content of research and news—and exert massive influence."

Most important, remember that replication is the cornerstone of good science. One study that claims that soft drinks are not linked to weight gain should not distract you from the fact that dozens of independent studies have found otherwise. Instead of being led astray by one clickbait headline, think about the larger body of research. If one sensational new study contradicts a large body of research and sounds too good to be true, then it probably is.

FOOD FIX: BIG FOOD AND SCIENCE SHOULDN'T MIX

It is fine for companies to carry out small studies looking at the potential benefits of their products. It makes sense for Pepsi to study whether the electrolytes in the Gatorade it sells can help athletes rehydrate more quickly, for example, or whether products like Quaker Oats might be more satiating than cornflakes. Food companies do research so they can use their findings to make marketing claims. Consumers should be aware that these claims are often exaggerated, but this practice pales in comparison to the problem of Coke, Pepsi, and other large junk-food companies publishing studies on public health matters like obesity and the diabetes epidemic.

Big Food is in the business of selling junk food. It should not be in the business of doing public health research. There's just no reason for it, and more important, food corporations cannot be trusted.

As my friend Dariush Mozaffarian at the Tufts School of Nutrition Science and Policy points out, there are ample reasons not to trust Big Food with public health research. Its documented tactics include "the promotion of harmful products, misleading marketing campaigns, targeting of children and other susceptible groups, corporate lobbying, coopting of organizations and social media with financial support, and attacks against science and scientists."[36]

At the same time, we must also face the reality that government funding for scientific research is already scarce and continuing to dwindle year after year. In the most recent NIH strategic plan, food was mentioned only once, in reference to the Food and Drug Administration. Academic jobs and research positions at universities are becoming more and more competitive, which is driving many scientists to work for the industry.

It's unrealistic to expect that not a single scientist, health professional, academic, or institution will ever accept any funding from the food industry. And not every company is nefarious. The food industry is not a monolith. Some companies recognize the growing demand for nutritious foods and have profited by catering to the health conscious with healthy, organic, and minimally processed foods. But if the food industry is going to be involved in funding studies, there are transparent principles they must follow to ensure that their research is untainted. Any engagement with the industry requires firm oversight and strict rules, like making sure that researchers have full independence to report and publish their findings, and that the companies they partner with have commendable track records of environmental and social responsibility. Some of the guidelines that Mozaffarian and other experts developed (e.g., vetting companies that want to fund studies, increasing funding for independent studies, forming an oversight committee for all studies) can reduce the problems that stem from food companies funding nutrition research. The companies should not be involved in any way in study design, data analysis, authoring of the manuscript, or even review or comments on the manuscript.

Another radical change would be to create a firewall between industry and science. This firewall would allow the food industry to fund important studies without biasing the researchers and their results. To make this work, companies would pool their donations into a common research fund. This pool of money—it could be called the Nutrition Fund, for example—could be managed and distributed to scientists by the NIH. Companies could get incentives to make donations to the fund through tax breaks and other benefits. This fund could then be used to support basic nutrition research on food, diet, and health, as well as food science research that could help companies develop products. A committee of independent scientific advisers could oversee the fund and review and approve research proposals. Ultimately, it could begin to restore the public's faith in industry-sponsored studies.

Such an idea would not be foolproof, of course. In fact, the USDA has actually created a fund from a levy on food companies. It is called the Checkoff Program and it is ostensibly to be used for research, but it is no more than a marketing program for Big Food. Remember the campaigns "Got Milk?" or "The Other White Meat" or "Beef. It's What's for Dinner"? They were all paid for by Uncle Sam to promote agricultural products, regardless of their health benefits. What's fascinating is that Congress introduced a bill to prevent FOIA (Freedom of Information Act) requests from accessing any information about the Checkoff Program. What are they hiding? Why is the government marketing food for the food industry?

Fixing Bad Science

Putting an end to Big Food's co-opting of scientists, academics, and health groups will only solve half the problem. The other problem is that nutrition science is in need of some big changes. Many of our dietary guidelines and health recommendations are based on what is known as nutritional epidemiology, which relies on easily manipulated observational studies. That's why Big Soda can publish study after study claiming that children who drink soft drinks aren't on a fast track to becoming obese and diabetic—they use observational data that can easily be molded to get the outcomes they prefer. Large observational studies also gave us the disastrous advice to eat low-fat diets and six to eleven servings of bread, rice, cereal, and pasta every day! The conventional nutrition wisdom has changed again and again over the years depending on the direction in which the winds of the latest observational studies are blowing.

To illustrate what I mean about observational studies being easily manipulated, consider these examples. If I did a study of women over fifty-five years old who had sex, I would conclude that sex never leads to pregnancy. It is 100 percent accurate, but 0 percent valid. Bruce Ames, one of the world's leading scientists, once said that if you ask epidemiologists who did observational population studies about Miami, they would conclude that everyone is born Hispanic but dies Jewish.

So what is the purpose of observational studies? It is quite simple. To generate hypotheses for future research, and to assess whether correlations are real or just noise. They *never* prove cause and effect. If the effect size is big, then it can be convincing and worth acting on. For example, the increased risk of lung cancer for smokers was 20 to 1. You can take that to the bank. But when a new study, for example, showed that eggs caused a "17 percent" increased risk of heart disease and an "18 percent increased risk of death," that sounds scary, but what it means is the increased risk is 17 and 18 percent, not 2000 percent as it was for smoking and lung cancer. If it is anything less than a 2-to-1 (or a 100 percent) increased risk, ignore it.[37]

Large reviews of observational studies found that less than 20 percent were later confirmed in actual experimental trials.[38] Asking people what they ate once or twice in 20 years and correlating that to health outcomes or death is highly inaccurate and confounding.[39] For example, some large observational studies have shown that eating meat increases the risk of heart disease, cancer, and death.[40] Sounds bad. But those studies were done in a time when we were all told to eat less meat to be healthy. The people who continued to eat meat didn't pay much attention to their health in general.

The problem with observational studies is that they are frequently subject to a phenomenon known as data dredging—scientists run repeated analyses on a data set to extract insignificant findings that might otherwise be meaningless and then amplify them. That's why nutrition science headlines can cause whiplash, with studies telling us one week that butter, cheese, and chocolate are bad for us, and then the next week new studies telling us that these foods are the key to weight loss and a slim waistline. Nutrition epidemiologists are notorious for squeezing trivial findings out of observational data sets and then transforming them into splashy and sensational research papers that attract headlines. It's the very opposite of the scientific method. And sadly, both the food industry and nutrition policy makers use it to their advantage.

The studies that I put more faith in are large randomized controlled trials, which are true experiments (although they too are subject to many limitations). In a typical randomized trial, scientists manipulate one variable—sugar intake, for example—and then assign people to different groups where they are exposed to high levels of sugar or low levels of sugar. Then researchers follow them and measure things like changes in their body weight, cardiovascular biomarkers, and appetite. This is how good science is done. A randomized controlled trial can prove cause and effect. An observational study can only suggest causality.

One great example was a study of 164 people that cost $12 million (yes, it is very expensive to do the right kind of nutrition research). It was an actual experiment where people got a low-fat, high-carb diet, then switched to a high-fat, low-carb diet. The study provided the food to participants and measured their metabolism and hormones. They found that the low-carb, high-fat group burned 300 to 500 more calories a day.[41] That is definitive. And if people paid attention, it would solve our obesity epidemic overnight.

"I think that much of the reason for the failures [of nutrition advice] we've seen is that we have over-trusted observational data," says John Ioannidis, the chairman of disease prevention at Stanford University. "I'm not saying that it's not possible for observational data to tell us something useful. Actually we have learned tremendous insights from observational data. But for nutrition that is so complex, and so difficult, we really need to use our best tools, our best methods, and our best safeguards before we can really trust these observational data."

Ioannidis and others have proposed a reasonable set of guidelines to reform nutrition science, which are badly needed. They include the following:

- **Focus on large randomized controlled trials.** Instead of publishing a million more observational nutrition studies that give us contradictory findings, the nutrition community should do large and rigorous randomized trials that give us definitive answers. According to Ioannidis, the randomized trials needed to answer critical questions in nutrition in definitive ways would add up to less than 1 percent of the NIH's budget.

- **Share raw data to increase transparency.** Journals should require that researchers share their raw data. This will increase transparency and reduce the likelihood of manipulation. All researchers should be able to access and analyze one another's data. Through Harvard, the NIH has funded some of the largest population studies, involving hundreds of thousands of people over decades. Much of our nutrition beliefs are derived from these studies, including the Nurse's Health Study and the Physician's Health Study. But even though taxpayers funded the studies, the researchers won't allow others to see or analyze their raw data. How does that make sense?

- **Enforce strict disclosure rules.** Every medical and nutrition journal should adopt strict conflict-of-interest disclosure rules, and they should impose penalties on researchers who violate the policies. First-time violations could result in a six-month to one-year suspension. Those who repeatedly violate the rules should face a lifetime ban from publishing in the journal. If all journals introduced a system of penalties for flagrant violations of disclosure rules, then researchers would take the policy more seriously. As Marion Nestle wrote in her book *Unsavory Truth: How Food Companies Skew the Science of What We Eat*, not everyone discloses, and many disclosures are incomplete. At the University of California, San Francisco, professor of clinical pharmacy Lisa Bero and her colleagues reported that one-third or more of authors in the studies they examined had undisclosed conflicts and that a similar percentage of published reviews omit statements of funding sources.

- **Media outlets should also be investigating conflicts of interest and report transparently on the food industry.** They should have strict conflict-of-interest policies and disclosures for any articles published. For example, an article in *Forbes* that targeted me made no mention that Monsanto funnels money to the industry front group behind the article—the Genetic Literacy Project. The same author, Kavin Senapathy, declared that breastfeeding is not always the best choice because it could lead to starvation and malnutrition. Sadly, most advertising is from the food or pharmaceutical industry, making tough, critical reporting difficult for media outlets.

Now you know what's really behind all those confusing headlines and reports. The fine print reveals who is funding a study and how the data might be manipulated for profit rather than for your health. So next time you read a nutrition headline, be wary, be thoughtful, dig a little, and ask these important questions: (1) Who funded the study and what are the conflicts of interest of the authors? (2) Is this a study that can prove cause and effect or just a correlation? If there is a correlation, is the increased risk or benefit over 100 percent? If not, move on.

For a quick reference guide on the Food Fixes and resources to help you decipher real science from fake news, go to www.foodfixbook.com.

CHAPTER 11

HOW BIG FOOD BUYS PARTNERSHIPS AND HIDES BEHIND FRONT GROUPS

The food industry strategy for controlling science, public health groups, professional health care societies, public opinion, schools, community organizations, the flow of information, political institutions, and policy is calculated, clear, and effective. And it is well hidden. On purpose.

When New York mayor Michael Bloomberg introduced his controversial ban on large, sugary soft drinks back in 2012, the soda industry promptly sued. The industry, led by the American Beverage Association, ultimately won that battle when a New York State judge struck down the ban in 2013. But the industry did it with the help of some surprising allies: Dozens of minority groups came to Big Soda's aid, filing "friend of the court" briefs in support of the soda industry's lawsuit.[1] These advocacy groups represent the very communities that have been hardest hit by the diabesity epidemic (the continuum from obesity to pre-diabetes to type 2 diabetes).

The NAACP and the Hispanic Federation were among the groups that came to Big Soda's defense. These groups are supposed to fight for the best interests of the communities they represent, which are plagued by chronic disease. African Americans and Hispanics have the highest rates of obesity and diabetes in America—and it is precisely because the junk-food industry preys upon them. Fast-food restaurants are often concentrated in black and Hispanic neighborhoods. Companies disproportionately target them with predatory advertising. And they are more likely to market their worst foods to minority children than to whites, plying them with ads for products laden with salt, sugar, and unhealthy fat.[2]

Researchers at the University of Connecticut found that junk-food companies spend the most on ads that target African Americans and Spanish speakers. Guess which products were most heavily advertised toward minorities—Gatorade, Pop Tarts, Twix, Cinnamon Toast Crunch, and Tyson frozen entrees. The worse the nutritional profile, the more heavily the products were promoted through advertising. Where are the broccoli ads? These findings, the researchers noted, "highlight important disparities in the food and beverage industry's heavy marketing of unhealthy foods to Hispanic and black youth, and the corresponding lack of promotion of healthier options."[3]

So why would groups like the Hispanic Federation and the NAACP support the soda industry in its battle against anti-obesity measures? Could it have something to do with the fact that Coca-Cola gave the NAACP more than $1 million in donations between 2010 and 2015? Or that it gave the Hispanic Federation more than $600,000 in the same time period? In fact, many of the black and Hispanic civil rights, business, and health advocacy groups that joined the beverage industry in opposing soda regulation in recent years have been the recipients of millions of dollars in gifts and funding from the soda industry. Soda companies sponsored NAACP scholarships, financial literacy classes offered by the National Puerto Rican Coalition, and programs from the National Hispanic Medical Association.

While these prominent groups and others cozied up to Coca-Cola, the soda industry has run roughshod over black and Hispanic communities. Things came to a head when two prominent African American pastors filed a lawsuit against Coke and the American Beverage Association in 2017, saying that the soda industry deliberately deceived Americans about the link between soft drinks, obesity, and diabetes—a practice that contributed to the devastating disease epidemic in minority communities. The pastors told the *Washington Post* that they filed their lawsuit because they were sick and tired of attending funerals for their parishioners whose junk-food diets gave them heart disease, diabetes, and strokes. One of the men, Delman Coates, the pastor at Mount Ennon Baptist Church in Maryland, told the *Post* that it was not uncommon for members of his church to give their babies bottles filled with sugary drinks.[4]

"It's become really clear to me that we're losing more people to the sweets than to the streets," he said. "There's a great deal of misinformation in our communities, and I think that's largely a function of these deceptive marketing campaigns." Pastor Coates pointed out that he was well aware that minority groups had been co-opted as well. "This campaign of deception has also been bestowed on the leadership of our major Latino and black organizations," he told the paper.[5] This is a form of legal racism practiced by the food industry. And it is effective. The communities most affected are completely unaware of this invisible, insidious form of oppression.

BIG FOOD'S MAFIA TACTICS: CORPORATE CO-OPTING AND MANIPULATION

While establishing links to minority groups is particularly insidious, the food industry uses corporate sponsorships and financial gifts to buy loyalty from a wide range of prominent organizations. In a report by the Center for Science in the Public Interest, called *Selfish Giving: How the Soda Industry Uses Philanthropy to Sweeten Its Profits*,[6] these nefarious tactics are extensively documented. Here's their strategy:

- Link their brands to health and wellness rather than illness and obesity
- Create partnerships with respected health and minority groups to win allies, silence potential critics, and influence public health policy decisions
- Garner public trust and goodwill to increase brand awareness and brand loyalty
- Court growing minority populations to increase sales and profits

This strategy of investing in "corporate social responsibility" can generate support, as we saw with the NAACP and the Hispanic Federation, and it can buy silence from groups that might otherwise criticize junk-food companies for their most shameful behaviors.

The seduction of soda money has created chilling conflicts for many influential organizations. We already saw in Chapter 4 how Big Food fights back against soda taxes; their tactics also include corrupting health groups. Save the Children, an international nonprofit that has long fought for children's rights, was once an outspoken proponent of soda taxes. The nonprofit group threw its endorsement behind soda tax campaigns in New Mexico, Philadelphia, Washington State, Mississippi, and Washington, DC. But in 2010, to the surprise of many in the public health world, Save the Children suddenly withdrew its support for soda taxes. It was perhaps no coincidence that around the same time the organization accepted a $5 million grant from Pepsi.[7] The following year it received $50,000 from Coke.

Sadly, Save the Children was not alone. When Mayor Michael Nutter of Philadelphia proposed a soda tax in 2010, the soda industry offered to make a hefty donation to the city if it would agree to abandon the measure. Eager to receive a windfall, the city council voted down the tax, and the American Beverage Association followed through with a $10 million donation—some might call it a bribe—to the Children's Hospital of Philadelphia for an obesity program.[8] Fortunately, years later, the tax passed on both diet and regular sugar-sweetened beverages. The reason the soda companies so aggressively opposed it is because taxes work. In Philadelphia after the tax, the rate of daily consumption of regular soda was 40 percent lower, energy drinks 64 percent lower, and bottled water 58 percent higher, and the thirty-day regular soda consumption frequency was 38 percent lower.[9] In a follow-up study of the 1.5 cents-per-ounce tax there was a 51 percent reduction in sugar-sweetened-beverage consumption, or 1.3 billion ounces less, over two years.[10] However, the American Beverage Association has spent millions fighting back against this tax, trying to get it repealed, and has even taken the city to court. The judge ruled in favor of the city, upholding the tax, and the revenue from the soda tax went to creating 4,000 pre-K slots and twelve new community schools and to rebuilding crumbling parks and libraries.[11]

These tactics are used across the country. In 2012, the Chicago City Council proposed a soda tax to help reduce the city's growing obesity rates—and you'll never guess what happened next. Coca-Cola donated $3 million to launch fitness programs in Chicago community centers—and the soda tax that had been proposed magically disappeared.[12] In the 2016 election, four cities in California had a soda tax on the ballot measure. The food industry spent $38 million in a campaign to defeat the measures. Former New York mayor Michael Bloomberg and the Arnold Foundation spent $20 million to pass it. It passed. But there are not that many billionaires who are willing to engage in heroic measures to defeat Big Food.

Thirty-three countries have enacted soda taxes, and seven cities in the United States. Studies show taxes work. If the United States passed a national penny-per-ounce tax it would save $25.6 billion in health care costs and produce $12.5 billion in revenue for community-based programs or programs to address obesity.[13] The beverage industry has not taken this lightly and is fighting back. Taking a page from the tobacco industry's playbook, they have launched a stealth strategy of preempting taxes. When tobacco was under the gun it launched a campaign to create state laws that would prohibit cities or municipalities from creating their own taxes. In effect, the state laws could preempt any city from passing a law restricting tobacco use, for example, in public places. It worked for tobacco.

The beverage industry launched two ballots to preempt taxes in the 2018 election. The one in Oregon was called "Yes on Measure 103, Keep Our Groceries Tax Free," supported by the Parents Education Association PAC (an industry front group). The American Beverage Association (Coca-Cola, PepsiCo, etc.) spent $7.63 million and public health groups spent $6.95 million, funded mostly by Michael Bloomberg. The measure did not pass. However, in Washington State, "Initiative 1634, Prohibit Local Taxes on Grocery Measure" did pass. Why?

The beverage industry spent $20.7 million to pass the preemptive measure, preventing any future soda taxes, while opposition groups were able to spend only $100,000.

In the face of a growing soda tax movement, the soda industry is making states an "offer they can't refuse." In California, the most liberal state in the country, where four out of the seven cities with soda taxes are, Big Food played dirty. They spent $7 million pushing a ballot measure that has nothing to do with soda taxes. It would force local governments to require a two-thirds majority to pass any local taxes. This would have effectively paralyzed local governments and limited their ability to fund public services such as schools, fire and police departments, and public libraries. In five days, before anyone knew what was happening, behind closed doors, the beverage industry told Governor Jerry Brown (formerly known as Governor Moonbeam for his liberal views) that if he signed a law prohibiting soda taxes for 12 years, they would withdraw the ballot measure that would cripple local governments.[14] He buckled and signed it. They have done the same in Arizona, Michigan, and Washington.[15]

INFILTRATING PROFESSIONAL MEDICAL AND NUTRITION ASSOCIATIONS

It is painful to see so many nonprofit groups and lawmakers neglect their principles and fall under the spell of soda industry money. But what is most vexing is how Big Food has commandeered some of the most influential health and nutrition groups in the world. It is one thing to see a politician make policy changes that favor his or her corporate donors. It is another thing to see a vaunted public health organization do the bidding of Big Food.

If we can't count on our leading health and nutrition professionals to do what is right for public health, then whom can we rely on? Public health groups are in many ways the last line of defense. We look to them for guidance and impartial advice. We count on their expertise. We expect them to do what is in the best interests of child, family, and societal health. And yet the evidence shows that many of these groups have far too often allowed themselves to end up in bed with Big Food. Take a look:

- **American Diabetes Association (ADA).** With diabetes maiming and killing millions of Americans every year, you would think that the ADA would take a hard stance against companies that peddle diabetes-inducing junk foods. And yet over the years the ADA has signed a number of major deals with more than a dozen companies, including General Mills, Coke, and Campbell's.[16] In one instance, the group signed a $1 million deal with Kraft Foods that allowed the company to slap the ADA logo on products like Snack-Well's cookies, Post Raisin Bran cereal, Cream of Wheat, and sugar-free Jell-O. The diabetes group signed another megasponsorship deal with Cadbury Schweppes, the world's largest candy maker, worth $1.5 million. In exchange, Cadbury was allowed to use the ADA logo on products that are terrible for diabetics, like Mott's applesauce, Snapple, and Diet Rite soda. Yes, diet drinks have been linked to obesity and type 2 diabetes through their effects on appetite, hormones,[17] and the gut microbiome.[18]

  I once gave a talk at the ADA. As I walked through the exhibit hall, I saw a big booth with the banner "Cure for Diabetes." It was a promotion for gastric bypass surgery. Yet the exhibit hall was a sea of processed food, junk food, and artificially sweetened products— things I would never let my diabetic patients near, ever.

- **American Academy of Pediatrics (AAP).** When it needed funding to create a website to promote children's health, the AAP turned to a company whose products have played a starring role in the childhood obesity epidemic: Coca-Cola. Between 2009 and 2015 the sugary-drink giant gave the academy roughly $3 million. The academy praised Coke for being a "gold" sponsor of its Healthy-Children.org website, calling it a "distinguished" company for its commitment to "better the health of children worldwide." For a while parents and pediatricians who logged onto the academy's website were treated to a picture of the Coke logo—a major coup for the world's largest soft drink manufacturer.[19]

- **American College of Cardiology and the American Academy of Family Physicians (AAFP).** Both have received millions of dollars in junk-food funding. The president of the American College of Cardiology carried the Olympic torch to help promote its CardioSmart initiative, which was funded by Coca-Cola.[20] In 2010 Coca-Cola spent $102 million to support charities, which sounds generous. But at the same time, it spent $2 billion marketing sugary drinks. The good news is that many leading family doctors resigned from the academy in protest over the AAFP getting into bed with Coca-Cola.

- **American Heart Association (AHA).** In 2017, the AHA received $182 million in industry funding from PepsiCo, Kraft, Monsanto, Cargill, Unilever, Mars, Kellogg's, Domino's, Subway, General Mills, and Nestlé, to mention a few.[21] And they are in charge of protecting our hearts? Trade groups and authors of guidelines that promote the use of more bean and seed oils, like soybean or canola oil, are consultants and receive funds from and sit on the boards of these groups or companies such as the Canola Council of Canada or Unilever. That is why the AHA came out hard against coconut oil despite the lack of evidence that saturated fat causes heart disease. One large review of seventy-two studies on 600,000 people in nineteen countries including randomized trials and observational studies found no basis for our current government recommendations to reduce saturated fat intake.[22] More than seventeen reviews of all the data on saturated fat and heart disease found no link.[23]

It is totally incongruous and offensive. Like a magic trick—look at the right hand doing something good, while the left hand does something destructive.

NUTRITION ASSOCIATIONS OR PUPPETS OF THE FOOD INDUSTRY?

Our most revered and respected nutrition societies are often in bed with Big Food. A prime example of the problems this can cause for both consumers and the public health community is the actions and policies of the Academy of Nutrition and Dietetics, also known as AND, the largest organization of registered dietitians in the world. Founded in 1917, the academy is considered one of the nation's preeminent nutrition groups, with more than 100,000 registered dietitians who work in hospitals, schools, universities, the food industry, and private practice. Its stated purpose is "empowering members to be the nation's food and nutrition leaders." It describes its mission as "optimizing the nation's health through food and nutrition."

The academy has annual revenues exceeding $34 million, much of it from membership fees and sponsorships. But 40 percent of its funding comes from the food industry.

Public health expert Michele Simon published an exhaustive and disturbing exposé on the academy entitled *And Now a Word from Our Sponsors: Are America's Nutrition Professionals in the Pocket of Big Food?* She found that in recent years AND underwent a radical transformation. In 2001 it had just ten food industry sponsors. But by 2011 that number had risen to thirty-eight. Among its most generous sponsors was a cast of characters that included some familiar names: PepsiCo, Mars, Kellogg's, General Mills, Conagra, Unilever, the National Dairy Council, and Coca-Cola.[24]

So what are the perks that companies get in exchange for their generous academy sponsorships? Mostly it is a way for them to buy access to nutrition professionals so they can indoctrinate them on how to get people to purchase their products. As Simon explains in her report:

For example, partners can co-sponsor "all Academy Premier Events," conduct a 90-minute educational presentation at AND's annual meeting, and host either a culinary demo or media briefing also at the annual meeting. Partner status also confers this benefit: "The right to co-create, co-brand an Academy-themed informational consumer campaign." Examples include the Coca-Cola "Heart Truth Campaign," which involves fashion shows of women wearing red dresses (also promoted by the federal government). Another instance of partner/sponsor co-branding is the National Dairy Council's "3-Every-Day of Dairy Campaign," which is a marketing vehicle for the dairy industry disguised as a nutrition program. The partnership consists of several fact sheets that bear the AND logo, demonstrating the value of the group's seal of approval. The National Dairy Council does not disclose that they paid for the right to use the AND logo.[25]

The thing is that AND's and the government's recommendations represent at best questionable science.[26] Turns out skim milk can cause weight gain, and milk can cause osteoporosis, cancer, allergies, digestive problems, and autoimmune disease. Oops.

Another practice the academy has engaged in is allowing food corporations to *teach* dietitians. The academy oversees the credentialing process for registered dietitians and requires them to obtain continuing education credits. The list of accredited continuing education providers includes industry outfits like the Coca-Cola Beverage Institute for Health and Wellness, Kraft Foods Global, PepsiCo Nutrition, Nestlé Healthcare Nutrition, and the General Mills Bell Institute of Health and Nutrition. The "education" sessions they provide to dietitians teach them, for example, that obesity is all about calories; that artificial sweeteners are safe for small children; and that health concerns about sugar are an "urban myth" and "a misconception."[27] All of it is unscientific nonsense and food industry propaganda that is passed off as fact.

The companies are also granted prime real estate at the academy's annual food and nutrition trade show. At one recent expo, the Sugar Association sponsored a booth where its representatives handed out flyers stating that mothers could placate kids who are picky eaters by sprinkling sugar on their vegetables. In her report, Michele Simon found that at one of these annual expos, many of the largest booths were occupied by processed-food companies. Among the largest expo vendors were:

Organization	Booth Fee
Nestlé	$47,200
Abbott Nutrition	$47,200
PepsiCo	$38,000
Unilever	$28,800
General Mills	$21,900
Cargill	$19,600
Kraft Foods	$19,600
Campbell Soup	$15,800
Coca-Cola	$15,800
Conagra	$15,800

These industry partnerships and financial arrangements hurt the academy's credibility and ultimately influence its policies. In 2015, the academy granted Kraft Foods permission to slap its "Kids Eat Right" logo on the company's infamous "Kraft Singles"—a product that is so ultraprocessed that Kraft by law cannot even call it cheese because it doesn't contain more than 50 percent cheese.[28] What's the rest of it? Instead, the label for Kraft Singles describes it as a "pasteurized prepared cheese product." Getting the academy to provide its seal of approval was a major coup for Kraft, which boasted to news outlets that the arrangement marked the first time the academy had ever endorsed a product. Health advocates across the country were understandably in disbelief. After a fierce public backlash, Kraft and the academy decided to terminate their deal to slap the logo on the product.[29]

"I am really shocked that this would be the first thing that the academy would choose to endorse," Casey Hinds, a mother of two who runs the blog USHealthyKids.org, told the *New York Times*. "It's confusing and just one more way that feels like as parents, there are so many forces working against us as we're trying to raise healthy kids."[30] The academy's behavior even drew the attention of comedian Jon Stewart, who lambasted the organization on *The Daily Show* for selling out to a food company that "wants the positive PR of going healthy but doesn't want the hassle of actually improving their product."

"Here's how you know Kraft has not changed their ingredients: Kraft is still not legally allowed to call their product cheese," Stewart scoffed. "It turns out the Academy of Nutrition and Dietetics is an academy in the same way that Kraft Singles is cheese."

Over the years AND and the soda industry became so entwined that it was hard to tell them apart. Coke and the American Beverage Association recruited some of the academy's most high-profile dietitians to act essentially as their public relations machine. The company paid them to:

- Promote mini-cans of Coca-Cola as a healthy snack.
- Write articles disputing the notion that sugary drinks play a role in the obesity epidemic.[31]
- Criticize soda taxes on social media. They paid more than $2.1 million to "independent nutritionists" to oppose soda taxes on social media.[32]

In 2017, the soda industry nearly took over the academy altogether, staging what many health advocates considered an attempted coup. That year, the academy held an election to select its next president. Two prominent dietitians ran for the position. But one of the two candidates, Neva Cochran, left some critical details out of her official bio that was circulated to voters: She failed to disclose that she had spent 27 years working as a consultant for Coke, McDonald's, Monsanto, the Corn Refiners of America, the Calorie Control Council (which promotes artificial sweeteners), and the American Beverage Association. She was also one of the registered dietitians whom the soda industry had paid to write social media posts opposing soda taxes and promoting beverage industry products. "Plain water isn't that appealing," she wrote in one social media post. In another, she encouraged parents to give their "active teens" soft drinks, lemonade, sweet tea, and chocolate milk and accompanied her recommendation with a vintage advertisement of a young cheerleader with the caption "Jenny needs a sugarless energyless soft drink like a Beatle needs a hairpiece. Two-four-six-eight, what does she appreciate? Sugar."

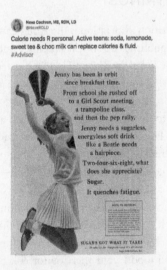

As Kyle Pfister, the founder of Ninjas for Health, a public health advocacy group, explained it: "Never before has an Academy's presidential candidate been so compromised by corporate conflicts of interest."[33] Cochran could have very easily won the election and been installed as the academy's new president, had it not been for Pfister and several courageous dietitians, who called attention to Cochran's deep industry ties. They sounded the alarm on social media, igniting a firestorm of criticism and embarrassing the academy leadership. Many dietitians who were already uncomfortable with the academy's cozy relationship with Big Food said that allowing an industry consultant to head the organization was simply beyond the pale. Cochran's opponent, Mary Russell, ultimately won the election, and a crisis was narrowly averted. As one nutritionist and academy member explained it, the election outcome showed that dietitians "want change and professional integrity, not more food-industry insiders."[34]

AMERICAN SOCIETY FOR NUTRITION: WHO PULLS THE STRINGS?

The other main nutrition association is the American Society for Nutrition (ASN), which publishes the world's premier nutrition journal, *The American Journal of Clinical Nutrition*. This "respected" society actively opposed sugar taxes. Could it be that its donors and sponsors include Coca-Cola, PepsiCo, Kellogg's, McDonald's, and Monsanto? Could that have anything to do with why they published a "scientific" article entitled "Processed Foods: Contribution to Nutrition" that concludes, "There are no differences between the processing of foods at home or at a factory."[35] Yes, cooking at home is processing—bake, broil, sauté. But is it the same as a processed Pop-Tart with forty-seven ingredients, most of which you would never have in your home? Sauerkraut is a processed food, but it's quite different from a Twinkie. Maybe the ASN didn't see the research that found that for every 10 percent of your diet that is ultraprocessed foods, your increase for risk of death goes up 14 percent. They also launched a Smart Choices Program to place their seal of approval on "healthy food," like Froot Loops. When questioned about this endorsement, their response was, "Well, Froot Loops are better than doughnuts." (Fortunately, the program didn't last; it shut down in 2010.) Is that really the advice we expect from the country's leading nutrition society? They have a long and sullied history of being in bed with the food industry, compromising science, and placing the welfare of their sponsors above public health.[36]

ASTROTURFING, FRONT GROUPS, AND OTHER TOOLS OF INDUSTRY DECEPTION

Not only does the food industry infiltrate and influence existing groups; they also create "grassroots" groups that are largely, or even entirely, funded by them to manipulate public opinion. One of the most insidious ways that Big Food controls public opinion is through benevolently named front groups, like the Alliance for Safe and Affordable Food, funded by the GMA and Monsanto, that pretend to promote the interests of citizens and the science. They fight GMO labeling and attack organic food. Another is the Center for Food Integrity, also funded by Monsanto, as well as the National Restaurant Association and the United Soybean Board. All of these organizations discredit organic food production, defend pesticides and antibiotics in animal production, and promote the benefits of artificial sweeteners, trans fats, and GMO foods. Some of the worst groups funded by Big Food, Big Ag, and Big Pharma are documented in a report by Friends of the Earth entitled *Spinning Food: How Food Industry Front Groups and Covert Communications Are Shaping the Story of Food.*

These groups have spent hundreds of millions of dollars to manipulate public opinion, discredit legitimate science, and influence policy makers. In just four years, from 2009 to 2013, four of the biggest trade groups spent more than $600 million to promote the benefits of pesticide use, GMOs, and the interests of Big Food. Fourteen front groups spent $126 million using stealth tactics to corrupt the truth. They attack journalists and scientists, pay "independent sources" like the *SciMoms* blog on evidence-based parenting, create propaganda disguised as editorial content, and employ covert social media tactics.

There are many of these groups. The American Council on Science and Health (ACSH) has one of the most striking names of any industry front group. The first time I heard their name I had to look them up to see if they were a legitimate public health agency. But make no mistake: The ACSH is a mouthpiece for some of the world's largest corporations.

Over the years the ACSH has received millions in funding from the likes of Big Food, Big Pharma, Big Oil, Big Tobacco, and other industries. According to the Center for Media and Democracy, their donor list has included names like Monsanto, McDonald's, Pfizer, Coke, Pepsi, ExxonMobil, and Dr Pepper Snapple.[37]

The ACSH portrays itself as an important defender of science. But it has proclaimed that smoking, pesticides, and sugar are not harmful. It routinely attacks people who raise concerns about drug side effects and toxic chemicals in food. It dismisses the benefits of organic produce and dietary supplements. And it defends things like GMO crops, high-fructose corn syrup, e-cigarettes, and artificial colors and sweeteners.

In 2015 a group from the ACSH wrote a letter requesting that Columbia University remove Dr. Mehmet Oz from the faculty after his show raised questions about GMOs. Dr. Gilbert Ross, one of the signatories on the letter, is the acting president and executive director of the ACSH. He is also an ex-convict who was sentenced to forty-six months in prison for defrauding Medicaid of $8 million and at one time had his medical license revoked for professional misconduct.[38]

There are literally dozens of similar groups. The innocuous or deceptive-sounding names mask their true intentions. Their aggressive tactics, and half-truths are an attempt to dupe the public. While food industry corporations create and pay for these front groups, they try to conceal that information to protect the public images of their funders. They do the dirty work of the food industry so that food companies can keep their hands clean. Don't be deceived by their pro-paganda. When you're tempted to believe the latest campaign ads or sensational headline, look at the tactics they use. A front group or astro-turfing efforts could be behind it.

FOOD FIX: ETHICAL SPONSORSHIP OF PROFESSIONAL SOCIETIES AND ASSOCIATIONS

Professional medical and nutrition associations like the ADA, the AHA, the ASN, and the AND should never accept money from junk-food companies. The practice is completely unacceptable. Dr. Ioannidis from Stanford University wrote an important review of corruption in these professional associations and recommended that they abstain from authorship of guidelines and disease definition statements.[39] In other words, they should not be in the business of giving "objective" advice or recommendations. Professional health organizations must face the reality that Big Food has a long history of lobbying against public health, influencing public policy to the detriment of society, and manipulating scientific research.

But much like researchers, health organizations cannot be expected to sever all ties with the food industry. Plenty of food companies have missions that align with professional health organizations. You don't have to look too far to see that in many cities a growing number of restaurant chains, grocery stores, health start-ups, and other food establishments are providing healthy, sustainable, and delicious options to consumers. Relatively new and popular farm-to-table food chains like Sweetgreen, Tender Greens, and Dig Inn are competing with McDonald's and Burger King. There are plant-based chains like Veggie Grill, Freshii, and Salad and Go (the drive-through salad chain). And stores like Whole Foods and Thrive Market make it easy to find wild, organic, and sustainable foods. Professional health organizations should be looking to promote, commend, and form partnerships with these food companies—not the ones that make all their profits from junk food.

To objectively determine what food companies are ethical to work with, there needs to be a set of guidelines that will help sort out worthy food companies from junk-food peddlers. In 2013, a group of registered dietitians who were frustrated with the AND and its ties to Big Food formed a splinter group called Dietitians for Professional Integrity.

They have been speaking out against Big Food's infiltration of the academy and demanding change. To a large extent, they've been successful: The academy has severed ties with Coca-Cola and reduced the amount of funding it takes from junk-food companies. The splinter group has also devised a set of guidelines to help ensure ethical and responsible industry sponsorships. The recommendations are so simple and sensible that there's no reason all professional health organizations shouldn't abide by them. Companies that sell alcohol, soft drinks, and confectionery are automatically disqualified from consideration, but beyond that, the guidelines work in part through a scoring system. Companies are awarded points based on how they do on the following criteria, with zero points awarded if they perform badly and 1 to 2 points awarded if their performance is good or excellent.[40]

- The extent to which they market their products to children
- Whether their products contain artificial colors and sweeteners
- How they rank on animal welfare and the use of hormones
- Their use of fair-trade ingredients
- Their organic production practices
- Whether they use trans fats
- Whether their meat and dairy products are grass-fed, organic, or conventionally raised
- Their fishing and aquaculture practices
- LEED Certification (a green building rating system)

Companies are scored in all applicable categories. In the event that a larger company owns a prospective sponsor, the parent company should be scored as well—which is important because most smaller good-for-you brands are owned by about nine Big Food companies. A company that attains a final average score of 1.5 or higher is considered an ethical and responsible sponsor.[41]

FOOD FIX: ETHICAL POLICIES IN MEDICINE

One of the reasons major conflicts of interest are so rife in the public health world is that many universities and medical centers do not have rigorous conflict-of-interest policies, nor do they impress upon future doctors and health professionals the importance of navigating potential conflicts. This is such a critical issue that the prestigious Pew Charitable Trusts convened an expert task force and published a report on conflicts-of-interest policies for academic medical centers.[42] If you work in a university or medical center, take these recommendations to your leadership team:

- Faculty members, staff, students, residents, trainees, and fellows should not accept any gifts or meals from industry.
- Faculty should be required to disclose to their institutions any industry relationships.
- Faculty should not accept industry funding for speaking engagements.
- Continuing medical education courses should not be supported by an industry.
- Faculty, students, and trainees should not attend promotional or educational events that are paid for by an industry.
- Pharmaceutical sales representatives should not be allowed access to any faculty, students, or trainees in academic medical centers or affiliated entities.
- Conflict-of-interest education should be required for all medical students, residents, clinical fellows, and teaching faculty.

It is a bit harder to ferret out the truth from fiction when professional associations, public health groups, and top scientists are co-opted by Big Food, Big Ag, and Big Pharma. Be a healthy skeptic. Get your information from independent nonprofits and public advocacy groups such as the Union of Concerned Scientists, the Environmental Working Group, and the Sustainable Food Trust, as well as academic institutions. Remember to follow the money and ask yourself when something fishy appears in the marketplace or media: Does it pass the sniff test? Is Froot Loops really a "Smart Choice" as our esteemed nutrition experts advise?

For a quick reference guide on the Food Fixes and resources to expose food industry partnerships and a deeper dive into front groups, go to www.foodfixbook.com.

PART IV

FOOD AND SOCIETY: THE DESTRUCTION OF OUR HUMAN AND INTELLECTUAL CAPITAL

"Structural violence is one way of describing social arrangements that put individuals and populations in harm's way," says Paul Farmer of Partners in Health. "The arrangements are structural because they are embedded in the political and economic organization of our social world; they are violent because they cause injury to people...neither culture nor pure individual will is at fault; rather, historically given (and often economically driven) processes and forces conspire to constrain individual agency. Structural violence is visited upon all those whose social status denies them access to the fruits of scientific and social progress."

The food industry is part of the story of structural violence that hurts minorities, the poor, and the food insecure. Those who consume our industrial diet suffer from cognitive and behavioral problems, violence, suicide, homicide, and more chronic disease and premature death and mental health problems. Many of these issues are related to lack of adequate real nutrition and an excess of ultraprocessed foods. Our children struggle with ADHD, learning challenges, and poor academic performance, due in large part to their ultraprocessed diets. Even our military has trouble finding healthy recruits. The food system also harms the very workers who farm and harvest our food. It's an injustice that we can no longer ignore.

Let's take a deeper look at the role food injustice plays in our current crises of obesity and chronic disease, our poor national academic performance, the perpetuation of poverty, the challenges facing food workers and farmworkers, violence, mental health, behavioral problems, and even national security. These are not separate problems.

CHAPTER 12

THE HIDDEN OPPRESSION OF BIG FOOD: SOCIAL INJUSTICE, POVERTY, AND RACISM

A few years ago, I had the opportunity to go on a whitewater rafting trip in Utah led by Waterkeeper Alliance, a nonprofit dedicated to protecting our waterways. The trip was designed to bring awareness to the tar sands mining of the Tavaputs Plateau at the headwaters of the Colorado River. Tar sands mining for fossil fuels will pollute the waterways critical for local and native populations and the long-term health of the Colorado River. On the trip was a Hopi chief and his wife. They were both severely obese and diabetic. While rafting, they mostly drank Coca-Cola. The chief got sick from his diabetes on the walk down to the river, vomiting and becoming weak. After a few days floating down the Green River on a raft together, I suggested to him that he could reverse his diabetes if he wanted. He asked what he had to do. I said he needed to eliminate refined carbs, starches, and sugars. He paused for a minute and said that it would be very difficult to do this, because it would be impossible to do the traditional Hopi ceremonies without their traditional ceremonial foods.

"What foods?" I asked.

He replied, "Cake, cookies, and pies."

How did this man come to believe that his traditional ceremonial foods were processed flour and sugar and refined oils? The story of the chief's answer is the story of sickness, poverty, social disenfranchisement, loss of food sovereignty, and internalized racism. It's what Paul

Farmer calls *structural violence*—the social, economic, political, and cultural factors that determine disease.

The chief's ancestors had no obesity, type 2 diabetes, or alcoholism. Now 80 percent of his people get diabetes by the age of thirty and life expectancy is fifty-three.[1] So, what happened? First, the Hopi were moved to reservations. Second, the water resources they depended on for drinking water and to grow their own traditional foods were usurped by the damming and diverting of the Colorado River to supply California and desert cities such as Phoenix. This pattern was repeated throughout Native American communities. Nearly 60 million bison were slaughtered by the US government to cut off the food supply of tribes on the plains. Buffalo Bill Cody once said, "Kill every buffalo you can! Every buffalo dead is an Indian gone."[2]

Unable to continue their traditional food systems, the Hopi received government-supplied commodities—white flour, white sugar, and shortening. They created new foods like "Indian fry bread." There is nothing Native American about deep-fried flour, sugar, and shortening. Their Hopi genetics were adapted to scarcity and a high-fiber, plant-rich diet. This is often referred to as the thrifty gene (or genes) because throughout history they were more threatened with starvation than with abundance and thus became efficient at storing excess calories. Flooding their bodies with starch and sugar made them obese and diabetic. The tribes have a word for the type of obesity caused by these highly refined processed commodities provided by the government to "help" their people. They call it "commod-bod."

This story is repeated over and over where our beliefs, attitudes, and policies perpetuate structural violence. This is a form of internalized racism. It is not as obvious as limiting voters' rights and employment opportunities, the bombing of churches, or hate speech and hate crimes. But it is far more pernicious and destructive, in part because most of the victims have not identified it as a problem to be fixed.

Of all deaths, 1.1 percent are caused by gun violence.[3] Seventy thousand people die every year from the opioid epidemic. Those problems are real and tragic and need to end. But 70 percent of deaths, or more than 1.7 million deaths, a year are caused by chronic disease such as heart disease, diabetes, cancer, high blood pressure, and stroke[4]—mostly the result of our toxic food system. More African Americans, Hispanics, and poor people are killed by bad food than anything else. Drive-through fast food kills far more people than drive-by shootings. Yet we remain silent about the role of the food system killing millions of Americans.

RETHINKING THE CAUSES OF DISEASE AND SOCIAL INEQUITIES: SOCIAL, POLITICAL, AND ECONOMIC CAUSES

It is clear what we are doing is not working. More and more people are chronically ill, as costs and suffering escalate dramatically. I first began to think deeply about this issue in 2010 when I had the opportunity to be one of the first doctors on the ground in Haiti after the earthquake. In Haiti, I met Paul Farmer, who cofounded Partners in Health. Partners in Health has created a powerful and successful model for treating drug-resistant tuberculosis and AIDS in the most impoverished nations in the world. Most public health officials had abandoned these nations and diseases as too tough to address.

The brilliance of Paul Farmer's vision wasn't coming up with a new drug regimen or building big medical centers, but a very simple idea: The missing ingredient in curing these patients was not a new drug, but addressing the structural violence that perpetuates disease.[5]

Recruiting and training more than 11,000 community health workers across the world, Farmer proved that the sickest, poorest patients with the most difficult to treat diseases in the world could be successfully treated. The community was the treatment. It was about providing clean water, access to food, and support from community members. The model is called "accompaniment," because the idea is that neighbors accompany one another to health.

I realized that this model was important not just for infectious disease, but for chronic "lifestyle" diseases as well. What determines your lifestyle? The community in which you live, your access to healthy food, the safety of your environment, your education, your family and your friends, and your level of income and employment.[6]

In Chapter 2, we discussed how "noncommunicable" diseases are mostly driven by our community and lifestyle. Only 10 percent of our health is determined by direct medical care. More than 60 percent is related to the social determinants of health. Your zip code is a bigger determinant of your health outcomes than your genetic code. But in health care we focus on the wrong end of the problem. Even though it is clear that the social determinants of health drive most disease, we continue to focus on the molecular pathways of disease, drug targets, and surgical innovation. We are promoting gastric bypass as the cure for diabetes even though it fails 25 to 50 percent of the time, because people go back to the same environment and culture without the health system addressing the real cause of their obesity or diabetes.[7]

Shifting our perspective from "blame the victim" to "change the system" is essential for addressing the social injustice that drives our chronic disease epidemic, obesity, poverty, food insecurity, and our toxic nutritional landscape, where making good choices is nearly impossible for many. Food is a social justice issue. Our industrial food system is an invisible form of oppression.

FOOD APARTHEID: POVERTY, DISEASE, AND FOOD INJUSTICE

A 2016 *JAMA* landmark study compared the difference in life expectancy between the richest and poorest 1 percent of the population. The difference between those two groups was 15 years for men and 10 years for women. That is equivalent to the loss of life expectancy that results from a lifetime of smoking.[8] More than 38 million Americans live in poverty and almost 100 million live in near poverty.[9]

Life on the other end of the spectrum is also shortened. The United States has the worst infant mortality rates of the top twelve richest industrialized countries.[10] But infant mortality among African Americans is two and a half times that among whites.[11]

Is there a reason that the highest rates of obesity, diabetes, and chronic disease are found in the African American, Hispanic, Native American, and poor communities? In the last decade, type 2 diabetes rates have tripled in Native American children, doubled in African American children, and increased 50 percent in Hispanic youth.[12] Native Americans, Native Hawaiians, Pacific Islanders, and Asians are also twice as likely as whites to get diabetes. If you are African American you are more than four times as likely to have kidney failure and three and a half times as likely to suffer amputations as whites.[13] Why are these numbers so staggering for our poorest citizens? Is this just bad luck, bad genetic cards, or something else?

Hundreds of thousands of African Americans, Hispanics, and the poor are killed every year by an invisible form of racism, a silent and insidious injustice. This is an often-internalized force of oppression that disproportionately affects the poor, African American, Hispanic, and Native American communities.

When we talk of racism we think of white supremacists, police brutality, job discrimination, limited opportunities, and hate speech, but rarely do we think of food as bigger than all those forms of racism. You've probably heard of food deserts—where the only food available is processed junk from convenience stores and fast-food outlets, the closest grocery store is more than a mile away, and it's hard to find fresh fruits and vegetables or other healthy food. How can we take care of our communities when 23 million Americans live in these food deserts? But the problem isn't only food deserts. It is food swamps— communities filled with fast-food chains and bodegas plying highly processed addictive foods. Food deserts imply a natural phenomenon, like an unfortunate desert somehow just occurred. Nothing is less true. It's hard to find fresh produce but easy to find gallon cups of soda and other sugar-loaded beverages, and fast-food chains peddling burgers, fries, and fried chicken are on almost every street corner. These toxic food swamps are more predictive of obesity and illness than food deserts.[14]

I remember when my friend Chris Kennedy brought his nonprofit, Top Box Foods, to the South Side of Chicago. Top Box buys real whole foods wholesale from distributors and brings them into makeshift markets in church parking lots in areas of food apartheid, so that the poor can buy a week's worth of real food for a family of four for $35. The local African American community came out in big numbers. Standing in the parking lot, I surveyed the landscape around me. As far as I could see was a sea of fast-food outlets. No real food in sight. The poverty, the limits on access to transportation, and the maze of fast-food restaurants and convenience stores that these communities live among all perpetuate disease, disability, and suffering.

In the 40 years since obesity and diabetes have exploded in America, the fast-food market has grown twenty times, that is, 2,000 percent. One in four Americans visits a fast-food restaurant every day. And Americans spend more money on fast food than on movies, books, magazines, newspapers, videos, and music *combined*.[15]

Black communities have almost twice as many fast-food restaurants as white neighborhoods.[16] The USDA found that only 5 percent of African Americans have a healthy diet.[17] That is a big change from the 1960s, when African American diets were twice as healthy as average diets, with more fruits, vegetables, fiber, and good fats.[18]

We talk of food deserts and food swamps, but perhaps a better term is "food apartheid," an embedded social and political form of discrimination that recognizes that these areas of food disparity are not a natural phenomenon like deserts. This term is increasingly used by affected communities to describe the lack of access to real food and the overabundance of disease-producing food-like substances. The history of sugar is closely linked to slavery. The slave trade served the growth of sugar production. Legal American slavery is over (although forms of slavery still occur on some farms with migrant workers). But today sugar, especially in its new form, high-fructose corn syrup, is connected to a new kind of oppression — food oppression, which makes people of color sick, fat, and disabled.[19] It is a form of apartheid in which the poor and minorities live in areas that lack healthy food and have an over-abundance of fast-food outlets and convenience stores.

STEALING LAND, SLAVERY, AND BROKEN PROMISES

Our country has a history of racism in agriculture and land ownership. We displaced Native Americans through Manifest Destiny and stole their lands. Our farming system and our nation's early prosperity were built in large part on the backs of slaves. After the Civil War, former slaves were promised forty acres and a mule by President Lincoln to start a self-sufficient life, but his promise was revoked by President Andrew Johnson, so former slaves were never allowed to establish a foothold in the economy and self-determination. If freed slaves had actually been given that land, today it would be worth $6.4 trillion.

Not surprisingly, at the turn of the twentieth century, blacks owned 14 percent of farms. This was a threat to whites, who stole black land via raids on black farmers, lynching, and murders. Now there are few black farmers, and fewer who own their land. And many African Americans have forgotten that their ancestors were brought to the United States (as slaves) to bring their agricultural wisdom and crops to the New World. Now many in the African American community equate farming with slavery.

As of 2017, less than 2 percent of farmers are black and less than 2 percent are Native American, according to the USDA Census of Agriculture.

The spread of fast-food and convenience stores in poor, urban, and minority neighborhoods—food swamps—has created a virtual food apartheid, an institutionalized form of segregation and racism embedded in the actions of corporations, business, and our government's policies.

The targeted marketing of the worst food to the poor and people of color compounds the problem. And children are the biggest targets.

Not only are they more susceptible to manipulation, but they also represent long-term investments for Big Food. Hooked young, they stay hooked.

Our health, our children, and many of our communities have been taken from us. It is time we take them back. It is time we address the institutionalized food injustice that is causing this slow-motion genocide. It is important to transition from a business model where corporate interests privatize the profits but socialize the costs of their products and the harmful consequences of their products are not taken into account. If these costs are not accounted for, we the taxpayers and our environment all pay the price. Historically corporations defined "value" as increasing shareholder profits, but times are changing. During a recent Business Roundtable, a group of the world's leading corporations, 181 CEOs agreed to redefine the purpose of a corporation to benefit not just shareholders but stakeholders including customers, employees, suppliers, and communities.[20] Omitted was any mention of the environment as a shareholder, but it is a step in the right direction, although transparency and accountability are essential to measure the impact of their intent.

FOOD INSECURITY

Even when food is available to disadvantaged communities, fresh whole foods can be expensive, which leads to the purchase of cheap, unhealthy junk food. Hawk Newsome, an African American community leader, shared his experience growing up in the Bronx, poor, hungry, and struggling. Hawk shared that many are food insecure in his community and struggle to get enough food on limited incomes. When the decision is between facing hunger and eating cheap processed food, the choice is inevitable.

Newsome grew up in a poor community where the only consideration about food was to feed the family as cheaply as possible to get them to the next paycheck. "You have to look at it from a perspective of people who are living in these conditions," Newsome says. "You have $20, and it's one or two days before payday. With a family of four,

McDonald's has a dollar menu that means you could get about eight burgers and four orders of fries for $12. It makes sense economically."

He explained, "My mother carried the family. She was extraordinary in her strength. But we always consumed unhealthy amounts of bad food. It was to the point that before my dad died, I would bring them healthy food and they would look at it like, 'I'm not eating that. Why would I eat that?' Not only is healthy food not available, but also the majority of us look at it like it's disgusting. My family is extremely intelligent. I went to law school. My sister went to one of the best universities in the country. We have a high IQ, but our food IQ is very low."

Food insecurity can also have incredibly detrimental effects on pregnant mothers. A colleague at work grew up in East Cleveland, a place with no job opportunities and even less real food. They don't even have a McDonald's. They have Rally's, a fast-food chain that makes McDonald's look like a gourmet restaurant. You can get two burgers for $3. Who knows if it is even meat? Through hard work she pulled herself out of her environment, something most women in that neighborhood can never do. She had a role model, her mother, who was a police officer. She recounted the story of one young woman of fifteen who begged my colleague to help the young woman find a way to get out of that neighborhood. The girl knew she would end up like her mother, on welfare, with multiple children, living in the projects with no way out. Yet getting pregnant made her eligible for $20-a-month subsidized housing in the projects, food stamps, health care, and social services. It was her only way to survive. How is this a just society?

Data shows that preterm labor and infant mortality decrease if we provide housing and food to pregnant mothers, and this reduces overall health care costs.[21] The same goes for the homeless. Provide housing and food, and health care costs plummet.[22] Pay now or pay more later. But the perverse financial systems in health care and social programs don't encourage us to do the right thing—the thing that will reduce costs, save lives, and protect our citizens.

The Food and Research Action Center produced a white paper in 2017 called *The Impact of Poverty, Food Insecurity, and Poor Nutrition on*

Health and Well-Being.[23] The consequences of our current food system for malnourished mothers are staggering. When children are born to malnourished mothers and grow up on a diet of artificially cheap sugar and processed and fast foods, they are stunted, developmentally delayed, and cognitively impaired, they suffer from learning disabilities, and they have behavioral and emotional challenges and increased rates of violence, obesity, and chronic diseases. The "food" they eat as children doesn't change when they grow older, and the malnutrition continues, perpetuating mental health issues and increased rates of obesity, type 2 diabetes, heart disease, depression, disability, and premature death, with a loss of an average of 10 to 15 years of life.

Living in poverty drives food insecurity, overconsumption of cheap processed foods, higher rates of obesity and diabetes, and a whole host of other chronic diet-related diseases. The risk of diabetes for any ethnic group is twice as high (100 percent increase) for those with less than an eighth-grade education. If you are food insecure, you are also twice as likely to be diabetic.[24] Diabetes rates are lowest in whites, at 8 percent; they are 16 percent among blacks and 22 percent among Hispanics, and much worse in the poor of all ethnicities. Education is also a huge determinant of health status, regardless of income.

It is both the overconsumption of bad food and the underconsumption of real food that drive this problem. Not surprisingly, the research shows that those who are the most food insecure use more health care services and have the highest health care costs. The cost of food insecurity is estimated to be $160 billion a year, not including the $70 billion a year in SNAP (food stamp) assistance.[25]

FOOD PUSHERS: HOW BIG FOOD SELECTIVELY TARGETS THE POOR AND MINORITIES WITH JUNK FOOD

Of course, the food industry welcomes those suffering from food insecurity with open arms, aggressively advertising unhealthy foods to them.

One day I was working in an urgent care center as a medical resident and a Hispanic woman came in for back pain with her seven-month-old baby in tow. The baby was sucking a bottle of brown liquid.

"What is that?" I asked.

"Coke," she replied, as if it were the most normal thing in the world. I asked her why she would give her baby Coke, and she said, "Because he likes it."

In Chapter 8, you read about Big Food's marketing ploys to reach children. That trend is amplified even more for minority children. In 2019, the Rudd Center for Food Policy and Obesity published a damning report entitled *Increasing Disparities in Advertising Unhealthy Food to Hispanic and Black Youth*.[26] The big food companies target black and Hispanic youth with their least nutritious products, including fast food, candy, sugary drinks, and snacks. From 2013 to 2017, food advertising on black-targeted TV increased by 50 percent. Black teens viewed 119 percent more junk-food-related ads—mostly for soda and candy—than white teens. The top ads came from Nestlé, Yum! Brands (like KFC and Taco Bell), Mars, McDonald's, and General Mills. The average teen saw more than 6,000 junk-food ads a year just on television. Even if you talk to your kid about healthy eating three times a day, there is no way to compete.

Food companies use cultural icons to influence minorities. Do you think LeBron James actually drinks much Sprite? McDonald's uses Serena and Venus Williams and Enrique Iglesias in their TV ads to attract black and Hispanic consumers. Is a Big Mac, fries, and a Coke really Serena's prematch meal? No matter, their dollars are well spent. Race-based advertising works.[27]

Our government is complicit in the perpetuation of these behaviors and the support of the production and sale of the very foods it tells Americans not to eat in its Dietary Guidelines. What may shock some is that government-guaranteed loan programs support fast-food outlets, which are far more prevalent in poor communities of color.[28] Why should government loans pay for the expansion of food that kills Americans?

CORPORATE SOCIAL RESPONSIBILITY OR
CORPORATE SOCIAL EXPLOITATION

In Part 3, we dug deep into the ways that the food and agriculture industries manipulate public opinion, co-opt public advocacy and public health groups, corrupt science, use illegal tactics to influence policy, and overwhelm the political process with billions in lobbying dollars. And we learned how these companies exploit and target the poor and minorities through "corporate social responsibility" in order to buy friends and influence opinions. That helps explain why the groups that are most affected by soda and processed foods from a health and social justice perspective are Big Food's best friends. The food industry employs nefarious tactics to squash opposition and prevent change to the status quo. They buy friends, silence critics, and sweeten their profits.

I was part of a documentary called *Fed Up*—a movie about how our food system makes us sick and fat with addictive sugary, starchy products. While on the road promoting the movie I met with Bernice King, Martin Luther King Jr.'s daughter, and she explained to me that nonviolence also includes nonviolence to ourselves. She was excited about showing *Fed Up* at the King Center in Atlanta. But a few days later I got a call to tell me that we couldn't show the film.

"Why?" I asked. The answer: Coca-Cola funds the King Center. Coca-Cola is busy co-opting other advocacy programs or groups throughout Atlanta. During the 2019 Super Bowl, Coca-Cola gave a $1 million donation to another group, the National Center for Civil and Human Rights, in Atlanta to provide free admission to visitors. How nice!

The dean of Spelman College in Atlanta told me that 50 percent of the entering class of African American women had a chronic disease— type 2 diabetes, hypertension, obesity. I asked her why there were Coke machines and soda fountains all over campus. Coca-Cola is one of the biggest donors to the college. In fact, Helen Smith, the vice president of global community affairs and president of the Coca-Cola Foundation, is on the board of trustees of Spelman College.

FOOD FIX: FOOD JUSTICE, FOOD SOVEREIGNTY, AND EMPOWERMENT

Often the people living in these circumstances are not aware they are victims of food oppression, food apartheid, and internalized food racism. The work of transforming this system of oppression must come from multiple sectors—changes in government policies at the local, state, and federal levels, regulation, litigation, health care reimbursement for food as medicine, nonprofits creating local programs to educate and empower people, and grassroots efforts of citizens working to change their communities and regain food sovereignty. In Atlanta, the Ebenezer Baptist Church—Martin Luther King Jr.'s church—started a 2-acre urban garden where parishioners participate in growing food for the local community. There are hundreds if not thousands of these stories of hope and empowerment.

One of the leaders in bringing health, food, and community to ravaged neighborhoods is Ron Finley, the Gangsta Gardener from South Central Los Angeles, a place of gangs, drugs, violence, and desperate poverty. He grew up in a food prison where he had to drive forty-five minutes to buy a tomato. Through a simple act, turning the dirt by the curb in front of his house into a garden, he started a small "horticultural revolution." The dirt by the curb was owned by the city, and he was cited for gardening without a permit. Finley persisted but ended up with a warrant out for his arrest for growing 12-foot sunflowers by the curb. He fought back, got the local laws changed, and started curbside gardens, turned lawns into food forests, and created raised-bed gardens in dilapidated vacant lots, helping gang members, ex-convicts, and drug dealers find a way out of their struggles. Finley wants to transform the food desert into a food forest and is leading a movement to bring the education and skills needed to the youth in his community and beyond.

These pockets of redemption and innovation are happening all across the country; they are models for breaking the cycle of food injustice. Here are just a few examples that we need to nurture and support.

- In West Oakland, California, a very poor neighborhood of 30,000 with no grocery store but fifty-four liquor and convenience stores, community members started the **People's Grocery**, a mobile grocery store (much like an ice cream truck), to bring produce to the local community. They expanded into urban farming and leased a 2-acre parcel of land near the city to farm, staffed by community members. And they started community cooking classes. They provide grocery bags full of fresh produce to people in their community.

- In the Bronx, Karen Washington founded **Black Urban Growers** to support black urban and rural farmers and help cultivate black leaders in the movement for food justice and sovereignty. Washington has helped turn abandoned lots in the Bronx into thriving community gardens, started farmers' markets, and engaged her community, bringing awareness to the intersection of food, poverty, racism, lack of health care, and unemployment.

- **Food Tank** is a remarkable organization whose mission is "building a global community for safe, healthy, nourished eaters." They showcase organizations in the food movement working for food justice[29] and for a better food system throughout the world.

- **Soul Fire Farm** was started in 2011 by Leah Penniman in Petersburg, New York, focused on ending racism, injustice, and food apartheid in the food system by raising life-giving food and providing training for troubled youth and activist farmers in sustainable agriculture. Understanding that one in ten people of color is hungry, that the top five killers of Latinos and blacks are diet related, and that these communities have been dispossessed of the land, Penniman focuses on the fact that our food system is rooted in racism and slavery. She has built a model to address food injustice.

Penniman and Soul Fire Farm highlight the power of farming to lift up poor communities, shifting their perspective and bringing pride back into farming for the African American community. Through the farm's community-supported agriculture program, Soul Fire Farm provides food to neighborhoods suffering from food apartheid and free food to refugees and families affected by incarceration. She even lobbied to allow SNAP benefits to be used for community-supported agriculture, which made it into the 2018 Farm Bill.

Faith and Food Justice

Increasingly African American pastors see the link between the plight of their congregations and food apartheid. They are helping their congregations link food and theology and improving their congregations' lives through food.

Methodist pastor Christopher Carter, who's also an assistant professor of theology and religious studies at the University of San Diego, focuses his work on helping link the health of humans, the treatment of animals, and the destruction of the environment to the food we eat and how it all connects to racial equity and Christian theology. He invites his congregants to ask: How was this food raised? Were the animals treated humanely? Were the farmworkers subject to harsh working conditions, underpaid, or abused? What is the impact of industrial food on the health of individuals and communities? He believes this is central to shifting deeply held notions that allow African American communities to be oppressed by the food they consume. He seeks to do what he describes as an effort to "decolonialize the plate" and reclaim old traditions. A friend was ridiculed by his family for eating "white people's food," not realizing that the current diet of most African Americans is actually white people's food. Carter's new book, *The Spirit of Soul Food*, seeks to redefine soul food.

Reverend Dr. Heber Brown III, the senior pastor of Pleasant Hope Baptist Church in Baltimore, Maryland, founded the **Black Church Food Security Network**. He recognized that in most food deserts (or areas of food apartheid) there was an abundance of churches, and he created a movement, not from farm to table but from "soil to sanctuary." His network empowers black churches to grow their own food and partner black farmers and urban growers to bring fresh produce to churches. They create pop-up farm stands at churches, start gardens on church-owned land, and lead lectures and small group meetings that focus on food justice and food sovereignty.

Imagine if black church leaders (or any affected minority group) collectively joined in a campaign to link the struggles of minority communities to food, to food apartheid, to racial targeting by the food industry, to the invisible form of oppression that keeps communities down, a form of racism that is internalized and insidious, that disables and kills more people of color than anything else, and created a call to action to change all that. Black lives matter. But black health matters too. What if African American churches boycotted soda or junk food, echoing Martin Luther King Jr.'s Montgomery bus boycott in the 1950s challenging segregation on buses? There is untapped power that could shift culture, shift the physical and economic health of communities of color across the country.

Art, Social Justice, and Food

Understanding the link between social justice, food, and disease, the University of California San Francisco Center for Vulnerable Populations and Youth Speaks (a youth development and arts education program) partnered to create the **Bigger Picture**, a public health campaign using spoken-word poetry and hip-hop music videos to call out the connection between the social injustice of stress, poverty, and violence and food insecurity, lack of access to whole foods, and a plethora of ultraprocessed and fast food in their communities.[30] The value teens place on social justice, their anger at manipulation by the food industry, and their witness to the death and destruction in their families and communities empowered them to create art that inspires awareness, agency, and change. It takes the blame away from individual choices and places it on the structural systemic problems that drive disease, disability, and poverty.

In his piece for the Bigger Picture, "Empty Plate," Anthony Orosco, age twenty, addresses the legacy of poverty of those who pick and pack the produce that we buy at Whole Foods but don't make enough money to buy the very food they pick. In her piece "The Longest Mile," Tassiana Willis, age twenty-four, a severely obese African American woman, highlights the toxic food environment that drives disease.

Whether through church leaders, activist farmworkers or farmers, or artists calling out social injustice, a growing awareness of food injustice attempts to correct the systemic conditions that fuel it. These are just a few examples of the movements happening across the country and the world, directed by local leaders and community organizers to reclaim the food system. It is a long road, with many obstacles, but we can drive change slowly from the margins. This is how all movements start. The abolitionists weren't deterred that it might take 100 years to pass civil rights legislation or 150 years to have an African American president.

Many other systemic problems perpetuate the food system's crisis of injustice; we need bigger, policy-wide reform. (Many of these ideas are also discussed in Part 3.) These reforms are very difficult to employ given our current political environment and campaign finance laws that make corporations able to contribute literally billions of dollars to influence policy and elections. The First Amendment protects speech, including apparently the right of corporations to target children and minorities with advertising. The most important reforms would be those akin to what we implemented for smoking and which have been effectively implemented in other countries such as Chile (see Chapter 3).

In fact, all the food fixes throughout this book are required to create a more equitable and just food system that serves individuals and communities, reforms agricultural systems, and protects our environment and climate.

For a quick reference guide on the Food Fixes and resources on combating structural violence and social injustice, go to www.foodfixbook.com.

CHAPTER 13

FOOD AND MENTAL HEALTH, BEHAVIOR, AND VIOLENCE

In 2009 I wrote *The UltraMind Solution*, linking diet, nutritional deficiencies, and lifestyle to mental illness, memory, and attention issues. These ideas were not widely understood at the time. Since then, mounting scientific evidence has made the clear link between diet, mood, behavior, and violence. As I treated my patients for a multitude of physical conditions, I saw changes in their diet that resolved their behavioral, mood, memory, or attention problems. One twelve-year-old boy, a patient of mine with severe ADHD, completely reversed his attention and behavioral problems after he got off processed and junk foods, ate a real-food diet, and added supplements to fix his deficiencies of omega-3 fats, magnesium, zinc, and B

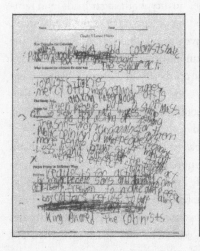
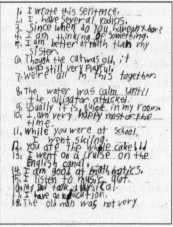

vitamins. Look at his handwriting before (previous page, left) and after two months (right) of improved nutrition and supplementation. What are the implications for all our brains if we can treat the root of the problem?

HOW FOOD CHANGES MENTAL HEALTH AND BEHAVIOR

Studies show that adults with many types of mental health issues and children with ADHD have very low levels of antioxidants (which come from fruits and vegetables),[1] such as the fifty-six-year-old man with lifelong crippling depression who improved by cleaning up his diet and taking a cocktail of B vitamins.[2] I remember one man who presented with severe panic attacks every afternoon. Turned out he was eating a diet very high in sugar and starch and had wild swings in his blood sugar, which triggered the anxiety. When he cut out sugar and starch, his anxiety and panic attacks vanished. These stories are not anomalies. They are predictable results from applying nutritional medicine.

In recent years, major medical journals have clearly shown the link between nutrition and mental health. *The Lancet Psychiatry*, a top medical journal, maps out just how nutritional medicine is a key to mental health and psychiatry.[3] Overall diet quality, high sugar loads, and rampant nutritional deficiencies (including omega-3 fats, zinc, magnesium, vitamin D, and B vitamins) all drive mental illness. In other words, the culprit is once again the American and increasingly global industrial diet. We have discussed the costs of obesity and chronic disease, but most don't connect mental illness to the costs of chronic disease. In fact, the cost of mental illness to the economic burden is far greater than the costs of heart disease, diabetes, and cancer.

Mental health issues may not lead to the same death rates as diabetes or heart disease, but they lead to more years of disability and lost productivity. For example, years of life lost to disability and loss of productivity from mental illness are more than eight times those of heart disease, in part because it affects younger people.[4] Population studies have found that more fruits and vegetables and less french fries, fast food, and sugar are associated with a lower prevalence of mental illness, and that junk food creates moderate to severe psychological distress.[5] The good news is that interventional studies have shown that treatment of mental illness with diet works well (especially since most medications for mental illness don't work that well, despite being the second-biggest category of drugs sold).[6]

EDUCATIONAL INEQUITIES: THE ACHIEVEMENT GAP

The disturbing news is that mental health issues are starting earlier and earlier. Is it any surprise knowing the state of nutrition in most schools? It's not uncommon to hear Americans lament our low global standing in academic performance. We are thirty-first in math, reading, and science in the world. To put that in perspective, Vietnam is twenty-first.[7] One in six children has a neurodevelopmental disorder. More than one in ten children have ADHD.[8] Depression, learning disabilities, and behavioral problems are rampant in schools. School nurses have to contend with boxes of prescription medications they have to dole out to kids during the school day. Academic performance is the worst in poor neighborhoods, but also declining in more affluent areas. Brain development is the worst in the poorest kids (who also have the worst diets), with brain sizes 10 percent lower and IQs an average of 7 points lower than developmental norms.[9] Why are so many children not graduating from high school? Why are kids in the most disadvantaged neighborhoods more likely to go to jail than college? There are many reasons for this, including social determinants such as poverty, crime, parenting, culture, and failure of government policies, but one of the biggest factors impacting cognitive development and behavior is nutrition.

To paraphrase President Clinton: It's the food, stupid.

This phenomenon of poor school performance in kids who face health issues, who consume poor diets, who are obese and often diabetic, is called the achievement gap.[10] A 2014 review of the science by the CDC entitled *Health and Academic Achievement*[11] documents the clear link between poor nutrition and academic performance, including lower test scores, lower grades, poor cognitive function with less alertness, attention, memory, processing of visual information, and problem solving, and increased absenteeism. Lack of fresh fruits and vegetables and vitamin and mineral deficiencies lead to the same problems. How can you expect kids to learn and function when they are hungry, skip breakfast, or go to school with a bottle of soda and a bag of chips? The result is that kids are inattentive, disruptive, late, or absent.[12] Food is driving many of these problems.[13]

The average kid in America consumes 34 teaspoons of sugar a day.[14] The cognitive and behavioral effects of sugar in children are well documented.[15] Kids literally bounce off the walls. Ever been to a birthday party where chaos ensues in the aftermath of a sugar binge? We are literally destroying the intellectual capital of our youth, with broad consequences for our whole society: less productive citizens who are more likely to earn less, suffer more, get sick early in life, and be incarcerated. We are raising the first generation of Americans who will live sicker and die younger than their parents.

Not only that, but special education costs are skyrocketing across the country. In San Diego, the cost for special education is $1 billion of a $5 billion overall school budget, an increase of 32 percent over five years.[16] The number of kids needing special education has grown 19 percent since 2012, while overall school enrollment has grown by 2 percent. There are multiple causes for this, but the majority of cognitive dysfunction in kids can be linked to poor nutrition. Iron deficiency is common, leading to lower dopamine function and impaired concentration.[17] Vitamin and mineral deficiencies including B vitamins, iodine, zinc, and vitamin E are linked to diminished cognitive abilities and poor concentration.[18]

CRIME AND NOURISHMENT: COULD OUR DIET BE THE CAUSE OF OUR OVERFLOWING PRISONS, BULLYING, AND CONFLICT?

The food we eat modulates all our biology, including our brain function. Food affects our hormones, brain chemistry, nutrient status, and other chemical and biological functions. What we eat affects our thinking, mood, and behavior. Food has also been linked to changes in behavior and violence. Consider the following research:

- Junk food makes kids act violently—bullying, fighting—and suffer more psychiatric distress, including worry, depression, confusion, insomnia, anxiety, aggression, and feelings of worthlessness.[19]
- In the article "Impact of Nutrition on Social Decision Making," scientists fed two groups different breakfasts.[20] One group got a high-carb breakfast, the other a high-protein, low-carb breakfast. The high-carb group was more likely to engage in "social punishment" behavior such as negative comments and actions toward others in structured behavioral experiments. Now consider that most Americans eat dessert for breakfast, full of sugar and carbs—cereal, muffins, bagels, sugared coffees, pancakes, French toast, oatmeal. This does not make for a very nice society.
- Those who consume high levels of refined oils (currently more than 10 percent of our diet and found in all ultraprocessed foods) and low levels of omega-3 fats from fish have higher rates of depression, suicide, and homicide.[21] Our consumption of these refined oils (mostly soybean oil) went up 248 percent from 1970 to 2010.[22]

Think about this: We incarcerate African Americans at five times the rate of white Americans. Thirty-seven percent of inmates are black, but black people make up only 12 percent of the population. That is the result of multiple complex factors. But it could be that a significant portion of violent crime is also the result of a diet that robs people of their minds and affects their thinking, judgment, and ability to make good choices. In fact, the communities with the highest rates of food insecurity and the worst food apartheid also have the highest rates of incarceration. Seems likely there is a relationship there. In fact, robust studies support this conclusion.

One day I walked into my office and found a handwritten letter from a violent criminal still in prison. He said he read one of my books, changed his diet, and realized that his whole life of violence was driven by his diet. Changing his diet in prison transformed him. Studies have shown similar results.

In one double-blind randomized controlled trial, researchers found a 37 percent reduction in violent crime in those taking omega-3 fats and vitamin and mineral supplements.[23] The author of the study said, "Having a bad diet is now a better predictor of future violence than past violent behavior.... Likewise, a diagnosis of psychopathy, generally perceived as being a better predictor than a criminal past, is still miles behind what you can predict just from looking at what a person eats."

One study of violent juveniles found that children given a vitamin and mineral supplement reduced violent acts by 91 percent compared to a control group.[24] These kids were deficient in iron, magnesium, B_{12}, folate—all needed for proper brain function. Researchers wired these kids up to EEG machines to look at their brain waves and found a major decrease in abnormal brain function after just thirteen weeks of supplementation. They also advised kids to improve their diets. The ones who didn't showed no reduction in violent behavior. The kids who improved their diets showed an 80 percent reduction in violent crime.

Another experimental study of 3,000 incarcerated youth replaced snack foods with healthier options and dramatically reduced refined and sugary foods. Over the twelve-month follow-up there was a 21 percent reduction in antisocial behavior, a 25 percent reduction in assaults, and a 75 percent reduction in the use of restraints. There was also a 100 percent reduction in suicides. This is stunning. As the world struggles to deal with the exploding rates of teenage suicide—suicide is the third leading cause of death in children ages ten to nineteen, and rates of suicide increased 33 percent between 1999 and 2014[25]—a simple diet change could be the key to a dramatic improvement.[26]

Another study showed the same thing. Violent behavior for incarcerated juveniles dropped by 47 percent with supplements.[27] They had lower rates of antisocial behavior in nine types of recorded infractions:

threats/fighting, vandalism, being disrespectful, disorderly conduct, defiance, obscenities, refusal to work or serve, endangering others, and nonspecified offenses. Depression, suicide, ADHD, and violent behavior are all linked to food.[28] The poor communities who live in food swamps and consume the most processed food and the fewest nutrients are often the ones who suffer from mental illness and violence and higher rates of incarceration.[29]

This is true not just in adolescent prison populations but also among adults. A rigorous randomized controlled trial of nutritional supplements in 231 adult prisoners found a 37 percent reduction in violent offenses. A Dutch study of 221 prisoners found a 47 percent reduction in violent crime with nutritional supplementation, and when drug offenders were removed from the analysis there was a 61 percent reduction in violent crime, comparable to a California study of 402 adult inmates.[30]

Clearly crime and antisocial behavior arise from a complex set of social, economic, and environmental factors. But what if a big part of the solution to our increasing social strife, exploding rates of depression, mental illness, ADHD, bullying, violence, and crime, and overflowing criminal justice system is fixing our food system? Maybe part of the solution is fixing the epidemic of broken brains by fixing the nutrition of those most at risk (and ideally all of us).[31]

Unfit to Fight: Food and the Threat to National Security

In a time of increasing global political instability, America is unable to find enough healthy recruits for military service. More than 70 percent of recruits are rejected as unfit to fight. In 2018, a group of retired admirals and generals from the organization Mission: Readiness published a report entitled *Unhealthy and Unprepared*.[32] Today the military cannot meet its recruitment goals. Plenty of people try to enlist, but most get rejected. Not only are recruits overweight and sick, but also active-duty soldiers are

73 percent more likely to be overweight than in 2011. Overweight soldiers are 33 percent more likely to suffer from musculoskeletal injuries. In fact, there were 72 percent more medical evacuations from Iraq and Afghanistan for injuries related to obesity and poor fitness than for combat wounds.

When one in four teenage boys is pre-diabetic or diabetic, solving the problem of military readiness, something that's critical for national security, is extremely complex and requires fixing the food system.

For active-duty overweight soldiers, the Department of Defense can transform food procurement. It can focus on food for performance enhancement, health, and fitness. This is essential to create and maintain a healthy military and save billions in taxpayer money required to address the high cost of taking care of overweight soldiers and veterans.

Our future as a nation, and as a global community, depends on preserving and enhancing the intellectual capital of our citizens. We are literally raising a new generation of children who are less able to learn, succeed, and contribute to society. We are threatening our global economic competitiveness. What is the cost of the loss of social, human, and economic capital because of poor diet and malnutrition? Isn't that alone worth addressing the failures of our food system?

FOOD FIX: HEAL MENTAL ILLNESS WITH NUTRITION

While not all mental illness is caused by food, poor nutrition can worsen mental health conditions. Solving this problem is complex and requires addressing poverty, inequities, trauma, violence, and more. But a few things can help integrate this into society and science.

First, if you suffer from a mental health issue, get help from a functional medicine or integrative practitioner to help you address the dietary needs that will improve the health of your brain. The eating guidelines in Chapter 2 will be a key component. You can also refer to my book *The UltraMind Solution* or my online documentary series *Broken Brain* (www.brokenbrain.com) for a detailed plan on how to fix your brain.

Second, the NIH should fund research to look deeply at the link between food and mental illness, especially clinical trials that help prove cause and effect. The focus can be on depression, anxiety, ADHD, autism, and bipolar disease. A lot of research already exists on nutritional psychiatry, but more is needed in order to provide more evidence for practitioners on how to treat the root causes of mental illness, not just the symptoms.[33]

We need reimbursement reform in health care to start paying for a food-as-medicine approach and programs to treat mental illness.

Health care systems should integrate a food-as-medicine approach to treat mental illness.

Medical education must be reformed so doctors can apply nutritional psychiatry with their patients.

FOOD FIX: GOOD SCHOOL NUTRITION MAKES KIDS SMARTER AND MORE WELL BEHAVED

We've already talked about the importance of a healthy school lunch in Chapter 8, so it's no secret that giving healthier food to children works, improving overall health and academic performance[34] and leading to healthier adults. Innovators and parents around the country are trying to create new ways to feed hungry kids in schools. In the poorest part of Washington, DC, a local philanthropist started a charter school and provided three meals a day of healthy whole foods to children. These children lived in extreme poverty, with food insecurity and unsafe environments. Children from this neighborhood rarely went to college and few graduated high school. They were destined to repeat the vicious cycle of poverty and disease from which they came. Yet simply feeding these children real food and providing a safe and supportive environment changed the trajectory of these children's lives. Most went to college instead of jail, and to good schools. Affluent families wanted to send their kids to this school because the academic performance on standardized tests was higher. It wasn't the children; it wasn't even poverty; it was access to real food essential for brain development, cognitive function, and emotional health.

The same experiment played out in the Academy for Global Citizenship on the South Side of Chicago, whose student body is mostly poor, minority, or immigrant children. At twenty-three years old, teacher Sarah Elizabeth Ippel started this charter school and figured out how to get the Chicago Public Schools food service program to provide real whole foods to her children at the same cost as the processed foods in most other schools. On the concrete playground were raised-bed gardens. I visited the school and saw the children ravenously eating all the vegetables and whole foods. I asked a seven-year-old Hispanic boy what his favorite food was, and he said broccoli!

Here are more examples of parents, chefs, and community leaders who are chipping away at the horrible school lunch landscape:

Brigaid, started by top chef Daniel Giusti, aims to reform school meals through building real kitchens, creating delicious recipes, and training food workers who are used to microwaves and deep fryers to cook real food from fresh whole ingredients.[35] He started in the Bronx, New York, and Connecticut and continues to expand.

Common Threads is a nonprofit that teaches low-income children and families in schools and the community how to cook real food on a budget as a way to lift themselves up from food scarcity, poverty, and social injustice. They view cooking as the key tool to fix the obesity and chronic disease epidemic. And it's true. We have raised generations of Americans who don't know how to cook.

Conscious Kitchen is a California nonprofit that partners with schools to address food equity, nutrition education, and access by changing school food service, linking local sustainable farm systems to the schools, and cultivating nutrition literacy in the schools. And they include kids in growing and making the food. They created a model for zero-waste kitchens and serve food that is local, organic, seasonal, and non-GMO. Once these conscious kitchens are built, the schools take over. The kids in the program are happier and healthier and have fewer academic and behavioral problems. Conscious Kitchen does this within the federal school lunch budget and nutritional guidelines. For those who say this can't be done, this model proves otherwise.

Big Green is a program started by Kimbal Musk to build school gardens and nutrition education in schools across the country at scale.

These programs need to be expanded and taken up as standard for all public and private school systems and local and federal policy. Real whole food should not be the privilege of a few schools and students. Real whole food that supports children's development and learning must be a right for all children. The legacy of not doing this for all children is a lifetime of struggle with obesity, disease, poverty, impaired cognitive development, and learning and mood disorders.

FOOD FIX: CHANGE THE FOOD IN PRISONS AND REDUCE VIOLENCE

Some aspects of the food system are going to be hard to fix, but prison food and its link to behavior, mood, and violence should be an easy target. The federal government, states, and cities all maintain jails or prisons and engage in food procurement and meal service. They can sign contracts with food service providers that have health in mind and on the menu. They can also mandate that private prisons provide healthy food. Some prisons have already started programs that teach inmates about healthy eating, growing food, preparing food, and other food education. Here are a few examples.

- **Bastøy Prison** in Norway provides monthly stipends for prisoners to buy and cook their own meals, and provides education about sustainable farming.
- **Harvest Now** in Connecticut, a nonprofit active in more than eighty-five prisons, links up underserved food-insecure communities with prisons. They provide prisoners with seeds and the education to farm. Most of the produce is then donated to local food banks, up to 24,000 pounds a year in some counties.
- **Michigan Department of Corrections** stopped buying food from Big Food service vendors and started buying from local farms and improved the nutritional quality of the food for 43,000 prisoners.
- **The Richard J. Donovan Correctional Facility** in San Diego has a Farm and Rehabilitation Meals program to address the link between prison violence and a poor prison diet. The prison buys farmland and hires inmates to grow and harvest the food, which is then fed to the prisoners.

Not only is our food system causing an economic crisis, spreading chronic disease across the globe, but it is also damaging the intellectual capital of our children, driving crime and violence and mental illness, and threatening our national security. These are not all separate problems. They are one big interconnected problem that can only be solved by multiple solutions across the entire food chain, from seed to fork and beyond.

For a quick reference guide on the Food Fixes and resources to help undo the damage of bad food to our mental health and behavior, go to www.foodfixbook.com.

CHAPTER 14

FARMWORKERS AND FOOD WORKERS: THE NEGLECTED VICTIMS OF OUR FOOD SYSTEM

My guess is that most of us don't think of farmworkers and food workers when we eat. Somehow cheap food magically shows up in grocery stores and in restaurants. While we may obsess over what we eat and whether it's healthy, and even think about how our food is grown and whether it's organic or grass-fed, we don't often think about who grows it, cooks it, or serves it. We may not fully grasp the impact of our food choices and the food system on the people who actually grow, pick, transport, and serve our food—the farmers and farmworkers, meat-packers, truckers, restaurant workers, and retailers.

Farmworkers and food workers are the largest sector of workers in America, numbering more than 20 million. Without farmworkers and food workers we wouldn't be able to eat. They rarely make a living wage and are subjected to harsh working and living conditions, including modern forms of slavery, sexual harassment, abuse, lack of health care, and exposure to toxic agricultural chemicals. And most of them are brown or black. Three-quarters of those living below the poverty line[1] and the 50 million food-insecure people in America are mostly black, Latino, or Native American.[2] And people of color suffer dispro-portionately from diet-related diseases, labor abuses, lack of access to resources, and the environmental consequences of our food system.

The issues of our global agricultural system are complex and inter-connected, and they affect everything from our health and our economy to climate change and the much-neglected plight of food workers and farmworkers.

FOOD SERVICE WORKERS AND THE OTHER NRA

More than half of all food workers and farmworkers are in food service. They are among the most exploited and underpaid workers in the country. According to the Labor Department, seven out of the ten lowest-paying jobs are in the food industry, all paying less than $20,000 a year.[3] The very people who grow and serve our food are often not able to feed their own families on the wages they receive. These workers have been left out of the protections afforded most other workers in our economy. In 1935, the National Labor Relations Act passed; a few years later the Fair Labor Standards Act, which established the minimum wage, excluded farmworkers and domestic workers from the most basic workers' rights.

These antiquated labor laws don't provide the protections afforded most other workers. Restaurant and other tipped workers' minimum wage is $2.13 an hour, unless state laws provide higher wages. Fifty-two percent of fast-food workers require food stamps and other government assistance costing taxpayers $153 billion a year.[4] More than 50 percent of workers reported illness or injury on the job, and the majority didn't have health insurance. Instead, they use emergency rooms or urgent care centers, offloading the cost of underpaying workers to the taxpayers. Workers of color make an average of $5,600 a year less than white workers in the food sector. Farmworkers have a sevenfold higher mortality rate than other workers. Pesticide exposure poisons 10,000 to 20,000 farmworkers each year and causes chronic health problems in millions more.[5]

The powerful trade lobby the National Restaurant Association, the other NRA, is one of the most influential lobby groups in the country. It vigorously opposes minimum wages and has been able to keep the minimum wage for food service workers at $2.13 an hour.[6] After the Civil War, the restaurant industry lobbied to hire the freed slaves, pay them nothing, and have them work for tips alone. Workers of color get paid $4 less an hour than white workers, and immigrant workers are subject to exploitation and fear of their employer's control over their visa status. Female workers often have to accept sexual harassment so they can feed their families on tips. Yet it has been estimated that if food workers received a minimum wage of $12 an hour it would increase the average household's food cost just 10 cents a day.

In 2013 One Fair Wage launched a campaign to raise the minimum wage for food workers to $12 an hour; they have had success in eight states and two municipalities and continue to raise awareness and advocate for change. These and other grassroots efforts can help raise awareness and create local change but must be scaled to become national policy. We need to be honest about the true cost of our food. The price we pay at the checkout counter or the restaurant is not the cost of our food or of the effects it has on humans, nature, and our economy.

THREATS AND VIOLENCE

Pay and working conditions aren't the only problems. Often through threats of violence and intimidation, workers are forced to work against their will, perpetuating harsh, unfair, and often illegal working conditions. More than 80 percent of female farmworkers in California's Central Valley have reported sexual abuse or harassment.[7] Much of our produce comes from Mexico and Central American countries, where workers suffer even worse abuses. The average farmworker in Mexico makes just $8 to $12 a day, and farming in Mexico "employs" 300,000 children. They are subject to slavery and violence. After protesting for reporting their employers' illegal wage deductions for food and housing, eighty Mexican farmworkers "disappeared."[8] In Mexico, our biggest source of avocados for our smoothies, guacamole, and avocado toast, many of the farmers are extorted and even murdered by the drug cartels, who sell their "blood avocados" to Americans, who consume 200 million pounds a year.[9] Might want to check where your avocado comes from. Local farmers in Mexico have fought back against the cartels, but it is often not enough.

These stories are pervasive in our food system, affecting the poor and disenfranchised, who are just trying to make a living. Chicken workers are a good (or bad) example. We Americans love our chicken, eating 89 pounds per person per year. The chicken production lines have doubled their speed in the last 30 years, and now workers have to process thirty-five to forty-five chickens a minute. Each worker does the same repetitive task, processing a chicken every two seconds for eight hours with one thirty-minute break. This causes repetitive motion injuries such as carpal tunnel syndrome, and poultry workers suffer five times the illness the average worker does. Chicken workers receive very low wages, $11 an hour. Often these are immigrant workers who live in a climate of fear of being fired, deported, or harassed. Workers are often denied bathroom or stretch breaks, forcing them to wear diapers to work. If you are eating your average chicken (90 percent of which has been processed into prebreaded, prefried, or preseasoned chicken-like substances), just imagine a poor chicken worker peeing into her diaper so you can have cheap chicken.

HEALTH RISKS

Being a farmworker is one of the most dangerous jobs in America. In Chapter 1, I mentioned their higher death rates and exposure to pesticides. The numbers of those who are poisoned are likely even higher if we account for the long-term effects of chronic toxin exposure, including cancer, type 2 diabetes, neurodegenerative diseases, and developmental disorders, among others.[10] Farmers' risk of Parkinson's is 70 percent higher than that of the average population because of pesticide exposure.[11] Vandana Shiva, an environmental activist, doesn't pull punches when it comes to characterizing the harm Big Ag causes—she calls them the "poison cartel." Chemicals known as herbicides and pesticides damage the brain, cause cancer, and disrupt hormones.

Many other countries have banned the chemicals we use in the United States, such as:[12]

- Atrazine, which disrupts hormones, damages the immune system, and is linked to birth defects
- Paraquat, which is linked to Parkinson's disease
- Neonicotinoids, which are linked to the disappearance of honeybees (which are essential for pollination)
- Glyphosate, which we have discussed at length and which is linked to cancer[13]
- 1,3-dichloropropene, which is linked to cancer and is one of the most widely used pesticides in California

These chemicals are also known as *obesogens* and can cause obesity and type 2 diabetes.[14]

The risks of injury and harm from agricultural chemicals are also borne by taxpayers. These workers, often living below the poverty line, have no health care and depend on emergency rooms and Medicaid. The food system disproportionately affects the poor, immigrants, and people of color who actually work in the food system.

The CHAMOCOS study of Hispanic agricultural workers in Salinas, California, found that these workers were 59 percent more likely to get leukemia, 70 percent more likely to get stomach cancer, and 63 percent more likely to get cervical cancer than the average population.[15] They also have about 40 percent more organophosphate pesticides in their urine, including pregnant and breastfeeding women. Babies exposed to these chemicals have lower IQ and cognitive function, behavioral issues, and attention deficit disorder. It is estimated that children younger than age five have lost 41 million IQ points because of exposure to environmental chemicals including pesticides, mercury, and lead.[16] What is the cost of that on future generations' happiness and productivity? *These kids are born prepolluted.* These chemicals are not regulated by the FDA for human safety like medication. They are regulated by the Environmental Protection Agency (EPA), also asleep at the wheel. Approve first, ask questions later (or not at all).

And it is not just farmworkers who are at risk. It's the food workers involved in the production, processing, distribution, and retail sectors of our food system. They are exposed to repetitive stress injury (remember the chicken processors who have to do the same motion thousands of times a day and wear diapers because they are denied bathroom breaks), physical risk, cleaning chemicals, biological hazards (from bacteria), and carcinogenic compounds.[17] Food workers have a 60 percent higher risk of occupational injury and illness than nonfood workers, and their risk of death is nine and a half times higher.[18]

FOOD FIX: THE VICTORY OF TOMATO FARMWORKERS

The story of the tomato farmworkers in Florida is one of tragedy as well as hope, possibility, and the power of grassroots efforts to transform communities and find a path to justice and fair food. Just outside Fort Lauderdale, Florida, in the small town of Immokalee, immigrant farmworkers grow and harvest 80 percent of America's tomatoes. The average backbreaking day of labor would yield the farmworkers $62 if they could pick 4,000 pounds, or 125 buckets, of tomatoes. That leads to an average of less than $10,000 a year with no benefits and few rights. These workers are also subjected to abuse including beatings, sexual harassment, child labor, forced labor, and lack of shade, water, and breaks.

A disparate group of farmworkers from Mexico, Guatemala, and Haiti banded together in 1993 to create the Coalition of Immokalee Workers to fight for better wages and working conditions. Appealing to the growers failed, so they went to the big purchasers of tomatoes like the Yum! Brands, including Taco Bell, Burger King, and KFC, and asked them to pay an extra penny a pound for their tomatoes. At first, they refused, but after the coalition launched campaigns like "Boycott the Bell" in 2004, they agreed, and other big companies followed suit, including McDonald's, Walmart, Whole Foods, Trader Joe's, Chipotle, Subway, and the big food service providers including

Aramark, Sysco, Compass, and Sodexo. (Wendy's and Publix super-market chain refused to participate.) These companies have agreed not to increase the price of tomatoes in stores or restaurants and to sign on to the Fair Food Program (see the "Food Fix" below). This coalition of farmworkers found a creative solution to injustice by creating the Fair Food Program, which mandates that growers provide basic protections for their workers.

"The Coalition of Immokalee Workers created a student/farm-worker alliance. And now their model is being replicated by folks in the dairy industry, and it might get translated soon to folks in the poultry industry," says Navina Khanna, director of HEAL Food Alliance. "They have set up a fair food standards council where they're the ones holding the corporations or the farms accountable and doing third-party verification."

The documentary *Food Chains* exposes the abuses of farmworkers and provides hope with the story of the Immokalee farmworkers. There is still much to be done across other farm systems and products, but this is a start.

FOOD FIX: EMPOWERING FARMERS AND FOOD WORKERS

That American workers should have basic rights would seem to be a given. But for farmworkers and many food workers it is not. Here's how we can change that.

1. Restaurant and food retailers must agree to the Fair Food Program[19] and pressure growers to adhere to its basic tenets for workers' rights:

- No forced labor, child labor, or violence
- At least minimum wage for all employees
- Pay workers for all their work
- No sexual harassment or verbal abuse

- Freedom to report mistreatment or unsafe working conditions without the fear of losing their job—or worse
- Access to shade, clean drinking water, and bathrooms while working
- Time to rest to prevent exhaustion and heat stroke
- Permission to leave the fields when there is lightning, pesticide spraying, or other dangerous conditions
- Transportation to work in safe vehicles

These rights are enforced through worker-to-worker education, audits, transparency, complaint resolution, and market-based enforcement. If restaurants and food retailers want to be part of the Fair Food Program, they must enforce those rights by the growers or stop buying from them.

2. Support Fairtrade products. Fairtrade International is an organization that supports farmers and farmworkers in dozens of poor countries while also working to protect the environment. Part of its mission is to promote fairness and justice in trade. Poor farmers in developing countries are frequently exploited. Fairtrade ensures that any product that carries its certified logo meets strong standards. The organization requires that products be sustainably sourced, that they be made in a way that doesn't pollute the land or waterways, and that farmers and workers receive fair prices. It's comforting to know this when you a buy a Fairtrade certified product. Look for their logo and support the important work they do.

3. Support advocacy groups ensuring safe and fair working conditions. A growing movement, exemplified by the Coalition of Immokalee Workers, is ensuring safe and fair working conditions for our food workers and farmworkers. The two groups most active in organizing and advocating around these issues are the Food Chain Workers Alliance and the HEAL Food Alliance.

The **Food Chain Workers Alliance** represents 370,000 workers in the United States and Canada, from farmers to farmworkers, from processors to packers to those who transport, prepare, serve, and sell food. They work to improve wages and working conditions for their members and to create a more sustainable and affordable food and agricultural system.

The work of the **HEAL Food Alliance** (HEAL stands for health, environment, agriculture, and labor) is focused on creating a platform for real food and bringing together diverse groups, including fifty organizations that represent farmers, farmworkers, and food chain workers, rural and urban communities, scientists, public health advocates, environmentalists, and indigenous groups. HEAL connects the dots across the whole food system and has laid out a ten-point plan for addressing the negative impact of our current food system on health, the economy, and the environment.[20]

"In general," says director Navina Khanna, "what we're trying to do is divest power from the stranglehold of corporations that are setting our policies and dominating the marketplace and that have bad practices around environment, worker health, animal health, and so on. We want them to invest their money into the kinds of systems that are more cooperative, that provide ownership opportunities for workers, that are ecologically sustainable. One of our campaigns is targeting the three biggest food service providers for school cafeterias in college campuses, prisons, and hospitals—that's Aramark, Sodexo, and Compass Group. Collectively, that's bigger than McDonald's. They do a huge amount of purchasing, so we have a set of demands for them around their carbon footprint and that they buy more from producers of color and from sources that treat their workers well. We're trying to move them away from those bad practices and then reinvest that money in local economies."

Their strategy includes providing a living wage for farmworkers and food workers by extending the protections of the National Labor Relations Act and the Fair Labor Standards Act, which haven't been updated since the 1930s. HEAL also recommends making agricultural supports extend to small farmers and independent producers, especially those of color, and supporting young farmers and regenerative agriculture. (More on this in Part 5.) HEAL also advocates for limiting junk-food marketing to children and treating junk-food and beverage companies like tobacco companies (from which they have taken their playbook), including taxes, warning labels, restricted advertising, and age limits for purchasing. The HEAL Food Alliance advocates for coordinating all our food policies and changing them to support the health of our citizens, our economy, and our environment.

While some of their proposals are difficult to imagine being implemented given the current corporate control of the political process, their platform is raising awareness of the problems and inequities that exist throughout the entire food system.

When taken as separate issues, the problems of poverty, racism, chronic disease, corporate manipulation of the poor and minorities, health inequities, violence, crime, suicide, mental illness, declining academic achievement, national security, and farmworker and food worker abuses seem overwhelming. But when filtered through the lens of food injustice and social justice, they are all connected to our modern industrial, ultraprocessed food and agricultural system. Through that lens, the fix seems clearer, but not simple. The actions required for a solution require individual awareness, collective action, business innovation, grassroots efforts, political will, changes in legislation, and regulation of and limits to corporate actions that allow abuses that perpetuate the current system. Defining the problem is the start of hope, of understanding the roots of the challenges that face us as a society and as a global community. The next place we will explore is the beginning of it all: the food we grow and the power of our agricultural system to be the solution to, rather than the reason for, our broken food system.

For a quick reference guide on the Food Fixes and resources to support food workers and farmworkers, go to www.foodfixbook.com.

PART V

THE ENVIRONMENTAL AND CLIMATE IMPACT OF OUR FOOD SYSTEM

Our food system isn't just making the world's population sick; it's making the environment sick. When we eat a hamburger, fries, and a soda, or even a green smoothie, it is hard to imagine the vast web that produced that food, and its potential to heal or harm humans, the environment, the climate, and the economy. We are insulated from the implications of our diet by the anonymity of our food. Where was it grown? How was it grown? What is the health of the soil and the impact of how the food was grown on nutrient levels in the food? Who grew it? What are their working conditions? What resources were used to grow it? What impact does our food have on our soils, our water, the biodiversity and survival of insect, animal, and plant species, the oceans, pollution, climate change, our health, and our long-term economic well-being as individuals and nations?

For many, the link between what we eat and its effect on the planet seems distant. You probably don't think about climate change, agricultural practices, or the potential for the extinction of our species when you chomp down on your dinner. It would be overwhelming. But each of us should know the food web we live in. We can no longer be complacent in the anonymity of our food.

Learning what we have done to create these problems and what we have to do to solve them is essential to our collective future. I wish this were just hyperbole, but sadly it is not. This is not so much about saving the planet as about saving humanity.

CHAPTER 15

WHY AGRICULTURE MATTERS: FOOD AND BEYOND

Since the dawn of agriculture in Mesopotamia 10,000 to 12,000 years ago, we have been growing food, which has allowed the rise of civilization. However, the history of agriculture is littered with our destructive habits born of a lack of knowledge of natural systems, resulting in vast ecological damage. The Roman Empire fell in part because of the demise of its agriculture, the result of destructive practices that depleted the soil.[1] Many other civilizations have suffered the same fate.[2] In *Sapiens: A Brief History of Humankind,* Yuval Noah Harari disabuses us of any notions of an idyllic past when humans lived sustainably on the Earth. In previous eras, however, the scale of our destruction was smaller, and there was more unspoiled territory, which meant new lands to farm.

Most of us don't think much about farming, except that it's fun to go to the farmers' market on a Saturday morning. At the turn of the twentieth century, half of all Americans were farmers; now it's only 1 to 2 percent. But while agriculture may seem like a distant concern best left to farmers, we must all come to terms with the fact that it is the most important aspect of our world today. Not only because we need to eat, but also because we need a planet to live on. Like it or not, we have to dig into the dirt of how we grow our food and its impact so we can find a new way to feed the world without destroying it.

Innovations in agriculture over the last century have allowed us to produce more food than ever, but at a serious cost. The methods we use to grow food are contributing to our future inability to grow food, by increasing greenhouse gas emissions, raising temperatures, and making current cropland unfarmable. As global temperatures rise we may have to grow corn in Siberia, not Iowa. Not to mention the extractive methods of farming, which deplete soil and water and create chemical pollution (from nitrogen fertilizers, pesticides, and herbicides), destroying species including pollinators, rivers, lakes, and oceans. The UN Food and Agriculture Organization report determined that we have only sixty harvests left before we run out of soil.[3] If we don't stop erosion and soil loss, by 2050 we will lose 1.5 million square kilometers of farmland—equivalent to all the farmable land in India.[4] Water scarcity is also a huge issue; at the World Economic Forum, I heard Jim Kim, the former head of the World Bank, say, "The wars of the future will be fought over water, not oil."

The good news is that the science of how to grow food that properly feeds humans, regenerates land, conserves water, and reverses climate change provides a path to fix it all. Whether we take that path remains to be seen given the powerful economic incentives to continue in our current ways—incentives present only because the true costs of farming and food are not paid by those perpetuating the destruction. If we harmed our world, we can heal it. And we must!

AMERICAN FARMERS: MORE THAN THE TOOLS FOR THE GLOBAL AG CARTEL

When we think of farmers, we imagine fiercely independent folk doing the hard work of feeding the population. But in reality, farmers are no longer independent, instead becoming subjects to the global consolidation of corporations at the top of the industrial food chain. Farmers are forced to grow food that harms human health, damages ecosystems, and drives climate change. The makers of seeds and agrochemicals and Big Food companies drive what is grown, how it is grown, whom it is sold to, and at what price, locking most farmers into a vicious cycle of less choice, less profit, and more environmental destruction. The farmers are the heroes, not the villains in this story. They just need a pathway to extract themselves from their current treadmill and retool their land as regenerative farms and ranches.

Recent megamergers have consolidated control of agriculture. Just a very few CEOs control most of our global food system, and their decisions impact every person on the planet:

- Three companies now control 70 percent of agrochemicals.[5]
- Large seed companies have bought up more than 100 seed companies since 1990, and now just four companies (Bayer [which recently purchased Monsanto], ChemChina, BASF, and Corteva) control more than 60 percent of the seeds sold to farmers (see figure below).[6]
- Ninety percent of the global grain trade is controlled by just four multinational corporations.
- Nine big food companies control what is sold and bought in retail outlets, including most health foods and organic brands.[7]
- Seventy-five percent of our food comes from just twelve plants (all controlled by Big Ag and chemical companies) and 60 percent comes just from rice, corn, and wheat.[8]
- Big fertilizer giants (Yara, Mosaic, and Koch Fertilizer) control most of the world's fertilizer market.

THE BIG 4: COMPANIES THAT CONTROL MORE THAN 60 PERCENT OF GLOBAL SEED SALES

These corporations' singular focus is on the economic bottom line. Ignoring the impact on human, social, and natural capital provides short-term profits, but it also threatens our collective survival. Their actions impact everyone along the food chain: producing poor-quality calories for the junk-food industry, driving down food prices, affecting the working conditions of migrant workers and food service workers, and increasing the cost of inputs for farmers for their proprietary seeds (soybean costs had risen 325 percent by 2012), pesticides, herbicides, and fertilizers, threatening the viability of farms across the world.[9]

Current large-scale agribusiness and the policies that support it are slowly harming farmers and the land on which they and we depend. As I write this, much of our 1.1 million acres of farmland is unplantable, the victim of extreme weather, tornadoes, and flooding, and the inability of degraded land to hold enough water.[10] In testimony submitted to the House Committee on Agriculture in May 2019, farmer Mike Peterson of Twin Oak Farms and the Minnesota Farmers Union spoke about farmers' dire financial conditions: "The last five years have been incredibly challenging on my farm and on farms across Minnesota," Peterson said. "Market consolidation and the increase of monopoly power has caused our input costs to rise dramatically. Overproduction has driven commodity prices low—a situation that is further exacerbated by the impacts of ongoing trade disputes. Our current environment is unsustainable."[11]

Rather than the farmers and ranchers calling the shots, a small number of corporate executives control the majority of agriculture and the food system. They hold the power to dictate what is grown, how it is grown, and who profits. "The American food supply chain—from the seeds we plant to the peanut butter in our neighborhood grocery stores—is concentrated in the hands of a few multinational corporations," agricultural economist Austin Frerick points out. "Because the supply, processing, distribution, and retail networks are controlled by only a handful of firms, farmers face higher costs for their inputs and lower prices for their goods. In the 1980s, 37 cents out of every dollar went back to the farmer.[12] Today, farmers take home less than 15 cents on every dollar.[13] This new economic reality forces farmers to survive on volume, creating a system where only the largest farms can make a living."[14]

Ranchers face the same economics. "The nation's meatpacking industry is now more concentrated than when Upton Sinclair wrote *The Jungle* more than a century ago," Frerick says. "Four companies, two of which are foreign-owned, now slaughter 53 percent of all meat consumed in the United States,[15] more than twice the market share that the four largest companies held in 2002."[16]

Farms that produce food in ways that are unsustainable in the long run—requiring large inputs of fossil fuels and water—drive soil erosion, climate change, and loss of biodiversity and are far less resilient than well-managed regenerative, organic, and sustainable farms (which now account for only 1 percent of agriculture).

In 2018 Monsanto's GMO seeds accounted for 90 percent of US corn, 91 percent of cotton, and 94 percent of soybeans grown.[17] It is more now. Monsanto, the company that brought you dioxin, Agent Orange, PCBs (industrial chemicals), and glyphosate (Roundup), recently merged with Bayer, which dropped the name Monsanto to protect the guilty. As of April 2019, Bayer stock lost $34 billion in market value because of successful lawsuits compensating cancer victims exposed to glyphosate. In 2018 and 2019 three large lawsuits against Bayer-Monsanto were successful, with one judgment of $2 billion for cancer victims. There are nearly 14,000 of these lawsuits pending against the makers of the herbicide glyphosate.[18]

The results are easy to see in economic data. The USDA Economic Research Service report *Three Decades of Consolidation in U.S. Agriculture* illustrates that over the past 30 years, the number of farms with less than 1,000 acres has fallen from more than half of American farms to roughly a third. The number of farms with at least 2,000 acres has more than doubled over that same time frame.[19]

HOW FARMS WENT DOWNHILL

How did agriculture get to this point? The short answer is government farm policy, changes in technology, and the unchecked power of corporate agribusiness.[20] The mainstream ideology was well summarized by Earl Butz, President Nixon's secretary of agriculture, in his infamous advice to farmers in the 1970s: Get big or get out. And that's exactly what happened.

Over the past century, as small farms gave way to larger farms, agriculture faced major environmental crises. In the 1930s, the introduction of mechanized farm equipment used without ecological knowledge of soil and erosion combined with eight years of drought created the Dust Bowl—one of the worst environmental crises in our country's history. Dark clouds of wind-blown soil covered the sky and forced thousands to migrate, leaving farmland abandoned. While some environmental programs like soil conservation districts came out of that experience, the dominant trend was to rely more and more on synthetic inputs, such as pesticides and fertilizers, mechanization, and more consolidation to remedy productivity and harvest. Seemed like a good idea at the time, but that was before Rachel Carson's *Silent Spring* sounded the alarm over pesticides like DDT, before deep understanding of the dangers of soil erosion and the value of organic matter in soil, before we faced water shortages, before we ever thought about climate change, before we knew the danger of ultraprocessed food to human health.

It's important to know that consolidation didn't happen for purely profitable reasons. Economic, political, and technological factors started the trend toward large-scale agribusiness. Changing agricultural technology—including machinery, fertilizers, and pesticides—made it possible to produce more food. Who would have thought that was a bad idea at the time?

Compared to 1900, fewer farmers produce more food today. But increasing productivity leads to falling prices.[21] Falling prices mean that farmers have to produce more to make ends meet, creating a self-perpetuating cycle. The result is that the United States produces more cheap grain and meat than ever, despite using substantially less labor and paying farmers less.

It's relatively easy for a small number of people to run a pesticide-drenched and synthetically fertilized crop field or operate a confined animal feeding operation (CAFO). However, the real cost of these operations is not factored into the price. We all pay the true cost of contaminated water, depleted soil, and catastrophic climate change—and those chronic diseases that stem from nutrient-depleted foods.

What corporate consolidation did was accelerate the practice of extractive agriculture—using up our natural resources to get as much profit as we could out of the ground. In other words, abusing the land with intensive mechanical plowing, diesel-powered irrigation, and other petrochemical-based inputs. Artificial nitrogen, pesticides, and herbicides dramatically increased after World War II as bomb factories and biological weapons like nerve gas were retooled into agricultural products. (If a biological weapon could kill an enemy, it could certainly kill a few insects, right?) The motivation was to improve yields and increase production. Yet those grand promises have failed to deliver. Chemical inputs are higher, yields are no better, and costs are higher than those for agricultural systems using regenerative practices, or even conventional agriculture in Europe that prohibits GMO crops and produces higher or equivalent yields with less fertilizer, pesticides, and herbicides.[22] In fact, according to a 1992 agricultural census report, small diversified farms produce twice as much food per acre as large conventional farms.[23] On degraded soils, higher chemical inputs may produce higher yields, but not on healthy soils. What has happened has led us to an agricultural and food crisis. Remember we have only sixty harvests left from our soil if we continue farming as usual. That should alarm you. It certainly shocked me.

Unfortunately, our government policies aren't helping. You read about the issues with subsidies and the latest Farm Bill in Chapter 7 (and will learn how they can be fixed later in this chapter), so it won't surprise you that the political power of the food system owners has greased the wheels of consolidation as well as changed the laws to benefit agribusiness (fertilizer, pesticide, seed, and machinery companies) and hurt independent small farms. The Farm Bill subsidizes monoculture crops like corn, wheat, soy, and CAFO meat, which deplete the land, making it harder and harder to produce crops and meat without chemicals, antibiotics, and genetic engineering. At the same time, these foods that produce disease and obesity are cheap and are in the highest demand.[24] Our government policies are not only promoting disease-causing foods but are also supporting agricultural practices that hurt the climate and the land.

"Despite the rhetoric of 'preserving the family farm,' the vast majority of farmers do not benefit from federal farm subsidy programs and most of the subsidies go to the largest and most financially secure farm operations," the Environmental Working Group reports. "Small commodity farmers qualify for a mere pittance, while producers of fruits and vegetables are almost completely left out of the subsidy game which allows the biggest farms to sign up for subsidized crop insurance and often receive federal disaster payments."[25]

American farmers are the victims, not the perpetrators, of the destruction of the American family farm and rural communities. Trade wars, severe weather driven by climate change, lower prices for farm commodities driven by globalization and farm policy shifts, and the rise of corporate farms have pummeled American farmers. The average farmer loses $1,600 a year (and many a lot more). Bankruptcies and farmer suicides are on the rise. Over 100,000 family farms disappeared between 2011 and 2018. Of the $16 billion President Trump provided in 2019 to compensate for losses from weather and trade policies, most went to corporate farms.

The results of the consolidation over the past century are stunning. We can't let our farm and ranch land continue to suffer. Food is a basic necessity for every human, so we must find a way to get farmers back to owning and running their farms with a holistic approach for our food supply.

THE GREEN REVOLUTION: SUCCESSES AND UNINTENDED CONSEQUENCES

Not too long ago, in the mid-twentieth century, we saw the rise of the promising "Green Revolution." The purpose was to use high-input (fertilizer, pesticides, herbicides), high-yield hybrid crops supported by mechanization, irrigation, and access to global supply chains. The "revolution" promised to boost agricultural yields, because the combination of these practices would allow farmers to increase the amount of food grown on a hectare of land in the hopes of addressing the world hunger crisis. It would be a win for small farmers and for the food insecure. While there are many valid criticisms of the Green Revolution, it made some real accomplishments toward reducing hunger. In fact, it succeeded in many of its goals. It is the unintended consequences of the overabundance of the raw materials for processed foods, too many calories, not enough nutrients, and the harm to soils, water, biodiversity, and climate that now must be addressed.

Agronomic scientists like Norman Borlaug made huge advances in plant breeding to take advantage of artificial fertilizer and irrigation. In places like Mexico, where Borlaug did his graduate research, the history of yield results is remarkable.[26]

In many developing countries, more people had access to food because of Borlaug and others. After World War II, Americans haven't faced crop shortages resulting in hunger (although poverty still perpetuates food insecurity). When asked about the criticism from environmentalists, Borlaug's reply was, "Some of the environmental lobbyists of the Western nations are the salt of the earth, but many of them are elitists. They've never experienced the physical sensation of hunger. They do their lobbying from comfortable office suites in Washington or Brussels. If they lived just one month amid the misery of the developing world, as I have for fifty years, they'd be crying out for tractors and fertilizer and irrigation canals and be outraged that fashionable elitists back home were trying to deny them these things."[27]

It's hard to argue against something that helped so many hungry people. While addressing hunger and food insecurity were crucial to the Green Revolution, the downsides are clear: polluted water from fertilizer and pesticide runoff, depleted soils, and loss of biodiversity (variety of plants, animals, insects, and soil microorganisms). It also contributed to about one-third to one-half of the global climate change that we've seen in the past half century, and to the consolidation of corporate power at the expense of small farmers and human health.[28] In the end, the Green Revolution didn't fulfill its promise of ending world hunger; 800 million people still go to bed hungry every night.

THE MYTH OF FEEDING THE WORLD

Big Food and Big Ag have pushed the myth that only they and their products can feed a growing world. The truth is we already produce enough food to feed the world, but that doesn't mean the hungry get access to that food.

"The world has long produced enough calories, around 2,700 per day per human, more than enough to meet the United Nations projection of a population of ten billion in 2050, up from the current seven billion," the food journalist Mark Bittman writes. "There are hungry people not because food is lacking, but because not all of those calories go to feed humans (a third go to feed animals, nearly 5 percent are used to produce biofuels, and as much as a third is wasted, all along the food chain)."[29]

The real problem is actually overproduction. "Though hunger and malnutrition are actually getting worse, we've been producing one and a half times more than enough food to feed everyone on the planet for half a century," writes Eric Holt-Giménez of Food First, author of *Can We Feed the World without Destroying It?*:

> The glut of food keeps prices low for grain traders and processors of animal feed and junk food. Competition drives these companies to out-produce each other, each coming out with cheaper and cheaper processed-food products. We end up with lousier food than the market can absorb and with meat fattened on grain in feedlots that hungry people can't afford. Prices drop and margins shrink, but "cheap food" hasn't ended hunger, and it comes at a tremendous social and environmental cost.... Overproduction results in monopolization up and down the food chain, giving agri-food corporations tremendous economic and political power to continue doing business as usual. These unregulated firms pay for none of the "externalities" they produce—we do.[30]

The truth is that the Green Revolution model didn't solve hunger through better seeds or increased chemical inputs or the increasing problems with corporate agriculture. And the Green Revolution also led to a more than 200 percent increase in the need for irrigation.[31] Even Dr. M. S. Swaminathan, the "Father of the Green Revolution in India," has since written scientific papers questioning the safety and sustainability of that very model. His main observation was that despite increasing yield, the quality of life for farmers was actually decreasing along with the health of the land.

"There is no doubt that genetically engineered Bt-cotton has failed in India: it has failed as a sustainable agriculture technology and has therefore also failed to provide livelihood security of cotton farmers who are mainly resource-poor, small and marginal farmers," he says.[32] Dr. Swaminathan and his colleague Dr. P. C. Kesavan also cited scientific evidence that the glyphosate-based herbicides, used on most genetically modified crops, have been found to cause birth defects, cancer, and genetic mutations.[33]

This recognition comes after years of warnings from social movements and scientists like Dr. Vandana Shiva, who have documented the human and ecological impacts of the Green Revolution including a wave of suicides by Indian farmers who become indebted because of the high costs of fertilizers, seeds, and pesticides. Their method of suicide, drinking pesticide, is a horrific reminder of the human consequences of the extractive model of agriculture.[34]

GMOS: SAFE OR HARMFUL?

GMOs came out of the Green Revolution. However, genetic engineering wasn't new even then. Humans have modified the genetics of plants and animals for thousands of years. Remember high school biology where we learned about Gregor Mendel breeding different pea varieties in the 1800s?

What is new is both the scale of genetic engineering technology and the proprietary profit logic that underlies it. For example, Pepsi is currently trying to sue Indian farmers for growing a "trademarked" potato.[35] In April 2019, CNN Business reported that Pepsi is demanding nearly

$150,000 each from four Indian farmers accused of growing the potatoes, which are exclusively used by the company for its Lay's potato chips. Really? They are suing over a potato? Local activists argue that the rural farmers were unaware of the trademark and their legal rights in the matter, and reportedly accused PepsiCo of sending private investigators posing as buyers to the farms.

If corporations control the seeds and plants that make our food, we disenfranchise the small farmers who feed most of the world's population, shift the profits to the top of the food chain, and perpetuate destructive agricultural practices, all of which ultimately threaten the stability of our food supply.

The promise of GMO crops requiring fewer chemicals to grow and resulting in higher yields has also failed, as demonstrated by comparative studies of agriculture in Europe (which prohibited the use of GMO seeds) and the United States.[36] In fact, GMO seeds have led to the rampant use of herbicides and pesticides, as pests and weeds became more resistant. Ironically, agriculture is now locked in a hubristic arms race against superbugs and superweeds, which have evolved to resist the very chemicals that are supposed to kill them.

As for the health effects of eating GMO foods, in an interview with Steven Druker from the Alliance for Bio-Integrity, he pointed out that while certain scientists have long rushed to declare GMOs safe, there has always been substantial disagreement among scientists about the health risks of genetically engineered (GE) foods. "In 2012, the board of directors of the American Association for the Advancement of Science went so far as to assert that 'every respected organization' that has examined the evidence has concluded that GE foods are no riskier than others. But these claims are demonstrably false. Eminent scientific organizations have not only critiqued the safety claims about GE foods, but have also cautioned about the risks and called for stricter regulation," Druker says.

The National Academy of Sciences, our nation's "independent" scientific advisers to the government, issued a report on GMOs and biotechnology, determining that they posed no risk. But in a damning investigative report by the *New York Times*, conflicts of interest on the expert panel were significant.[37] Seven of the thirteen members had significant ties to the GMO and biotech industry, calling into question their findings. And a few had conflicts that violated the National Academy of Sciences' own conflict-of-interest policies yet were allowed to remain on the panel. Just as food companies infiltrate scientific bodies and taint research, so do Big Ag and biotech companies.

Although proponents of GE foods also routinely claim that none has ever been associated with harm, a substantial body of research in peer-reviewed journals has demonstrated adverse effects on laboratory animals that were fed GE food, and some of those harm-linked foods have been in the human food supply for years. The Public Health Association of Australia has repeatedly issued warnings about GMOs and called for an "indefinite freeze" on the commercial growing of the crops and their importation until long-term testing can prove their safety.

Relying on industry data for a product's safety, whether it's tobacco "science" proving cigarettes don't cause cancer or aren't addictive, or the soda industry data that sugar doesn't cause obesity or artificial sweeteners are safe, is not a good bet. History has been full of "advances" like DDT and trans fats that turned out to be deadly after 50 or 100 years of use.

ROUNDUP OR COVER-UP?

Even if it turns out that consuming GMO products is not so bad, their use is currently a large uncontrolled experiment on humans, and there is no doubt about the harmful effects of pesticides and herbicides. David Bellinger of the Harvard School of Public Health has shown that American children under the age of five have lost 17 million IQ points because of the harmful effects of pesticides.[38]

Take glyphosate (or Roundup), for example. Before they're plucked and fed to animals or sold to humans, GMO crops are routinely sprayed with toxic herbicides, the most famous of which is glyphosate, sold under the brand name Roundup. In the four decades since Monsanto released its blockbuster weed killer, the amount of it sprayed on the nation's crops has risen more than a hundredfold. According to the EPA, some 220 million pounds of Roundup's active ingredient were used in the United States in 2015. In California alone, more than 10 million pounds of glyphosate are applied to crops every year. Glyphosate now is the world's most commonly used herbicide and accounts for almost 72 percent of all pesticides used around the world, and since 1974, 1.6 billion kilograms (more than 3.5 billion pounds) have been used on crops in the United States.[39]

According to the EPA, glyphosate is sprayed on more than seventy different food crops. It is used on corn, soy, canola, and wheat. If you eat a slice of bread, a bowl of Cheerios, a sushi roll, a plate of pasta, a slice of pizza, or a chicken nugget, there's a good chance one or more of its ingredients was doused in Roundup before it left the farm. In fact, it is sprayed on all wheat just before harvest, even though wheat is not a GMO product. Glyphosate defoliates the plants, making the wheat easier to harvest. That's why Honey Nut Cheerios have more glyphosate per serving than vitamin D and vitamin B_{12}, which have to be added to enrich the cereal.[40] Glyphosate has even been found in jars of commercial honey.[41]

We are all exposed. Even though I am careful about what I eat, choose organic at home and when I can when eating out, and don't eat GMO soy or corn, when I tested my glyphosate levels, they were in the fiftieth percentile. It is everywhere, from our lawns to our plates.

Glyphosate is increasing our cancer risk, according to a report by a working group of seventeen experts from eleven countries published by the International Agency for Research on Cancer.[42] Glyphosate also harms our microbiome, causes negative behavior changes in animal models, and causes epigenetic changes that lead to disease.[43] Studies clearly show harm in animal models, including birth defects, low sperm counts, low testosterone, ovarian and uterine abnormalities, and liver damage, among other harmful effects.[44] It also damages the microbiology of the soil on which we all depend.[45]

Even more concerning was a 2019 study that glyphosate can have transgenerational effects.[46] When you eat your GMO soy burger, or your Cheerios laced with glyphosate, it may not just be affecting your health; it may also be putting your grandchildren and great-grandchildren at risk. In this study of rats, direct exposure to glyphosate had negligible effects on the mothers and their offspring, but significant effects on little grand- and great-grand-rats that were *never* directly exposed to glyphosate. This effect is driven by changes in epigenetics, tags on our genes that are carried forward to our offspring. What did the study find? Pretty scary stuff. The unexposed little grand- and great-grand-rats suffered from prostate disease, obesity, kidney disease, ovarian disease, and birth defects. Yes, these were rats, not humans. But this massive use of glyphosate is essentially an uncontrolled experiment on humanity. Shouldn't we be thinking about the effects of our actions on future generations?

THE NEXT GENERATION OF AGRICULTURE

We need a new generation of farmers and ranchers to transform agriculture. The average age of farmers in America is fifty-seven and a half. The problem is that corporate consolidation creates monopolistic control and expensive land and prevents a new generation of young farmers from entering farming.

Jennifer Dempsey, director of American Farmland Trust's Farmland Information Center, projects that ownership of 40 percent of the forty-eight states' 991 million farm and ranch acres will change hands from 2015 to about 2035.[47] The question remains: Who will be the farmers of the future? How will the land be farmed? What policies are needed to encourage a new generation of farmers who can solve the challenges of our current agricultural system?

Young people who want to become farmers, or even people in inner cities and in suburbs becoming urban farmers, immediately run up against the problem of land access. Land is too expensive and is often worth more for its financial value than its agricultural value. The corporate profits from overproduction have gone into buying up land. Millions and millions of acres, an area about the size of France, have been bought up as a repository for excess capital because there's been no regulation on land purchases. The result is inflated land values around the world that prevent people from being able to go into agriculture as a livelihood. We need to change the incentive structures across the scale from federal to state to local initiatives that support young farmers and ranchers. We should also consider creating a federal program, a "Farmer Corps," to support a new generation of regenerative farmers.

FOOD FIX: CONNECTING THE DOTS— REIMAGINING FOOD SYSTEMS AND AGRICULTURE FOR HEALTH AND SUSTAINABILITY

The unintended consequences that emerged from our agricultural industrial revolution and the policies that supported it and the food system it created were hard to foresee. But now that we know, we can't unknow it.

Changes across the board from farmers, corporations, and government policies can help shift the entire system. We must move away from an extractive, destructive, fossil-fuel, chemical-dependent model to one that understands and restores natural systems and employs agroecological and regenerative practices.

In Chapter 7, we talked about the importance of implementing a national food policy. Instead of working within dysfunctional silos, the solutions need to integrate all aspects of the food system and build policies and initiatives based on solving the big problems of healthy nutrition, sustainability, social equity, and economic benefit. In fact, these are not separate problems; they are one problem. Thankfully many groups of very smart people are tackling this complexity and mapping out a new vision for our food and agricultural system.

1. Among the most coherent comprehensive attempts to connect the dots for a common policy is the report from iPES Food (International Panel of Experts on Sustainable Food Systems) entitled *Towards a Common Food Policy for the European Union.* The iPES report has key objectives that require coordinated effort across all sectors of policy agencies, businesses, and farmers, including shifting to regenerative agriculture, shortening supply chains (i.e., emphasizing local food), and fixing trade policies to support local agriculture. Read the executive summary or full report at www.ipes-food.org under "Reports." If its principles were implemented at scale, we could solve our food, climate, and health crises.

2. In 2018, the UN Environment Program hosted an initiative called TEEB, or **TEEBAgriFood**,[48] that brought together more than 150 scholars from thirty-three countries to assess the impact of and solutions for our food and agricultural systems (visit teebweb.org). According to the TEEBAgriFood report, our food system accounts for 43 to 57 percent of human-created greenhouse gas emissions when you include soil loss, factory farms, deforestation, food waste, food transportation, refrigeration and freezing, and processing and packaging.[49] Their Scientific and Economic Foundations report mapped out a very different future that addresses some of the biggest global challenges today linked to food and agriculture—climate change, environmental damage, and loss of biodiversity, among others. No small task.

3. Another important report, *Fixing Food 2016: Towards a More Sustainable Food System*,[50] focused on how to address sustainable agriculture and food loss and waste. The authors created a Food Sustainability Index that ranks twenty-five countries on fifty-eight indicators: environmental, societal, and economic. Sustainability is defined as the ability of our food system to not deplete or exhaust natural resources or compromise health. The United States was ranked eleventh, followed closely by Ethiopia and China. Not the best company in terms of sustainability. France, Japan, and Canada topped the list. This tool can help countries assess their progress in meeting benchmarks for building a sustainable food system.

4. In the United States, there are voices of change in Congress. For example, Earl Blumenauer, an Oregon congressman, has laid out a road map called *Growing Opportunities: Reforming the Farm Bill for Every American*[51] to address the problems of our current agricultural system through Farm Bill reforms. Incremental changes won't be sufficient to address the magnitude of the problems in our current food system. The current bill undermines human health, carbon reduction, economic development, land conservation, and animal welfare. More than 88 percent of our agricultural production comes from only 12 percent of farms.[52] Eighty-five percent of subsidies go to the biggest 15 percent of farms,[53] including more than fifty billionaires,[54] while those wanting to shift to regenerative agriculture don't get much support. Our current Farm Bill encourages farmers to behave in harmful ways—1) to grow more commodity crops used not for humans but for animal feed, biofuels, and the building blocks of ultraprocessed (aka deadly) food; 2) to grow more and more crops, regardless of supply or demand, on marginal land or sensitive lands; and 3) to ignore the environmental consequences of their actions or be penalized for growing food that actually nourishes Americans, like fruits and vegetables.

The road map for a new farm bill would focus on reforms to crop insurance, incentives and support for regenerative agriculture including more research, and investment in local food systems and urban farming, and would address food waste. Imagine if farmers were incentivized by the amount of soil organic matter on their farms. If they didn't create more good soil, then they would have to pay higher insurance rates. Good soil helps reverse climate change, reduce water use, build resistance against droughts and floods, and increase ecosystem biodiversity.

Visit blumenauer.house.gov/growing-opportunities for Congressman Blumenauer's full report and guiding principles for reform.

An exhaustive catalogue of the solutions proposed is beyond the scope of this book. Smart scientists, policy makers, and stakeholders all across the food system are chewing on how to create a food fix. There are major efforts to shift our food system to one that is more sustainable and regenerative. Some are specific to US policies; some are more global in nature. It's a tall order, but solving these problems is the most urgent task of our generation and the generations to come.

Old technologies will fade, and new ones will emerge that focus on a triple bottom line—economic, social, and environmental profits will all be counted and measured in the calculus of success.

I will map out more of these ideas, strategies, policies, and innovations in the next two chapters because they impact all the challenges of modern agriculture, including soil, water, biodiversity, the environment, and the climate.

For a quick reference guide on the Food Fixes and resources on supporting small farms and combating corporate consolidation, go to www.foodfixbook.com.

CHAPTER 16

SOIL, WATER, BIODIVERSITY: WHY SHOULD WE CARE?

Our food doesn't just magically show up in the grocery store; it emerges from a complex set of natural processes that we ignore at our peril. Unfortunately, we do ignore those natural cycles. Man conquering nature has always been our operating paradigm. We can plow the earth with machines, fertilize plants with nitrogen, kill weeds and pests with poisons, dominate nature, and use fossil fuels to supercharge the agricultural machine. It has worked for a while. Sort of. But along the way it has drained our natural bank account built up over millions of years—the soil, water, microbes, insects, and living systems that produce food.

We are in debt. Our natural capital is near exhaustion. Every five seconds a soccer field's worth of soil erodes because of bad land management practices.[1] At the current rate of soil erosion, we have only sixty harvests left before our soil is too depleted to grow food.[2] Seventy-five percent of the world's fresh water that is used by humans is used for intensive methods of crop and livestock production, depleting it faster than it is being replenished. Even industrial organic agriculture uses lots of water from deep aquifers and rivers. The water from these deep aquifers brings up salt and selenium. The salt damages the soil and the selenium kills birds. Most of that water cannot be stored in degraded soils, so it is wasted, running right past the roots of the plant. Nearly half of the sea-level rise since 1960 is due to irrigation water flowing straight past the crops.[3] Pollinators, on which 75 percent of our agricultural production depends, are disappearing because of the pesticides, which also kill bees. Without this natural capital, no food. No food, no humans. There are very real solutions that can stop and reverse this trend—and all the side effects are good ones.

IT'S THE SOIL, STUPID!

We must treat the whole problem of health in soil, plant, animal and man as one great subject.

—SIR ALBERT HOWARD, *SOIL AND HEALTH,* 1947

Soil is the most ignored and most important solution to almost everything that's wrong with our food system. In fact, could soil even be the solution to climate change? Let's take a little science lesson.

I spent the summer of 1979 in the mountains of northern Vermont studying soil, taking courses in "biological agriculture," or what we would now call regenerative agriculture. Probably not what my mother had in mind when she sent me to Cornell. But I was interested in natural systems, in growing food, in health and sustainability. In that idyllic summer, we made compost, built raised-bed gardens, planted marigolds to repel bad insects, and planted crops together that were mutually supportive, just as Native Americans grew corn, beans, and squash together. The beans provided natural nitrogen fertilizer and the squash, cover for the soil to retain water.

I read classic books on soil and agriculture including *Soil and Health* by Sir Albert Howard, the original tome on organic agriculture that implored us to work with natural systems rather than against them. The book was written in 1947. We are slow learners. But those lessons are now more important than ever. Understanding the problem of the health of soil, plants, animals, and humans is critical to our survival.

Soil is everywhere, but increasingly, our agricultural practices are turning our soil into dirt. Dirt is dead. Soil is alive. Plants thrive in soil, not dirt. Healthy soil rich in organic matter retains water, which reduces floods and the effects of droughts, puts carbon in the soil, which feeds all the microbial life that makes nutrients available to the plants (and to the humans who eat them), detoxifies pollutants, and more. Soil is rich in fertility, microbes, fungi, and nutrients. Dirt needs fertilizer, pesticides, herbicides, nutrients, and water to grow food. Soil doesn't. Dirt causes climate change. Soil reverses it. The top meter of soil contains three times as much carbon as the entire atmosphere.[4] Building healthy soil allows plants to put down deeper roots, pulling carbon from the air deep into the soil. The rich microbial life in healthy soil also helps keep the carbon in the soil, creating a virtuous cycle. Soil is our ace in the hole to reverse climate change, if we use it.

Healthy soils also provide healthy, nutrient-dense food. Our current plant breeding and loss of soil organic matter have produced plants lower in nutrients,[5] higher in carbohydrates, and lower in protein. Research shows that by 2050, increasing CO_2 levels and poor soil quality will worsen the nutrient composition of the food we grow, which could result in zinc deficiency for 175 million people, protein deficiency for 122 million, and iron deficiency in 1 billion.[6] There is less calcium, magnesium, iron, and other minerals in food today compared to 100 years ago. Just as you can't get blood from a stone, you can't get nutrients from dirt.

Soil is a renewable resource we have squandered. We have lost 430 million hectares of arable land to soil erosion, which is one-third of the world's available farmland. We have mined the land, turned it to dust, and lost the 60 to 80 feet of topsoil that existed in some areas of the Midwest. Through tillage and erosion, soils have lost 133 billion tons of carbon into the atmosphere since we started farming, driving global warming.[7]

Across the globe, farmland becomes desert at alarming rates. The UN's Food and Agriculture Organization says 12 million hectares of arable land (or about 23 hectares a minute), enough to grow 20 tons of grain, are lost to drought and desertification annually, which affects 1.5 billion people in more than 100 countries.[8]

According to President Obama's 2016 initiative "The State and Future of U.S. Soils: Framework for a Federal Strategic Plan for Soil Science," it is estimated that the United States will run out of soil by the end of this century.[9] That's a terrifying projection for a nation that is such an important exporter of grain and soybeans.

Experts say we have globally lost 50 to 70 percent of our topsoil. Soil degradation is caused primarily by

- Livestock overgrazing (poor livestock management)
- Industrialized agriculture
- Deforestation
- Urban industrialization
- Overfertilizing
- Monocrop agriculture
- Tilling
- Bad crop rotation
- Bare fallows (leaving bare ground) and not using cover crops

In other words, industrial agriculture has strip-mined our rich organic soil. We ran mechanized plows through the soil for years, rupturing these biological and chemical cycles. Then we added chemicals and started killing off organisms. Big fertilizer conglomerates such as Yara, Mosaic, and Koch Fertilizer (yes, those Koch brothers) produce 20 million metric tons of fertilizer a year using fossil-fuel-intensive processes. When that fertilizer is applied to farms, the damage is wrought on the soil, and it weakens plants, pollutes water systems, and drives huge external costs, as we reviewed in Part 1. The bacteria in the soil convert the nitrogen fertilizer into huge amounts of nitrous oxide, which is released into the air, a greenhouse gas that has 300 times the heat-trapping potential of carbon dioxide.[10] Adding nitrogen fertilizer to soil paradoxically makes the soil less fertile because it depletes the soil organic matter, which then results in the need for more fertilizer.[11] Good for big fertilizer companies, bad for the soil, for us, and for the climate.

Halting land degradation has become an urgent global imperative.

There is a way to fix all of this. We have the technology, it's low cost, it's available globally, and it has been proven and tested (for billions of years). It is called photosynthesis, the magic cycle plants use to turn water and carbon dioxide (which they breathe from the air) into carbohydrates, which we eat (called "carbo" hydrates because they are built from carbon in the air), and that also feed the microbes in the soil, which in turn feed the plants nitrogen, phosphorus, and minerals. It's a great barter system that makes the world go around, and it's one of the foundations of regenerative agriculture.

On the Great Plains of North America, tens of millions of bison, elk, and deer used to feed on deep-rooted perennial grasses. As these bison moved through the landscape, their hooves pierced the soil and their waste nurtured the soil biology and their saliva increased the growth rate of grasses.[12] Native Americans participated in this process by periodically burning the prairie to encourage new growth. The plants, in turn, bartered some of the carbohydrates they made through photosynthesis with soil microbiology to make minerals and nutrients in the soil available to the plants.

Regenerative agriculture aims to restore soil by farming with those same principles in mind. That means using no-till methods that don't disturb the ground, cover crops that protect the soil, and crop rotations that keep pests and weeds under control. The use of livestock in managed holistic grazing plays a critical role in stimulating plant growth, root structures, and soil fertility by adding manure, saliva, and urine. Some estimates are that this practice can draw down enough carbon from the atmosphere to result in a 15 percent[13] to 100 percent[14] reduction in all carbon released since the industrial revolution (from all causes). That big range relies on different estimates on the scalability of soil carbon capture throughout the world's varied ecosystems. Regardless, it's a lot of carbon—1 trillion tons. Not bad for just soil. Experts suggest that this is the most important untapped, low-cost solution to reversing global warming. Five billion acres of agricultural land have been degraded through industrial, chemical-intensive farming practices. According to UN climate scientists, if we spent $300 billion (the total global spending on military for sixty days, or less than the annual amount the United States spends on type 2 diabetes—$327 billion) on restoring 2.2 billion of the degraded acres through regenerative agriculture, we could stop the rise of greenhouse gas emissions. That would delay climate change by twenty years, providing more time to innovation climate solutions.[15]

The good news is that some big players in the food industry are recognizing this. The former vice chair of PepsiCo Mehmood Khan told me he was invited to speak at the USDA about regenerative agriculture. Big Food knows that if there is no soil and no water, they can't make their products. Danone, Nestlé, and Kellogg's are among nineteen food companies with revenues of $500 billion that formed a coalition called One Planet Business for Biodiversity, launched September 23, 2019, at the United Nations Climate Action Summit in New York to support regenerative agriculture, biodiversity, eliminating deforestation, and the restoration of ecosystems.[16]

The international initiative "4 per 1000," launched in 2015 by Stéphane Le Foll, then French minister of agriculture, agri-food, and forestry, includes more than 300 partners (governments, NGOs, foundations, farmers, scientists, and industry). The goal is simple: to increase carbon in the soil by 0.4 percent (4 per 1000) every year by scaling regenerative practices to the more than 500 million farms and 1 billion farmers worldwide.

DIRT TO SOIL—FROM TRAGEDY TO TRIUMPH

Several farmers have shown that we can do better farming with cheaper production, better-quality food, fewer or no chemical inputs, more yields and more profits to the farmer and lower costs to the consumer. Gabe Brown, a North Dakota farmer trained in land-grant colleges (funded in part by Big Ag) on the merits of industrial agriculture, assiduously applied these conventional methods to his 5,000-acre farm. After four seasons of crop failure from destructive hail, storms, and heat waves, he was about to go bankrupt.

Brown then discovered the principles of regenerative agriculture, and now 15 years later he has created a thriving, highly profitable, highly diversified carbon farm that lets nature do the work. Brown's farm has created 29 inches of new topsoil, and his farm is healthier, more productive, and far more profitable than his neighbors' farms. He says that his soil used to hold only half an inch of rain per hour; now it can hold 8 inches. Rather than buying fertilizer, by planting nitrogen-fixing plants and grazing cattle on those plants, which put down more nitrogen into the soil with manure and urine, Brown said he actually makes money from his "fertilizer," instead of having to buy it. He produces 20 percent more food than his neighbors on the same land and makes up to twenty times more money from his diversified regenerative farm. Now he travels the country teaching other farmers the false promise of industrial farming and the true power of regenerative agriculture to help farmer, nature, and eater.

Allen Williams, PhD, a sixth-generation Mississippi farmer, bought a depleted 100-year-old cotton plantation, which had been overgrazed by cattle, then turned into hunting grounds, then sold for pennies to Williams because there was no life on the land. In five years, he created 5 inches of soil with regenerative agriculture. He has taught more than 4,000 farmers how to transition their farms and ranches. He is part of a group of ranchers and farmers known as the Soil Carbon Cowboys.[17] They make more money with less effort and time and fewer inputs, and in tougher conditions, and are more resistant to climate stress than conventional farmers.

> I encourage you to watch the short video on what the Soil Carbon Cowboys do at https://vimeo.com/80518559.

WATER: ARE WE RUNNING OUT?

Soil loss is one of the many crises on the planet. We can add to that the depletion of the world's freshwater supplies. Seventy percent of human use of fresh water (which is only 5 percent of all water on the planet) is used to grow food, much of it to feed animals for human consumption on factory farms, not rangelands. It is also used heavily in crops like almonds and cotton. The World Economic Forum declared water scarcity the fourth-biggest global threat right after weapons of mass destruction, climate change, and natural disasters (which are linked).[18] Time to binge-watch reruns of *Game of Thrones* and forget about it all?

Remarkably, as I have mapped out in *Food Fix*, these issues are connected by food, and they are fixable.

Water is something most of us take for granted. Turn on the tap; buy a case of bottled water; take long, hot showers. Sadly, water is not so plentiful in much of the world. Cape Town, South Africa, recently almost completely ran out of water.[19] Californians couldn't water their lawns and were forced to limit water use because of droughts. About 2 billion people face water scarcity one month a year; half a billion face it all year round. Half of all major cities experience water scarcity.[20]

Sucking the Earth Dry

Groundwater is drawn out from our aquifers for irrigation of agriculture faster than it can be replenished. Water overdraw from irrigated agriculture is expected to increase with growing populations. Overuse (such as through pumping for irrigation or fracking) can mean that sources that were previously renewable get so low that they can't recover. For instance, Saudi Arabia decided it wanted to grow its own food and used its ancient fossil aquifers. They were successful for five years, until all their water ran out.[21] Forever. Closer to home, the 174,000-square-mile Ogallala Aquifer lies underneath the Great Plains and irrigates America's breadbasket. It is also being pumped dry. We are currently taking out 1.3 trillion gallons a year more than can be replenished by rainfall.

Fortunately, innovations in farming and regenerative agriculture build soil, which acts as a sponge for rain, reducing the need for irrigation. Some farmers are changing their practices. Kansas farmer Rodger Funk now farms without groundwater. Today he pumps almost no water on his 6,000 acres, which are planted largely with wheat and grain sorghum. "We decided to go dryland," he says.[22] "Dryland" means growing crops without irrigation. Instead of plowing his fields after harvest, he leaves the stubble in the ground and plants a new crop in the residue. Leaving the roots and stems intact not only reduces soil erosion but also decreases evaporation and catches more blowing snow than bare ground. Leaving crop residue in the field can reduce moisture loss by the equivalent of an inch or more of rainfall annually, scientists say.[23] Funk aims to capture every bit of the 18 inches of precipitation that fall on southwestern Kansas. "Got to," Funk says. "It's all we've got around here."

MAKING SOIL A GIANT SPONGE FOR WATER

In some regions the issue is not enough water, while in other areas it's too much. For example, in 2019 the Missouri and Mississippi Rivers flooded fields all the way from Minnesota to Louisiana. Some farms had millions of dollars in damage. While floods may sound like they create extra water for the farms, most of that water runs off or through the soil and can't be retained. Soil rich in organic matter can help farmers make their land more resilient to floods by improving the health and spongelike qualities of their soils. Although they can't prevent floods, they can do damage control. In fact, a 1 percent increase in organic matter in the soil can hold up to 27,000 gallons of water per acre. Regenerative practices can increase soil organic matter 3 to 8 percent, creating a virtuous cycle. Allen Williams, a Mississippi regenerative rancher, didn't suffer the damage his neighbors did from the floods. The water went right into the soil. More soil, more water retention, more drought resistance, more water in soil, more plant growth, more evaporation from plants, more rain. Ever wonder why it rains in the rain forest and not the desert? It's the evaporation of water from plants!

Overflowing Manure Lagoons, Poisoned Aquifers, and Dead Zones

In addition to using up valuable water resources, agriculture can also pollute the water it doesn't use. Industrial livestock farming manages to do both.

It is rightly said that it takes about 1,800 gallons of water to produce a pound of meat. But all water is not created equal. In fact, water in agriculture comes in three shades: green, blue, and gray. Pasture-raised beef uses mostly green water that comes from rain falling on grasslands that otherwise wouldn't be converted into food. Feedlot-finished cattle (currently 95 percent of all beef cattle) use significantly more blue water (irrigation from groundwater sources, rivers, or lakes) than grass-finished cattle, but still most of the water is green water. Gray water is polluted water that comes from giant toxic manure lagoons full of antibiotics, hormones, pesticides, heavy metals, nitrogen, and toxic bacteria, which seeps into the ground, polluting aquifers and surface water and creating big dead zones in rivers, lakes, and oceans.

Confined animal feeding operations (CAFOs) are industrial farms where thousands of animals are crowded into massive barns and fed cheap grains and soy. The manure and urine from these barns are stored in nearby lagoons that can leak into waterways and aquifers and create air pollution for people who live nearby. The massive corn and soy operations that provide feed for CAFOs, ethanol, plant oils, and other uses in a biobased economy deplete our water reserves through irrigation and pollute our water supplies.

CAFOs: The Atomic Bomb of the Twenty-First Century

In the report *CAFOs Uncovered*,[24] the Union of Concerned Scientists exposes the dark underbelly of animal feeding operations in America and their hidden costs. The growth of factory-farmed meat (including beef, pork, and chicken) in CAFOs is one of the most destructive industries on the planet. The cheap price of meat exists only in the context of the taxpayer and the environment paying the cost. These operations are a significant contributor to greenhouse gases, deforestation, water and air pollution, and depletion of water resources from irrigation to grow feed crops, which require subsidies, and a significant portion of which are used for feed. CAFOs also lead to the overuse of antibiotics to prevent disease in overcrowded feeding operations, resulting in antibiotic-resistant superbugs. Property values around CAFOs are also depressed. Who wants to live near a toxic, smelly feedlot? And the oft-cited refrain from Big Ag that we can't supply the world's meat demands without CAFOs has been proven false.[25]

In 2018, Trump's Environmental Protection Agency rolled back regulations, deprioritizing water–quality enforcement around CAFOs.[26] Then Hurricane Florence hit, dumping 9 trillion gallons of water on North Carolina in four days. CAFO lagoons overflowed with waste containing E. coli, salmonella, Cryptosporidium, and other harmful bacteria into surrounding rivers and streams. The people who live in this area now face contamination of the wells they rely on for their daily drinking water.[27]

The overuse of pesticides and fertilizers also pollutes our water. Conventional farmers use large amounts of nitrogen fertilizer to grow large crop yields, and that fertilizer runs off fields and into the groundwater, rivers, lakes, and ocean. It destroys aquatic life in places like the Gulf of Mexico, Utah Lake, Lake Erie, and 400 other dead zones around the world.[28] If those chemicals are killing fish and plants, then what are they doing to us through the food we eat?

Much of the drinking water in America is contaminated.[29] Toxins, including pesticides, herbicides like glyphosate, plastics, prescription medicines, nitrates, and more, are in our water supply. Many of these toxins cause cancer, birth defects, cardiovascular issues, and reproductive problems, as well as other harmful effects. The food industry has a solution, though—bottled water! Not so fast. Water from plastic bottles contains phthalates or bisphenol A (BPA), which are also toxic. Purchasing bottled water puts a huge burden on our environment. The Great Pacific Garbage Patch (of plastic) between Hawaii and California is 1.6 million square kilometers (twice the size of Texas) and contains 1.8 trillion pieces, or 79 million tons, of plastic.[30] We need clean public water for everyone. To best protect ourselves, we should drink filtered water. We need better public water safety and infrastructure.

Innovation in farming and regenerative agriculture and in water conservation, repurposing of gray water (wastewater), better stormwater management, and other innovations all can help avert a water crisis. But CAFOs and traditional farming techniques are a significant part of the problem and the best targets to address.

THE LOSS OF BIODIVERSITY: WHY SHOULD YOU CARE?

If the bee disappeared off the face of the Earth, man would only have four years left to live.

—ALBERT EINSTEIN

In recent books like *Growing a Revolution* by David Montgomery and *Kiss the Ground* by Josh Tickell, and films like *The Biggest Little Farm*, the importance of rebuilding soil is being shared with new audiences. What we are learning is the crucial biological elements of soil health: the critters living there. These critters include the familiar earthworm as well as ones that may be new to you: arbuscular mycorrhizal fungi, soil bacteria, protozoa, nematodes, and arthropods. Together they form complex ecosystems that build soil structure, prevent erosion, and absorb water and carbon from the atmosphere. Living creatures are central to decomposition, nutrient cycling, and plant growth. Working together, these ecosystems can nurture crops and protect them from pests and diseases. The soil is home to a large proportion of the world's genetic biodiversity. There are more microbes in a handful of soil than all the humans that ever lived. The soil food web is the whole life cycle of the Earth. When soil is depleted, small insects die, then larger insects that eat the small ones die, and then the birds, small mammals, and amphibians that eat the insects die, which is why these populations are crashing around the world.

In 2019, the UN Intergovernmental Science-Policy Platform on

Biodiversity and Ecosystem Services (IPBES) released the most comprehensive report of biodiversity to date, estimating that 1 million species are on the verge of extinction because of human activity. That includes 40 percent of amphibian species, 33 percent of coral reefs, and 10 percent of insects.[31] According to the Living Planet Index, we have seen a 60 percent decline in species since 1970.[32]

Why should you care? Aside from just the idea of destroying the natural world, what does it really matter if we lose species, insects, forests, plants, and microbes and damage oceans and kill coral reefs? It matters because biodiversity is essential to grow nutrient-dense (or any) food, to have coral reefs that support our fisheries, to protect our coastlines and control floods, and to have fresh drinking water filtered by wetlands, medicines from wild plants, and even building materials and breathable air. Economists estimate that these ecosystems provide services worth $125 trillion a year in benefit to humanity (the total global GDP is $80 trillion).[33] In the end, saving nature is not about saving it for its own sake (which should be enough), but about saving it for our sake.

According to the UN report on biodiversity, "The health of ecosystems on which we and all other species depend is deteriorating more rapidly than ever. We are eroding the very foundations of our economies, livelihoods, food security, health and quality of life worldwide," said IPBES chair Sir Robert Watson. "The Report also tells us that it is not too late to make a difference, but only if we start now at every level from local to global. Through 'transformative change,' nature can still be conserved, restored and used sustainably—this is also key to meeting most other global goals."[34]

We are witnessing massive insect population collapses due to pesticides and land use changes such as converting land into monocrop agriculture.[35] But it is not just soy fields and cornfields that are the problem. Massive almond orchards in California require "slave" bees to be shipped in from around the world, and local bee populations are dying because once the almonds are pollinated, there is no other food to eat.[36] We have seen a 75 percent decline over 30 years in flying insect biomass.[37] Just the decline in pollinators is putting $577 billion of food crops at risk. No pollinators, nearly no food. Insects are crucial to the web of life. Their demise ripples up the food chain; bird populations are declining because they have less food. It also has huge economic implications for us. Bees, butterflies, and other insect pollinators contribute $29 billion to US farm income.[38] There is no doubt that our well-being is interconnected with biodiversity on farmland.

Many causes contribute to the biodiversity loss: climate change, pollution, invasive species, human encroachment on natural habitats, and excessive harvesting through fishing, hunting, and poaching. However, regenerative agricultural practices at scale can stop the destruction. This is not some hippie fad, but the position of the UN, the European Union, and every major scientific and governmental assessment of our current state of affairs.

FOOD FIX: REGENERATIVE AGRICULTURE— WHAT IS IT?

There are so many labels for our food it's a bit overwhelming and confusing: factory-farmed, grass-fed, organic, sustainable, pasture-raised, and now regenerative. This simple concept is relatively new but is based on ancient principles to restore and enhance natural systems. While it can be organic (and ideally should be), it goes beyond organic by laying out the principles for building soil, enhancing biodiversity, and reducing outside inputs. Large-scale organic farms can use methods that, while better than conventional agriculture, still can deplete soil, require extensive inputs, and drain water resources. Michael Pollan refers to this as "industrial organic" in his book *The Omnivore's Dilemma*. Even small organic farms that don't use regenerative practices can contribute to the problem through tillage and leaving land bare instead of planting cover crops to protect the soil and build organic matter.

Regenerative agriculture on farms, grasslands, and rangelands is the most powerful force for fixing much of what's wrong with agriculture while producing more and better food. And the practice can be adapted across diverse and global environments. These are the foundational principles:

- Regenerative agriculture is a system of farming principles and practices that increases biodiversity, enriches soils, improves watersheds, and enhances ecosystem services.
- Regenerative agriculture aims to capture carbon in soil and aboveground biomass, reversing current global trends of atmospheric accumulation.
- It offers increased yields, more nutrient-dense foods, resilience to climate instability, and improved health and vitality for farming and ranching communities and consumers.
- The system draws from decades of scientific and applied research by the global communities of organic farming, agroecology, holistic management, and agroforestry.

We need to quickly and radically change how we grow food and change the food we eat. But our systems and policies make it hard for farmers who want to do the right thing. Farmers growing healthy food, using sustainable, organic, or regenerative methods, often impoverish themselves to grow food for the rich, while conventional corporate farmers supported by our government get rich growing food for the poor. This must change and is changing.

The good news: It turns out that regenerative agriculture is more profitable (for farmers, not Big Ag or Big Food) and produces higher yields and better-quality food, even when used to grow commodity crops (soy, corn, wheat), all while reversing climate change, conserving water, and increasing biodiversity![39]

There are extraordinary examples of conventional farmers who turned to regenerative agriculture to save their farms after hail and drought destroyed them and now have more productive and profitable farms than their conventional-farming neighbors. There are "soil farmers" like Joel Salatin from Polyface Farm, who use animals as a method for building soil, increasing productivity and the nutrient density of food. Their mission statement is to "develop environmentally, economically, and emotionally enhancing agricultural prototypes and facilitate their duplication throughout the world." They say they are in the redemption business, healing land, food, economy, and the culture. They are grass and soil farmers. The amazing-quality food created is a natural by-product of a soil farm!

Three longtime farmers—Dave Brandt, Gabe Brown, and Allen Williams—are teaming up with the government's Natural Resources Conservation Service soil champion Ray Archuleta to help farmers and ranchers across the world apply soil-health-focused, regenerative agriculture systems.[40]

Their consulting focuses on ecological principles that can be applied practically and profitably in any farming operation:

- Limiting the amount of soil disturbance, preferably using no-till methods. Tilling turns over soil, disturbs root structures, and leads to soil erosion and loss. A number of effective alternatives to digging up the soil, such as seed drills or strip-till plows, minimize soil disturbance.
- Leaving no bare soil. This means leaving some plant material, such as roots and stalks, on top of the soil or planting cover crops during fallow periods, which help reduce soil and water loss and increase soil organic matter, soil biodiversity, and nutrient content.
- Maintaining diversity in what is planted in the fields. Rotating between crops prevents diseases and pests. In fact, regenerative farms have far fewer invasive insect pests than conventional farms that use insecticides. Using diverse cover crops can help break up soil compaction and bring nutrients like nitrogen into the soil.
- Integrating livestock into the farming operation. Cycling animals through the land means that their manure, urine, and saliva fertilize the soil, building soil the fastest. This must be done correctly by moving a diversity of animals around the farm ecosystem. If it's done incorrectly, overgrazing can harm the farm. There is no regenerative agriculture without animals as part of the ecological cycle.

FOOD FIX: THE GUATEMALAN AND THE COWBOYS—FOREST-FED CHICKENS!

In a room full of cowboy hats, Regi Haslett-Marroquin cuts a contrasting figure. As the native Guatemalan takes the stage to address the hundreds of farmers and ranchers who have gathered in Albuquerque, New Mexico, for the 2018 Regenerate conference, his humble brilliance electrifies the room. "We are not food producers," he says, softly smiling at his paradoxical challenge. "We are energy managers."

Regi is one of the architects of the Main Street Project (MSP), a poultry-centered regenerative agroforestry system that aims to equip farmers to solve our nation's food crisis. It's not enough to just blame Big Ag, he says; we need to create new ways of thinking and doing when it comes to food production.

MSP starts with a regenerative farming model that is built not on a nearsighted drive toward maximum profit, but on a *triple* bottom line. Agriculture must be ecologically, economically, and socially viable.

Regi says their methods are informed by indigenous knowledge, supplemented by farmers' own experiential learning, and validated by scientific testing. When he tells the story of chicken, he speaks of their origin as jungle fowl, living under the canopies of forests. This origin is a long way from the cages of today's factory farms. Regi and MSP are designing a system that mimics this origin by raising chickens in food forests that produce the food sources that the chickens eat. MSP's free-range poultry are raised in paddocks planted with a "stacking function" combination. This type of farming is called "silvopasture," or raising animals in forests or trees. Hazelnut trees provide shade, food for the chickens, and an additional source of income from selling the nuts. And the trees protect the chickens from aerial predators such as hawks. Cover crops like legumes, along with the manure from the chickens, help to put nitrogen into the soil. A variety of grains grown on-site provide more chicken feed, which reduces the amount of money farmers have to spend on outside feed sources. The chickens also eat tons of insects. The farm is built as a living ecosystem, and Regi jokes that it's easier to work with nature rather than fight it.

With their quick growth, chickens, whether for meat or eggs, provide a positive revenue stream at a low cost of entry. Think of this type of farming as a mutual fund versus an individual stock. There are multiple crops, livestock, and multiple streams of revenue, creating a healthier farm and more stable economics for the farmers. Chickens are at the center of MSP's system because they work so well with the crops, farmers, and environment. They are a "one-stop weed-eating, bug-killing, soil-enhancing replacement for the counter-productive synthetic pesticides, herbicides, and fertilizers destroying conventional farms and their communities."[41] This type of agriculture—diversified, intensive, integrating animals, trees, and plants in a natural ecological restorative cycle—is resilient and low impact, protects and builds soils, conserves water, and draws down carbon from the atmosphere, all while producing healthy, nutrient-dense food.

This is quite a contrast to the factory-farmed horror that is the majority of American chicken production: massive buildings where thousands of chickens are crammed into cages, are fed imported grain and antibiotics, and pollute the environment. Tyson Foods dumped 104 million pounds of pollutants into waterways, more than Exxon, and is the second-biggest industrial polluter after Big Steel.[42] Which chicken would you prefer to feed your family? The antibiotic- and arsenic-laced industrial chickens? Eggs that are pale yellow, devoid of nutrients? Or forest- and bug-fed chickens, and eggs with deep orange yolks dense in phytochemicals and nutrients?

MSP helps farmers incubate their own enterprises with a goal of developing regional food systems. They are building a poultry-production system that can also help immigrant communities move from laboring in an exploitative system to owning a small business. At the same time, the community benefits from the increased access to local, healthy food and the economic boost of thriving local markets. After years proving their concept, MSP is expanding from their central farm into a regional cluster of farms in southeast Minnesota. Their blueprint is also being applied to partner farms in Mexico, Guatemala, Honduras, and South Dakota. Everybody wins when the goal is regenerating human and environmental health rather than simply extracting a profit at any cost. If the true costs of food production were included in the price, these methods would provide much cheaper food.

Regi's story is one thread in an expanding tapestry of regenerative agricultural innovation that is occurring across the world. Efforts are underway to convert millions of acres of land to these types of integrated regenerative farms and ranches. While this innovation has developed on the margins, it's making its way to the mainstream. General Mills, one of the nation's largest food companies, has pledged to "advance regenerative agricultural practices" on 1 million acres of farmland by 2030.[43] That's a huge step in the right direction. Other companies such as Danone and Nestlé are also committing to shift their supply chain to regenerative agriculture. Purdue Farms has also responded to consumer demand by removing all antibiotics from their chicken farms, and shifting toward more organic, regenerative, and pasture-raised animal farming.

OTHER INNOVATORS

Other business start-ups are increasingly focused on regenerative agriculture, not only because it is the right thing to do, but because it is more profitable. Investors are getting in on the action.

Big start-ups like Pivot Bio (supported by investors such as Bill Gates, Jeff Bezos, and Richard Branson) and Joyn Bio (supported by Bayer) are solving the nitrogen problem using natural principles such as applying nitrogen-fixing bacteria to seeds, which eliminates the need for fertilizer. Some suggest, however, that this is just another way for big companies to control seeds with patents and intellectual property protections. And there are other ways to do this with natural biostimulants, which are biological or biologically derived fertilizer additives, and similar products that are used in crop production to enhance plant growth, health, and productivity. Bio-Integrity Growers farm in Australia, for example, uses biostimulants.[44]

One investment fund, Farmland LP, buys conventional commodity-farmed land and converts it to regenerative agriculture, turning conventional farms with profits in the single digits into regeneratively farmed land with profits of 40 to 50 percent, while increasing productivity, biodiversity, resiliency, soil carbon, and water conservation, and reducing pollution and agrochemical inputs. These are called ecosystem services. Transitioning farms to regenerative agriculture with their first fund produced a 67 percent return and $21.4 million in benefits to the environment and local communities, while those same farms continuing business as usual would have caused $8.5 million in harm to the environment.[45] It takes time to transition farms from conventional—three to five years—but once the transformation is complete, a regenerative farm outperforms a conventional one in every metric.

Exciting innovations in technology (like using bacteria to fertilize plants) and global recognition of the need to reverse the harm of our agricultural practices are cause for hope.

Leading groups like the **Carbon Underground** are working with big businesses like Danone, governments, and grassroots groups globally to educate and support them to transform harmful systems of food production into healing systems.

A large study of 163 million farms using regenerative or sustainable practices shows that they are actually more productive than agrochemical-dependent farming.[46] So much for Big Ag needing to feed the world. It's propaganda. And Big Ag's front groups, like CropLife, and initiatives like "Climate Smart Agriculture" seek to confuse policy makers and consumers. It sounds good, but think of it like "clean coal."

Join the Carbon Underground's campaign to Adopt-a-Meter of soil for $5, which will go toward initiatives that support regenerative agriculture (https://thecarbonunderground.org/adopt-meter/).

The **Soil Carbon Initiative** has developed metrics that can be used to measure the performance of every part of the food chain and its contribution to soil health. Imagine if we as consumers could have front-of-packaging labels that provided transparency that showed how our food affects soil health and its impact on sequestering carbon, reversing climate change, improving biodiversity, and protecting our water resources. Wouldn't that be nice to know? This initiative can push farmers and food companies to shift their practices toward regenerative agriculture.

FOOD FIX: THE ROLE OF GOVERNMENT AND POLICY MAKERS

As individuals we can advocate for change, drive changes in the marketplace, hold our representatives accountable, elect members with values we share, and engage in individual choices that don't contribute to the problems we face. "The only remedy for the threats we face at the scale at which they confront us is massive political and economic change," Dr. Daniel Aldana Cohen, assistant professor of sociology at the University of Pennsylvania, says. "By far the most meaningful thing an individual person can do is join a social, political, or cultural movement aimed at transforming our political economy. No individual's consumer choices and no group's consumer choices are significant in the absence [of] structural change."[47]

Here are key policy levers that can move us to a saner approach to our agriculture and food system. In the United States these reforms must happen across agencies, but the most important instrument of change is the USDA's Farm Bill. Much more has been mapped out in the reports I have mentioned in this chapter, among others.

1. Establish a national food policy and a national food policy advisor[48] and reinvent the USDA as the US Department of Food, Health, and Well-Being to align our agricultural and food policies with economic and public health goals, coordinating policy across all agencies that touch any aspect of our food system, from seed to fork to landfill. Much can be done with regulation, executive action, and enforcing existing laws, even in the absence of legislative changes (which are desperately needed). We need to stop incentives for growing the wrong stuff, which makes us sick and poisons the planet, and support growth of food that focuses on quality of calories rather than quantity.

2. Re-solarize agricultural production. Shift the energy input to farms from fossil fuels to the solar inputs of photosynthesis, which will improve our diets and reverse climate change.

3. Increase publicly funded research on sustainable, regenerative agriculture to improve practices, build soil, determine best regional practices, and address water issues. Much research is done through publicly funded land-grant agricultural colleges, which now receive funding from Big Ag, helping them generate private profits from public investment. That needs to stop. Future studies should focus on evaluating reductions in concentrations of toxic runoff such as nitrogen, phosphate, and organic carbon from integrated crop and livestock systems.[49]

4. Start a Farmers Corps to enlist a new generation of farmers in regenerative agriculture and help them overcome the financial and education barriers to joining our food production system. Provide training and funding to access land and resources for converting conventional farms to regenerative farms. Think of it as a Peace Corps for regenerative agriculture.

5. Create incentives and support for regenerative agriculture through the USDA (and global agriculture ministries and departments) including financial support for farmers to transition from industrial, chemical-intense agriculture and to integrate animals into farm ecosystems. New Zealand ended all agricultural subsidies, and as a result, its farms are more diverse, productive, and profitable.[50] Support for regenerative agriculture will increase productivity, reduce soil and water loss, reduce fertilizer, pesticide, herbicide, and antibiotic use, and promote the production of healthier foods and the creation of healthier ecosystems. **Kiss the Ground** is an education and advocacy nonprofit advancing initiatives across four distinct programs: advocacy, farmland, education, and media. One of their programs provides training and support for farmers to transition to regenerative agriculture. I was able to connect Kiss the Ground with a venture philanthropist who could provide up to $1 billion in funding for farmers to transition to regenerative agriculture.

6. End the ethanol mandate. The Energy Independence and Security Act of 2007 mandated that US farms grow corn for ethanol to decrease reliance on foreign energy sources. This led to 33 million acres producing 40 percent of our corn crops being used for ethanol.[51] It takes more energy to produce ethanol (from all the fossil-fuel inputs needed to grow corn from fertilizer, pesticides, herbicides, etc.) than the energy that is provided by the ethanol, according to Cornell scientist David Pimental.[52] Environmentalists and oil companies both oppose the ethanol mandate. Agricultural policies could be implemented that simultaneously protect the farmer who grows the corn and convert those 33 million acres to regenerative agriculture, creating more and better food, restoring ecosystems, and helping reverse climate change.

7. Create a safety net of credit and risk management tools for farmers who practice sustainable and regenerative agriculture, not just for commodity farmers who produce corn and soy. The farmers are pawns in the big game of agribusiness and food conglomerates. If we reduce or eliminate subsidies for commodity crops, it won't be enough to protect farmers. The subsidies encourage overproduction of corn, soy, and wheat, leading to low prices, which hurt farmers. The real beneficiaries of the subsidies are the factory farms, food processors (like Cargill and Archer Daniels Midland), manufacturers, and meatpackers that buy the cheap raw materials from the farmers. Rather than taxpayers helping Big Food and Big Ag buy cheap food, farmers should be protected, and industry should pay the true cost of the food. I once asked the vice chair of PepsiCo why the company uses high-fructose corn syrup in their beverages. "Mark," he told me, "it's because the government makes it too cheap for us not to."

8. Pay for ecosystem services.[53] Many countries have created systems to support farmers and corporations who restore ecosystems through reforestation, soil restoration, better water management practices, and improvements in biodiversity. Costa Rica has been a pioneer in this. Payment for ecosystem services (PES) incentivizes farmers and corporations to solve the problem of climate change, water shortages, biodiversity loss, and soil degradation rather than contribute to it.

9. Consider a "nitrogen tax" levied on fertilizer companies to account for the greenhouse gases and the destruction of our soils, waterways, and fisheries and provide funds for the cleanup of our lakes, rivers, and oceans and fund transition to regenerative practices. Shouldn't big fertilizer companies be accountable for the harm they cause?

10. Implement mandatory municipal and institutional (and even personal) composting and provide the compost to farmers and ranchers.

11. Have Congress fund, and the USDA implement, programs that help farmers grow more fruits and vegetables, or actual food. Support the development of "specialty crops" such as fruits and vegetables, whole grains, beans, nuts, and seeds. This could create 189,000 new jobs and $9.5 billion in new revenue for healthy foods.[54]

12. End penalties for farmers who receive crop insurance so they can create diverse farms that include fruits and vegetables. Research has shown that if farmers in six midwestern states shifted some of their cropland to fruits and vegetables it would create 6,724 new jobs and $336 million in additional income.[55]

13. Include environmental and sustainability guidelines in the US Dietary Guidelines. The 2015 scientific advisory group recommended including this in the guidelines, but the politicians took it out under pressure from Big Ag and Big Food.

14. Ensure that the next farm bill helps break up monopolies and addresses consolidation of seed companies, seed patents, grain trading, animal feeding, meatpacking, agrochemical companies, and supermarkets.[56] This will create a fairer and more sustainable marketplace. Antitrust legislation would break up these monopolies, encouraging open access to and use of seeds, supporting local farming systems, and increasing the diversity of our food by supporting diverse seed libraries. Remember that 75 percent of our food comes from just twelve plants (all controlled by Big Ag and chemical companies) and 60 percent comes just from rice, corn, and wheat. This is not good for humans or the planet.

We need to enforce and strengthen antitrust laws to establish fair and functioning markets by breaking up the massive consolidation in the seed, agricultural chemical, fertilizer, and food industries. There is enormous control of the food system by a few dozen companies across these sectors, with very little oversight, which prevents fair competition in the marketplace. They control what is grown, how it is grown, what seeds and chemicals are used, what's manufactured, and even what ends up where on the grocery store shelves. The first antitrust laws were established to break up the railroad, oil, and steel conglomerates in the 1890s. Senator John Sherman, author of the first antitrust law, said, "If we will not endure a king as a political power we should not endure a king over the production, transportation, and sale of any of the necessaries of life." These laws were established to protect consumers, ensure fair competition, and rebuild the infrastructure to link farmers to eaters in their region. The harm done by today's monopolization of the food industry is far greater than any impact of the railroad, oil, and steel industries 100 years ago. Yet the laws are not enforced.

15. Build local and regional capacity to transition the food system from extractive agriculture to regenerative agriculture. While it could take years for land reform and a new farm bill to go into effect, consumers, farmers, and state governments can still do plenty to stem the tide of the environmental fallout and build better farming and better food. As you'll see in the next chapter, regenerative agriculture is absolutely essential. And it will take more than farmers to make that transformation.

16. Align all agricultural and public health policies by providing incentives for purchasing healthy foods and limiting harmful foods in all federal, state, and local programs.

17. Support urban agriculture and vertical farming to both improve food access and food quality and revive impoverished urban communities. A real food fix will align agriculture with nourishing people, repairing our environment, stabilizing our climate, and taking hidden costs out of the system. This alignment is one of the most important challenges of our lifetime.

18. Create federal, state, and local food procurement standards and practices to ensure that tax dollars are spent only on health-promoting foods. This initiative could be modeled after the Good Food Purchasing Program, whose mission is to transform "the way public institutions purchase food by creating a transparent and equitable food system built on five core values: local economies, health, valued workforce, animal welfare, and environmental sustainability. The Center for Good Food Purchasing provides a comprehensive set of tools, technical support, and verification system to assist institutions in meeting their Program goals and commitments" (www.goodfoodpurchasingprogram .org). This should also apply to public hospitals and health care institutions with any government funding (which essentially includes every health care institution that receives money from Medicare or Medicaid). And of course, it must apply to all schools and universities with government funding, the military, prisons, universities, community colleges, day care centers, government offices, and any other government organization or organization that receives government funds.

FOOD FIX: GRASSROOTS AND CITIZEN ACTION

> *Never doubt that a small group of thoughtful, committed citizens can change the world: indeed, it's the only thing that ever has.*
> —MARGARET MEAD (ATTRIBUTED)

If we're not farmers or policy makers, or don't run a Big Ag or Big Food company, can we influence change in agriculture and our food system?

Here's the truth: The deck is stacked against us by the corporate control of government.

But that doesn't mean our actions, our voices, and our votes don't matter. They do. Change happens from the margins to the center. Did Harriet Tubman believe that ferrying a few slaves to freedom was fruitless? Did Emma Goldman believe there was no point marching because the Equal Rights Amendment would not pass even decades after women got the right to vote? They were radicals, on the sidelines, but their voices and actions carried, inspired, and changed an entire entrenched agriculture system based on slavery and delivered women from second-class citizenship.

Your daily food choices absolutely matter, and we all must work together to make agriculture work for producers, consumers, animals, and the land that grows everything we eat.

Here's a list, by no means exhaustive, of what you can do to be part of the solution.

1. Look for the regenerative organic certified label. In 2019, a coalition of groups launched a pilot program to develop Regenerative Organic Certification (ROC).[57] These guidelines should seem self-evident but are not; they are aspirational. ROC is a "beyond organic" certification that involves three areas: soil health, animal welfare, and social fairness.

Learn more about what brands are certified at regenorganic.org /pilot/. It's a start and creates awareness of issues that matter.

2. Join a community-supported agriculture (CSA) program in your area for local organic produce. Go to www.localharvest .org to find one in your area. They will deliver a box of organic vegetables every week at low prices. Get a cow share from a regenerative farm. For example, you can get grass-fed meat for an average of $8 a pound from Mariposa Ranch[58] and other regenerative farms and ranches across the country. That's $2 for a 4-ounce serving or about half the price of a Big Mac. Certainly, this is doable for most families.

3. Shop at farmers' markets. The popularity of farmers' markets is growing, and they support local food systems. While the impact may be small, it provides a foothold into innovations in agriculture that eventually will spread.

4. Start a home garden (even a windowsill of herbs is great). Or reserve a plot in a local community garden. Turn your lawn into an edible garden or orchard. Plant fruit trees and avoid the use of glyphosate herbicides like Roundup and pesticides.

5. Create a community garden. Do it with your church, school, or company or as a family project. Even the CDC determined that community gardens can help rebuild broken communities and reduce violence in urban areas.[59]

6. Educate yourself and your community about regenerative agriculture. Films like *Kiss the Ground* and *The Biggest Little Farm* are a good start. Check out the Carbon Underground to learn more.[60] Take a tour of a regenerative farm to see how it all works.

7. Change your banking and investment strategy to support regenerative and sustainable business solutions. Check out Good Money digital banking (www.goodmoney.com) to learn more about how to put your money in a banking system that aligns with your values. Seek out other social investment companies and options. Most big investment firms now offer this. The Jeremy Coller Foundation in the United Kingdom aggregated institutional investors with $12 trillion in assets and got them to agree to change their investment policies to end factory farming of animals.[61] Their first step was to get the largest twenty fast-food companies to agree to end the use of antibiotics in animal feed by a certain date. They simply told those companies they would divest all their investments if they didn't do what they asked. Who knows? Their next target may be to force Big Food to source from regenerative agriculture. That would be a game changer. Not all of us have that power, but all our little choices matter.

8. Avoid GMO foods as much as possible. Everyone can do this to some degree. In Chapter 6, I mentioned buying non-GMO foods as a way to support grassroots efforts to support non-GMO labeling, but it's also a way to support better agricultural practices through your food choices and avoid potential health issues from the pesticides and herbicides like glyphosate used on GMO foods. You may want to check your urine levels of glyphosate. One test is offered by Great Plains Laboratory; ask your health care provider to order one for you.

9. Vote with your vote. The truth is that if we had an active voting citizenship, much could change. Only 55 percent of Americans vote in presidential elections, and even fewer do in midterm elections, while an average of 70 percent vote in most other democracies.[62] The Food Policy Action network created "An Eater's Guide to Congress" scorecard,[63] rating each member on how they vote on food and agriculture policies. In the 2018 election, two congressmen with dismal scores on food policy were defeated by a targeted social media campaign focused on low-turnout voters.

These are just a few ways to push the rock up the hill. Buying local, organic, and regenerative food is a start. Consider joining or starting a food policy council, through which local people can educate one another and advocate for better food policies.[64] Petition anchor institutions like hospitals and schools to buy locally sourced, regenerative food.[65] Support farmworkers and the organizations, such as the HEAL Alliance, fighting for their rights.[66] Small steps add up to big change if we all participate.

For a quick reference guide on the Food Fixes and resources to restore our natural resources and promote regenerative agriculture, go to www.foodfixbook.com.

CHAPTER 17

THE FOOD AND AG INDUSTRY: THE BIGGEST CONTRIBUTOR TO CLIMATE CHANGE

When you hold an apple (or anything you eat) in your hand, you are connected to a global climate system. The tree that produced the apple takes in carbon dioxide, sunlight, and water to create the fruit. The nitrogen fertilizers, pesticides and herbicides, the truck that transported the apple, and the refrigerator that kept it cool all emit greenhouse gases (GHGs), which trap heat in our atmosphere. Human agriculture is able to exist because of a balance in the carbon cycle. The problem is that the world is heading toward a dangerous destabilization of this balance with carbon dioxide, methane, and nitrous oxide reaching concerning levels.

We may not realize that the corn-sweetened soda we drink, the juicy cheeseburgers raised on factory farms, the chicken breast sandwiches from giant poultry factories, or our GMO soy-based burger drive climate change in a way that is completely unsustainable. Our food system as a whole is the biggest contributor to climate change, even more than the energy sector. And in turn, climate change is threatening the future of food production. Reimagining how we grow, produce, consume, and waste food is the number one solution to reversing climate change. The good news is that it is not too late, but to understand why fixing our food system is so critical to our survival, we have to brace ourselves and focus on the bad news first. Yes, fixing our food system will make us healthier; result in economic abundance; help our kids learn better; improve our nation's mental health; reduce poverty, violence, and social injustice; and even improve national security. And, yes, it will help us conserve our limited water resources, restore healthy soils, and make working conditions better for farmers and food workers, but none of that really matters if we become extinct. And that, my friends, is what most climate scientists believe is happening. The sixth extinction. NASA scientist James Hansen estimates that the amount of heat released into the atmosphere is the equivalent of atomic bombs the size of the one dropped on Hiroshima going off 400,000 times every single day, or about five every second.[1] That is what is happening right now, even if it doesn't seem that way. Understanding how food, agriculture, and climate are all linked may be daunting and depressing, but it is also ultimately hopeful. Many scientists, governments, international agencies, business innovators, agricultural and climate visionaries, and activists understand the intersection of these problems and are building solutions on multiple fronts. And we can all be a part of that with our choices, our voices, and our votes.

IS CLIMATE CHANGE REALLY THAT BAD?

The speed of change of our climate is increasingly evident. Octopi are found in strip mall parking lots as Miami floods. In 2019, we had 500 tornadoes in thirty days, flooding agricultural lands in the Midwest and impacting the ability of the Farm Belt to grow our food. We have once-in-500,000-years rains in Houston. In the Arctic, ice melt is destroying habitat for polar bears and raising sea levels. In May 2019, the global level of carbon dioxide crossed the threshold of 415 parts per million (each part per million equates to 2 billion tons of carbon). The last time Earth saw this level of carbon in the atmosphere (about 800,000 years ago) humans didn't exist and oceans were 100 feet higher, there were hippos swimming in swamps that have become London's Thames River, and trees grew in the South Pole.[2] We're already experiencing the crop failures, droughts, floods, heat waves, and extreme weather associated with climate change.

In David Wallace-Wells's book *The Uninhabitable Earth: Life after Warming*, the first sentence is, "It's worse, much worse than you think." His *New York* magazine article of the same title laid out the threats in bold relief.[3] Hold your nose. This is hard medicine to swallow. But ignoring it won't make it go away. And facing it just might herald our redemption from extinction at worst, or catastrophic disaster at best.

Fifty percent of GHGs now in the atmosphere have been released by humans in the last 25 years, and the rate is accelerating. If GHG emissions continue to rise at current levels, we can expect temperatures to rise up to 4 degrees Celsius or more, and extreme weather to intensify and damage life, infrastructure, and our food system.[4] It may feel like slow change, but we will soon pay the price if we don't reverse the trends. Within 20 years, temperatures are likely to rise more than 2 degrees Celsius. What does that world look like? The polar ice would significantly melt in the summers; coral reefs (on which we depend for our fisheries, which feed 500 million people) would disappear; extreme heat would make much of the South uninhabitable. Severe water scarcity would threaten more than 400 million in urban areas. Rising seas would wipe out island nations and coastal communities. Tropical diseases would migrate north, with 5.2 billion at risk for malaria. Air would increasingly become unbreathable, as it was in China in 2013, when melting arctic ice changed weather patterns, increasing pollution, which led to one-third of deaths that summer. Violence and wars would increase. We would have at least 100 million climate refugees, destabilizing countries around the world. Food would become scarce, with crop failures from heat, drought, and floods. We may need to grow crops at the North Pole rather than North Dakota. Global economies would be threatened by projected costs of more than $50 trillion.

According to the October 2018 report by the UN Intergovernmental Panel on Climate Change[5] we must keep warming to just 1.5 degrees, so that means we have only 12 years to cut our emissions in half and 30 years to cut them to zero. According to the IPCC report, to achieve that, governments would have to radically transform the global economy, energy system, and food systems in ways that do not seem politically likely. Nearly all the countries that signed the Paris Accord are not meeting their pledges to reduce emissions.

"There is no status quo. Change is coming one way or another," climate scientist Dr. Kate Marvel says. "But the fact we understand what's causing climate change gives us power. We can choose the change we experience."[6] The biggest offenders? Farms and food waste. Fixing our food system on the front and back ends is one of the most effective ways to improve our changing climate. Even if we reduce our fossil-fuel use in the near future to zero through electric cars and more solar and wind power, the expansion of CAFO meat production and conventional agriculture with the loss of soil organic matter and soil erosion and ongoing deforestation could still produce enough GHG emissions to raise global warming by 2 degrees Celsius, the level the UN IPCC considers catastrophic.[7]

There is a slim possibility that new technology such as carbon capture machines can help. This suits the fossil-fuel industry and investors because they assume it means we can still pollute and just "capture the carbon," and because it requires huge investment and infrastructure and can be very profitable. The scale needed and costs of this technology are staggering; the technology's ability to draw down enough carbon is unproven; and even if it works it will not fix deforestation, desertification, draining of wetlands, soil loss, or the water cycle, which requires plants to create rain, or restore ecosystems. There is only one thing than can draw down enough carbon fast enough to matter: soil. No sector has more power to reverse global warming and climate catastrophe than our food system. It is the only solution that doesn't just reduce emissions, but also sequesters carbon from the environment through the ancient technologies of soil, plants, and animals.

And while we need to convert to renewable energy, it will not save us. In fact, the only thing that can save us is the Earth itself—and rapid conversion of our current extractive, destructive food and agriculture system to a regenerative one.

INDUSTRIAL FARMS: MASSIVE PLAYERS IN CLIMATE CHANGE

Industrial agriculture contributes to climate change through the over-production of the three main GHGs: methane, nitrous oxide, and carbon dioxide. Here's how:

- Carbon dioxide gets released from the soil through tilling the land (causing loss of organic matter) and through deforestation to grow soy and corn for CAFOs. The world's soils contain three times the carbon contained in the entire atmosphere and can suck up a lot more.
- Methane is released from factory-farmed cattle. It is also released by grass-finished cattle, which some suggest may produce more total methane because it takes longer for those cattle to grow to be market ready. However, this fails to account for the quality of feed (grasses), which leads to less methane production, or methane-fixing bacteria in the soil on rich grasslands, or that the net greenhouse gas emissions on regenerative ranches is negative (meaning more GHGs are stored than released into the environment, actually helping reverse climate change).[8]
- Nitrogen fertilizer pollution turns into nitrous oxide (far more potent than carbon dioxide).
- Food waste in landfills is responsible for off-gassing of GHGs (methane).
- Food transportation, processing, and refrigeration use fossil fuels all along the food chain.

Globally, agriculture and related deforestation are responsible for about a quarter of GHGs, but when every aspect of the food chain is included, it may be more like 50 percent.[9] We must transform our agriculture and food systems to avoid dangerous damage to the climate. In fact, our very survival as a species may depend on it. If we are smart enough, if we act now, we can avert it.

SHOULD WE ALL BE VEGAN OR IS GRASS-FED MEAT THE MOST VEGAN THING YOU CAN EAT?

You've probably read or heard that meat is bad for the climate (and your health) and that we should adopt plant-based diets in order to lower our carbon footprint and prevent disease. The idea goes that if we all become vegans, or close to it, we can save the world and ourselves.

Meatless Mondays, cow farts, plant-based lab meat, and Impossible-brand plant-based GMO soy burgers are all buzzwords swirling around these days. I'm all for eating lots of vegetables, fruits, nuts, seeds, real whole grains, and beans. In fact, I have spent most of my career as a doctor telling people to do just that. We clearly should all be eating a plant-rich diet for our health. And there is no argument that feedlots are anything other than an unmitigated disaster for the cattle finished in them, the humans who eat them, and the planet. Case closed, right? Well, Nicolette Hahn Niman, the vegetarian cattle rancher who wrote *Defending Beef*, put it this way: "It's not the cow; it's the how," a catch-phrase she borrowed from Russ Conser, one of the Soil Carbon Cowboys.

First let's talk about CAFOs and how and why they are so bad for our climate. According to a UN Food and Agriculture Organization figure, using a full life-cycle assessment, livestock are responsible for 14.5 percent of human GHG emissions, more than all transportation emissions.[10] Eighty percent of these emissions come from ruminants (e.g., cattle, sheep, goats), half being methane, a quarter nitrous oxide, and the rest carbon dioxide.[11] The feed required for these operations is often grown with the worst agricultural practices: annual tilling combined with pesticides and fertilizers, often accompanied by deforestation and use of native grasslands to grow food for the animals. Native grasslands are being lost faster than our forests, with dire consequences for the climate and the environment.[12] Preserving grasslands through regenerative livestock integration is essential and profitable.[13] In fact, 70 percent of available agricultural lands are used to grow feed for animals in feedlots for human consumption. A report released by the Institute for Agriculture and Trade Policy calculated emissions from the entire supply chain. Their study found that the world's top five meat and dairy producers combined—Brazil's JBS, New Zealand's Fonterra, Dairy Farmers of America, Tyson Foods, and Cargill—emit more GHGs than oil companies ExxonMobil, Shell, or BP. If these meat and dairy companies continue to grow conventional meat and dairy based on current projections, by 2050 they will be responsible for 81 percent of global emissions.[14]

It should end. Period. Full agreement on all sides.

So, the logical answer, it would seem, is to all become vegan. Not so fast. Not all farms and ranches are the same, nor are all cattle. Grass-fed beef, managed the right way, is good for animals, humans, the environment, and the climate. In fact, properly managed livestock on grasslands and on diversified farms can convert inedible grasses on land unsuitable for crops into healthy protein and nutrients for humans. Well-managed grazing is the most important strategy to create the new soil required to suck carbon out of the atmosphere and save us from extinction.

IT'S NOT THE COW; IT'S THE HOW!

Ranchers who raise grass-fed beef under holistic management (a very specific method of grazing) actually do a lot of good. This term, holistic management, is used interchangeably with "adaptive multi-paddock grazing." Cattle can stimulate the growth of grasses in a way that sequesters, or absorbs, carbon. When cattle are managed through techniques like mob grazing, which mimics the behavior of natural herd animals, they eat some of the grass and then are moved, giving the grass a chance to regenerate. This regeneration draws down carbon through photosynthesis and pushes it through the grass's roots to stimulate the soil biology, as we discussed in the previous chapter.

Other research claims that the amount of methane released into the air from ruminants such as cattle surpasses the amount of carbon those animals sequester on rangelands. The *Grazed and Confused* report, writ-ten by Tara Garnett, a vegetarian, from the Food Climate Research Network found that ruminant methane emissions outweigh the carbon sequestration capacity of grasslands.[15] This is important because methane is a powerful GHG and over the last decade, methane emissions have been rising. Rice cultivation also contributes to climate change and accounts for 10 percent of GHG emissions globally and up to 19 percent of methane emissions. No one says to cut our rice consumption by 90 percent, although innovative methods of rice cultivation can dramatically reduce those emissions. Methane is also produced from poor manure manage-ment on CAFOs, and, yes, cow burps (actually it's fermentation from bac-teria in ruminants' guts). Turns out that fracking for natural gas along with the production of synthetic nitrogen used to fertilize commodity crops (like corn) release more methane than animal agriculture.[16]

Many cite *Grazed and Confused* as proof that even grass-fed cows are harmful to the environment. However, while many of Garnett's find-ings are accurate, there are major flaws in the report.[17] Sadly, ideology often mixes with science, leaving the average reader or policy maker dazed and confused. The flaws in Garnett's report were detailed in a report from the Sustainable Food Trust.[18]

Studies debunking the idea that grass-fed beef can help reverse cli-mate change focus on old-style continuous grazing, which damages the land, not on holistic management, which uses adaptive multi-paddock grazing. Short-term studies Garnett relied on weren't long enough for the benefits of increasing soil carbon to be measured. It takes time to regenerate land and bring it back to life. Looking at carbon cycles over four years, a recent study of using adaptive multi-paddock grazing (which rotates livestock around multiple paddocks to avoid overgrazing and stimulate plant growth) in the Midwest found that approach put more carbon back into the soil (where we need it) than into the air (where it does harm),[19] taking into account methane produced from grass-fed cows. The few papers on which Garnett's assessment was based didn't actually review holistic management, making her assessment of the soil and climate impact of grass-fed cows irrelevant.[20]

Another recent life-cycle analysis of regenerative methods on the White Oak Pastures farm in Georgia also found net carbon sequestration,[21] meaning their farming practices are actually reversing climate change. The degree of sequestration depends on the quality of the soil to start with. Poor soils when rehabilitated will sequester more carbon than soils already in good shape, but much of our soils are depleted to varying degrees and the promise of regenerative agriculture at scale is significant.[22]

CARBON FOOTPRINT BREAKDOWN FOR WOP BEEF

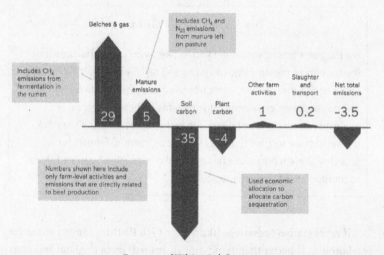

Courtesy of White Oak Pastures

So holistically managed animals can actually be part of a regenerative system that draws carbon out of the atmosphere by building healthy soil and offsets methane emissions as well.[23] In fact, high-quality forage in these actively managed pastures is easier for cattle to digest and reduces methane production. The net benefit of this type of management is carbon sequestration.

The Marin Carbon Project studies "carbon farming" and through meticulous research on grasslands in California also proved that properly managed grasslands remove carbon from the atmosphere. The animals are not optional but essential to the cycle of carbon sequestration.[24] It's a complicated ecosystem. Not accounting for the full cycle and all the players could easily lead to a misinterpretation of the data. In a robust study comparing feedlot beef to adaptive-multi-paddock-raised grass-fed cattle, including all the outside inputs and methane, the grass-fed operations reduced net carbon by 170 percent and the feedlots increased net carbon emissions.[25]

THE BENEFITS OF GRAZING

For the geeks among you, I refer you to twenty-six papers documenting the benefits of the right kind of grazing and regenerative farming for restoring the environment, water retention, increased biodiversity, and soil carbon sequestration, among other benefits.[26] These are known as ecosystem or environmental services. In the report *Greening Livestock*, the benefits are so great that they suggest payment to farmers for providing these services, much like carbon credits, allowing more farmers to transition to regenerative agriculture.[27]

If regenerative operations like White Oak Pastures can net sequester carbon, this is better than removing all animals from the land and converting it to the monocrop soy that is used to create the plant-based Impossible Burgers. While some studies seem to show that regenerative agriculture doesn't produce a net benefit, they are flawed because they examined only conventional (over)grazing and assumed 50 percent of the land was irrigated.[28] True holistic management doesn't require irrigation and builds more soil that holds more carbon. In fact, a comparative analysis of true regenerative practices (from White Oak Pastures) compared to those used to grow GMO monocrop soy for Impossible Burgers found that you would have to eat one 100 percent grass-fed burger to offset the GHG emissions produced by one Impossible Burger.[29] The life-cycle analyses for both the grass-fed burger and the Impossible Burger were done by the same research organization, Quantis.

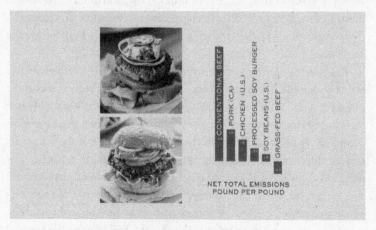

CONVENTIONAL BEEF
PORK (CA)
CHICKEN (U.S.)
PROCESSED SOY BURGER
SOY BEANS (U.S.)
GRASS-FED BEEF

NET TOTAL EMISSIONS
POUND PER POUND

Courtesy of White Oak Pastures

We should be cautious of anyone trying to sell a simplified food solution that requires eliminating cows from the planet or eating only vegan. The suggestion to completely cut out meat also means we'd be cutting out essential amino acids, high-quality protein, and highly bio-available nutrients such as preformed vitamins A_1, K_2, D_3, and B_{12} from our diet. If we ditched meat, where would the alternative plant-based protein come from? Nuts and soy still have an environmental and climate impact if grown with conventional methods. We can't convert rangeland used for livestock into cropland because it is often "marginal," meaning the soil quality and/or moisture won't allow crops to grow. Additionally, the tilling and irrigation required to convert rangeland into cropland to grow more soy, corn, and wheat winds up producing more CO_2. So, without livestock, we would forgo the use of rangeland that could do two very important things: (1) generate high-quality, nutrient-dense protein, and (2) restore ecosystems and biodiversity and store large amounts of rainwater and carbon, creating a virtuous cycle of fertility, food, and environmental restoration.

The best solution for rangelands is managing livestock in ways that sequester carbon, help prevent floods and droughts, and promote biodiversity. On top of that, water consumption by animals on rangelands is mostly rainwater, so it doesn't contribute to depletion of the earth's fresh water the way the irrigation required to grow feed for feedlot cattle does.

Regenerative grazing restores the land and supports livestock and all forms of wildlife—a beautiful ecological cycle. Land regenerates as the soil is restored. With better grazing practices, where cattle eat only half the forage before being moved, the root mass is retained. And the roots continuously pump carbon into the ground. This causes the soil structure to improve and thus more water infiltrates and is retained. The nutrients from the soil are more available. There's more plant growth and forage, which in turn transpire both water vapor and monoterpenes, molecules created by forests that form aerosols, which create clouds, create more rain, and cool the climate. Soil science, botany, and atmospheric science are all closely interconnected. The circle of life!

It is often pointed out that grass-fed meats are expensive and elitist and can't be scaled. But they can, and then some. Allen Williams, PhD, has done the math.[30] There are 29 million grain-fed cattle consumed from factory farms in America every year. By using idle grasslands, including existing USDA Conservation Reserve Program land unsuitable for farming but good for grazing, and converting corn and soy monocrops used for fattening feedlot cows, we could produce 52.9 million grass-fed head of cattle a year, which is almost double what's produced in feedlots today. Those grass-fed cattle would help revitalize rural communities, reverse climate change, increase biodiversity, reduce water use, and improve soil health. Similar approaches can be used globally. While we don't need that much meat, the argument that this is simply an elitist, limited strategy is clearly false.

Agriculture is massively destructive—and not just factory farms. Even growing beans, grains, and vegetables is inherently harmful because the natural ecosystem and animal habitat supporting wild animals such as rabbits, rodents, turkeys, bees, earthworms, and insects is destroyed, not to mention the living, breathing system that is soil and all its trillions of inhabitants. A 2018 study entitled *Field Deaths in Plant Agriculture* estimated that 7.3 billion animals are killed every year from plant agriculture. Even organic vegetable farms use bone meal and oyster shells to enhance soil and plant health.[31] I respect the moral choice of being a vegan, but the idea that it is saving animals and the planet and even improving our health is unfortunately not true. Turns out a cornfield is much more destructive than a grass-fed beef regenerative farm or ranch.

THE EAT-LANCET COMMISSION REPORT ON HEALTHY DIETS AND SUSTAINABLE FOOD SYSTEMS

The good news is that there is increasing awareness and extensive science on the links between our current food system, how and what food it produces, and the links to health, the environment, and climate. The EAT-Lancet Commission report was a notable attempt to highlight these issues.

The report got a lot right:

- The need for plant-rich diets
- Reductions in sugar and processed foods
- Reduction or elimination of factory-farmed meat
- Highlighting the importance of transitioning to sustainable agricultural systems that address environmental degradation and climate change and the need to feed a population of 10.5 billion by 2050 in a sustainable way for the planet
- Providing flexible guidelines for diet that match cultural and geographical needs
- Providing the first-ever scientific modeling connecting diet, environment, and climate to create healthy humans, environment, and climate

While there are always challenges in modeling and the underlying science that informs any attempt at developing guidelines, the report takes a big leap forward in defining the issues and spurring further research and policy actions. However, many scientists have taken issue with the science, the omissions, and the conclusion that we should dramatically reduce meat consumption (the average American man consumes 68 grams of meat a day, or about 10 ounces, while the EAT-Lancet advises only 7 grams a day, or one ounce — one once of protein is about 7 grams), which can produce a nutritionally deficient diet.[32] The EAT-Lancet Commission does acknowledge that the sick, elderly, malnourished, and young have higher protein needs that cannot be met by a plant-based diet and that low consumption of animal-based foods in children results in stunting, anemia, and malnutrition, while increased consumption of those foods results in improved growth, nutritional status, cognitive performance, motor development, and health.

The data on the harmful effects of meat used in their analysis is from population-based studies fraught with problems, the biggest of which is that cause and effect cannot be determined from those studies. It is an association that can and does have many other explanations. In rigorous reviews, up to 80 percent of these conclusions from population-based studies turn out to be false when subjected to proper clinical trials. These are the other issues that have been identified with the EAT-Lancet Commission report:

- No explicit recognition that well-managed holistic farm and rangeland ecosystems require animals to sequester carbon
- Calls for increased use of chemical inputs, which is perplexing considering the toxicity of nitrogen pollution to the soil, water, and climate, to support growth in developing countries, which may be better served by more local, regenerative practices that don't depend on outside chemical and seed inputs
- Contradictory mention of managed grazing and the use of manure as part of the solution but no acknowledgment of the profound difference between CAFO meat and grass-fed regeneratively raised meat

- Thirty-one out of thirty seven scientists behind the report have published records in favor of vegan or vegetarian diets or against meat
- No external peer review, and conflicts of interest not reported
- Members of their corporate partner FReSH (Food Reform for Sustainability and Health)[33] hail from big seed monopolies, fertilizer giants, agrochemical companies, Big Pharma (seven companies), and food behemoths including Bayer (Monsanto), DuPont, Syngenta, Yara (the biggest nitrogen fertilizer company), PepsiCo, and Cargill[34]

Twenty of the largest Big Food companies signed up to support the report. Why would they be supporting this platform? Hidden within it is the implicit need to grow more grains and beans and food products using industrial agriculture, seeds, fertilizer, and chemicals that drive profits for all these companies.

Physicist and agroecologist Dr. Vandana Shiva says that the EAT-Lancet report evades the "glaring chronic disease epidemic related to pesticides and toxins in food, imposed by chemically intensive industrial agriculture and food systems."[35] She says, "Instead of recognizing the role of organic farming and agroecology for providing sustainable ways for repairing the broken nitrogen cycle, the report recommends 'redistribution of global use of nitrogen and phosphorus,' which in effect is saying chemicals should be spread in the Third World."[36] We've already exported our ultraprocessed foods to developing countries to the detriment of their health. Should we really harm them even more by exporting our chemicals, and expanding extractive, fossil-fuel, and chemical-industrial agriculture to grow more grains and beans?

It is true that the developed world eats too much meat, and the wrong meat. But eating less meat and better meat is good for you and the planet. Meat can be responsibly raised and ideally should complement a plant-rich diet.

BUT ISN'T MEAT BAD FOR OUR HEALTH?

The question of whether meat is bad for our health has been extensively debated, sadly mostly along ideological lines, not accurate scientific data. Nearly all studies on the harm of meat studied only factory-farmed meat, and they are population-based studies that cannot prove cause and effect. Meat eaters in those studies were an unhealthy lot. They smoked more, drank more, ate less fruits and vegetables, exercised less, and ate 800 more calories a day than the non–meat eaters.[37] Many other studies contradict those findings as well. The PURE study of 135,000 people found those who ate animal protein and fat had fewer heart attacks and deaths than those who ate more cereal grains.[38] Another study of food consumption patterns in forty-two countries showed a lower risk of heart disease and death in those who ate animal fat and protein and higher risk in those who ate cereal grains and potatoes.[39] A 17-year study of vegetarians and meat eaters who shopped at health food stores found mortality dropped in half for both groups.[40] Other studies point to the nutritional benefits of grass-fed meat, including higher levels of omega-3 fats and CLA (a metabolism-boosting anti-cancer fat) and high levels of minerals, vitamins, and antioxidants.[41]

I have reviewed this subject extensively in my book *Food: WTF Should I Eat?* I also recommend, for those who want to take a deep dive into the research, Chris Kresser's online review of the science, called "Why Eating Meat Is Good for You."[42] Read the data. Decide for yourself. Avoid relying on inflammatory documentaries or others' interpretation of the science (including mine).

FOOD FIX: ADAPTING FOOD SYSTEMS TO CLIMATE CHANGE

The worse climate change becomes, the harder it will be to grow crops in hotter, more unstable climate conditions. The faster we can transform the food system, the better we will be in terms of buffering the effects of climate chaos.

It may seem complex to transform agriculture. And it is. We need overall change of the economic, political, and agricultural systems that cause environmental destruction. We need to build systems that can address regeneration of soil, water, climate, biodiversity, and human communities. Luckily, efforts are already underway.

You may have heard about Project Drawdown, a quantified study of the eighty most effective solutions to climate change. Paul Hawken started Project Drawdown to change the climate narrative from doom and gloom and to focus on solutions that currently exist. *Drawdown: The Most Comprehensive Plan Ever Proposed to Reverse Global Warming* (because no other plan has been proposed) lays out all the solutions that are scientifically established. This is not just about slowing emissions, converting to renewable energy, climate mitigation, or carbon taxes or credits, which are most of the solutions proposed in the Paris Accord. Those measures are necessary but not sufficient. What's required is literally to massively reduce or draw down carbon from the atmosphere.

Project Drawdown collected proven, data-driven, economically viable, commonly available solutions that remove carbon from the atmosphere while saving billions of dollars, far offsetting the costs of implementing the solutions. Nothing new needs to be invented, though innovation will drive more solutions over time. Hawken brought together a team of seventy scientists from twenty-two countries that analyzed the data and mathematically modeled the most effective ways to reduce GHG emissions as well as take carbon out of the atmosphere and put it back into the soil. Each solution is measured by gigatons of CO_2 reduced, the cost to implement, and the billions saved. Guess what tops the list. Food-related solutions collectively were the number one solution to reverse global warming. We also need to draw down fossil-fuel extraction worldwide while scaling up renewable energy.

The data is clear: Our food system as a whole is the number one cause and the number one solution to climate change. Project Drawdown outlines the food-based strategies that collectively will make the biggest difference for human and planetary health.[43]

- Support regenerative agriculture, optimizing farmland irrigation and managed grazing, which is estimated to reduce CO_2 by 23 gigatons and save $1.93 trillion on an investment of $57 billion.
- Shift agriculture to support a plant-rich diet that is ideally regeneratively grown (which doesn't mean going vegan, just eating mostly plants).
- Restore depleted farmland and protect the Amazon rain forest from expanding cattle ranching and monocrop soy production for CAFOs. Deforestation is also driven by land speculation because land without trees is worth 100 to 200 times more than land with forest.
- Address food waste, including mandated food composting. Composting addresses food waste while improving soil health.
- Reduce fertilizer use and improve nutrient management to draw down 1.8 gigatons of CO_2 and save farmers $102 billion.
- Improve rice cultivation (which now accounts for 10 percent of GHG emissions and 19 to 29 percent of global methane emissions).
- Intercrop trees and crops to reduce inputs and create healthier crops and higher yields.
- Develop silvopasture, lands that integrate trees with pastures for cattle or livestock that forage in the forests.
- Scale no-till farming and conservation agriculture.
- Plant more tropical staple food trees such as avocados, coconuts, and tree legumes to provide food and sequester carbon.
- Create government financial incentives for new enzyme and algal technologies that greatly reduce methane emissions from cows.

All these practices have been scientifically quantified in both cost savings and gigatons of carbon that would be reduced.

To learn more, read *Drawdown: The Most Comprehensive Plan Ever Proposed to Reverse Global Warming*, edited by Paul Hawken (www.drawdown.org).

ENDING FOOD WASTE: A SOLUTION FOR HUNGER AND CLIMATE CHANGE

Imagine throwing away a third of your paycheck. Ridiculous, right? Well, a third to half of the food we grow does not make it from the farm to your fork to your belly. To grow the food we waste in the United States, it would take 780 million pounds of pesticides and 4.2 trillion gallons of water on 30 million acres of cropland.[44] To grow all the food we waste around the world—about 1.6 billion pounds' worth— it would take the entire landmass of China![45] And the loss of all that food costs our economy $2.6 trillion a year, or about 4 percent of global world product.[46]

This is an obvious waste of resources at every stage. Think of the labor, seeds, water, energy, land, fertilizer, and money that end up in the landfill. Even worse, when this wasted food sits in the landfill, it undergoes anaerobic decomposition (decomposition without oxygen) and generates methane gas—a powerful GHG. If you are worried about cow burps, you should be much more worried about the consequences of your veggies ending up in a landfill. Under the current system, the food we waste is responsible for roughly 8 percent of global emissions. If food waste were a country, it would be the third-largest emitter of GHGs after the United States and China.

The new UN Sustainable Development Goals have called for cutting food waste in half by 2030.[47] Food waste can happen because prices are too low, and farmers leave food to rot in the fields because it is not worth selling even though it is perfectly good. Food waste can also come from food that is ugly, misshapen, or not "perfect," like the 800 million pounds of sun-bleached watermelons that are thrown out every year.[48] Food service companies, restaurants, retailers, and consumers waste food at each step, and much ends up in landfills. Grocery chains police their garbage to make sure dumpster divers don't get their slightly overripe food—which, by the way, is still safe to eat. Restaurants overorder to be sure not to run out of anything and disappoint their customers.

Rich and poor countries waste food for different reasons and need different solutions. While poor countries struggle with lack of refrigeration, bad roads, heat, humidity, and lack of proper packaging, they waste almost no food once it enters the home. But rich countries throw out massive quantities of food. Americans throw out 35 percent of the food in their fridge.[49] "Best by" and "sell by" dates are related not to food safety but to when the food will taste best, which only confuses customers and leads to massive food waste.

A family of four throws away $1,800 in food every year,[50] and in the United States we spend $218 billion a year, or 1.3 percent of our GDP, growing, processing, transporting, and disposing of food that is never eaten.[51] We have more than enough food to feed all 7 billion humans. We grow enough food for 10.5 billion. But more than 40 percent (some estimate more) is wasted at every step in the food chain.[52]

METABOLIC FOOD WASTE: HOW THE OBESITY EPIDEMIC CONTRIBUTES TO CLIMATE CHANGE

Is there an environmental and climate cost to obesity? It turns out the answer is yes, and it's a big cost. Ten percent of the world's population doesn't have enough food to eat, while 30 percent of the population is overweight. Big Food and Big Ag have produced about 500 calories more a day per person in the United States than in the 1970s, and we have eaten them. That's about 170 billion extra calories a day just in the United States. The energy, water, and soil needed, and GHGs produced, in growing all that excess food (which makes us sick and fat and has been pushed on us by the food industry) globally equates to about 140 gigatons of carbon a year.[53] To put that in perspective, the total annual emissions of CO_2 from the fossil-fuel industry are 9.7 gigatons. The explosion of obesity across the globe, it turns out, is not only damaging human health, but also driving climate change.

FOOD FIX: FOOD WASTE INNOVATIONS

No one is for food waste. The US government has made addressing it a priority. In October 2018, the USDA partnered with other agencies on the Winning on Reducing Food Waste Initiative. This is big! The government is focused on research, community investments, education and outreach, voluntary programs, public-private partnerships, tool development, technical assistance, event participation, and policy discussion to end food waste. Reducing our GHG emissions and our food waste will require all hands on deck working with local governments, national policy makers, farmers, distribution chains, grocery chains, restaurants, food service providers, and every citizen in their kitchen. Wherever I have lived for the past 40 years, I have had a compost pile. Even in New York City I can drop off food scraps at a farmers' market in Union Square to be composted. Some cities and countries mandate a zero-waste policy for food scraps. A few key innovators are worth mentioning.

- **France.** The French have a law that grocery stores cannot throw out any food. It must be composted or given to food banks or charities. Grocery store owners must pay a $4,500 fine or go to jail for two years if they throw food in the garbage.[54]
- **San Francisco.** San Francisco turns garbage into profit with their new composting law, the Mandatory Recycling and Composting Ordinance, which makes composting mandatory, even for tourists. The city provides the bins for every citizen. This is a win-win solution. Not only do they avoid food in landfills, which causes climate change, but they also contribute to the solution of building healthy soils.
- **Apeel Sciences.** This company has created an edible, safe, vegetable-derived coating for produce that more than doubles shelf life, protecting it from the farm to your fridge.
- **Imperfect Produce.** Twenty billion pounds of perfectly good produce are thrown out on farms because they are not perfect or they are funny-looking. Who wants a carrot with two legs, or a weird-looking potato? I do. Imperfect Produce solves this problem

by taking millions of pounds of ugly food thrown out at farms, packaging them up, and shipping them directly to your door. Buy ugly food. Save the planet; feed yourself.

Food activists have pointed out that Imperfect Produce's strategies take food waste from industrial agriculture and resell it at a discount, undermining the economic base of local farmers and community-supported agriculture.[55] Imperfect Produce is doing good and giving conscious consumers a chance to do the right thing, but we need educated and critical conversations about the effect innovations will have across the spectrum of agriculture and consumers.

- **WTRMLN WTR.** The founder of this company turns 800 million pounds of ugly watermelon that are thrown out every year into the most delicious, nutrient-dense, low-sugar beverage, which beats out coconut water in minerals, nutrients, and electrolytes. It's the Gatorade replacement.
- **Food Maven.** This company takes oversupply from grocery stores and imperfect or ugly food and produce from local farmers and ranchers who have a hard time getting their food to market and provides a marketplace for restaurants to buy the food at 50 percent off.

FOOD FIX: WHAT YOU CAN DO

Here's how you can join the movement to save our planet and transform the food system.

1. Eat at restaurants that serve organic, farm-to-table, and/or regenerative food. Restaurants all over the world are putting sustainability on the menu, supporting local food systems, preserving lost varieties of vegetables and animals, and more. Restaurants across the world are embracing sustainability and healthier eating. Find ones in your neighborhood.

2. Look for food labels that identify sustainable, humane food sources including American Grassfed Association, American Humane Certified, Animal Welfare Review Certified, Global Animal

Partnership, Certified Sustainable Seafood MSC, Biodynamic, and Bird Friendly, among others.

3. Support innovation and policies for food and agricultural practices that help to reverse climate change. Elect leaders who are committed to implementing policies that support regenerative agriculture and reduce the use of fossil fuels and bring us closer to 100 percent renewable power.

4. Start and support businesses that draw down carbon through agroforestry, silvopasture, holistic grazing, and composting operations. Learn more from groups like Land Link, LandCoreUSA, and Regeneration International.

5. Reduce your own food waste. Use Fresh Paper, a simple piece of paper infused with herbs that keeps your produce fresh three to four times longer, or use produce protected by Apeel, the plant-derived coating that keeps produce fresher longer. Make soups or stews from veggies that are a little wilted. Cook just enough for your family, and make sure to eat all your leftovers.

6. Start a compost pile. That way, whatever waste or food scraps you produce don't end up in a landfill. No more produce, grains, or beans in landfills. Composting allows food scraps to biodegrade aerobically by exposing them to oxygen, rotating the food scraps, and mixing them with brown matter (such as sawdust, cardboard, or leaves). This turns it into a nutrient-rich organic material that can be used to help build soil in gardens, farms, or your backyard.

Studies found that when compost is applied to rangelands, the compost increased production between 40 and 70 percent, increased soil carbon sequestration, which pulls carbon dioxide from the air into the ground, allowed soil to hold more water, and provided nitrogen and other nutrients to improve soil quality.[56] Your garbage can help reverse global warming.

If you live in a city, consider advocating for a municipal-level composting program. Find out if there is an urban compost drop-off center in your city or town. If you have a backyard, create a compost pile there. If you live in an apartment, get a kitchen composter. You might even consider starting a community or city compost program like the one in Sacramento called BioCycle. Or petition your local government to start one.

Most important, don't forget to eat well, thank your farmers and ranchers, and remember that fixing our food system is a choice you can make every day. You have patiently waded through a deep, long lesson on the environmental and climate impacts of our food and agriculture system, and what policies, business innovations, and you can do about it. Understanding is the first step in shifting our food system to one that is good for humans, animals, the economy, communities, and the planet. Action at every level is needed to transform our food system. It's time.

For a quick reference guide on the Food Fixes and resources to reverse climate change through food-related solutions, go to www.foodfixbook.com.

THE FUTURE OF FOOD, HUMANS, AND THE PLANET

Where are you going to leave your one grain of spiritual sand on the universal scales of humanity?

—COMMON (PARAPHRASED)

Facing the facts of our food system is sobering. But after years of research and after speaking to dozens of experts, scientists, and policy makers about the solutions, I am left with a sense of hope and possibility. Understanding the problems and challenges we face sets the foundation for the solutions. It is also the beginning of reimagining a food system that provides real, whole, nutrient-dense food across the globe, addressing hunger and obesity. A food system that saves trillions of wasted dollars every year that could be redirected to solving our most intractable problems of disease, poverty, violence, lack of education, and social injustice. A food system that restores ecosystems, builds soil, protects our scarce water resources, reduces pollution, increases biodiversity, and reverses climate change. A food system that builds rather than destroys communities. A food system that is not extractive and destructive to everything that matters but is restorative and regenerative. A food system that is redemptive rather than rapacious.

We need to think about these issues as one interconnected, intersecting set of challenges that we can and must address if we are to reverse the crises we now face and avert the disasters just over the horizon. As Donald Rumsfeld once said, this is a "known known." We may not be able to end war or achieve immortality, but this is a solvable problem. Yes, it will take enormous effort from every stakeholder, but first we must be able to see the problem in its entirety, draw the map, connect the dots, embrace the dangers we face as a species and a planet. That is the hope of *Food Fix*. This is just the beginning, a vision and call to action for fixing our food system.

This affects all of us, whether you are the CEO of Bayer or Coca-Cola or the head of the Sustainable Food Trust or the Environmental Working Group, or Republican, Democrat, Muslim, Christian, Jewish, any race or any ethnicity. This is the defining problem of our time and as yet has not been clearly recognized as a threat or addressed in a global, coherent, coordinated, strategic way.

We need new ideas, strategies, policies, and business innovations to fix these problems and bring diverse groups together to solve them together. Imagine if the groups at odds with one another come together to fight a common problem. It is possible. Solutions exist. They are achievable, and we need the push up from grassroots efforts and from the top down to shift public opinion, to create a movement that forces legislatures and policy makers to take notice and take action.

Remember that the campaigns for abolition, suffrage for women, civil rights, women's rights, and gay rights didn't start in Congress. They ended in Congress. These massive shifts in laws occurred because we voted with our voices, our actions, and our ballots. We can vote with our forks and vote with our votes. Our collective actions and behaviors will move things in the right direction, and our children and their children might enjoy a sustainable future of good food and a safe climate.

The work has begun across the globe, illuminating a hopeful way forward. These nuggets of innovation and creativity restoring land and communities and inspiring new policies are the seeds of a new future. The nonprofit Beacons of Hope: Transforming Food Systems gathers these stories, learns from them, and has created a pathway for future change.[1]

Food Fix is just the beginning, the outline of the future of food pointing to solutions for citizens, grassroots organizations, advocacy groups, philanthropists, businesses, and governments. These are just a few of the many innovations and ideas moving from the margins to the center and providing a road map for fixing our food system. It is the great work of our time. And it depends on all of us.

We need a national (and ultimately global) campaign to fix our food system. If you're interested in helping transform our food system and want to learn more, please join our campaign and prescription for a new food system at www.foodrxcampaign.org.

FOR MORE INFORMATION

For a quick reference guide to all the Food Fixes in this book, visit www.foodfixbook.com.

To learn more about any of the issues that stem from our food industry, take a look at our online resource guide for articles, studies, reports, books, videos, companies, and organizations that are raising awareness and changing the conversation at www.foodfixbook.com/resources.

Acknowledgments

This book was inspired by the work of an endless list of individuals dedicated to transforming the food system starting from the farm and extending all the way to our fork and beyond. There are thousands of people who are fighting this good fight along with me, and I would like to take this opportunity to thank them, specifically those who helped to bring this labor of love to life. And any whom I didn't mention, all the tireless workers, warriors, farmers, health activists, food leaders, and voices of truth, without your inspiration, teaching, and support, this book would never have come to be. Thank you.

I'd like to thank my patients, who will always be my greatest teachers and the reason behind my passion for creating a happier and healthier world.

I'd also like to thank my book team: Andrea Vinley Converse for her insights and for keeping this project organized while constantly keeping my vision in mind. Will Munger and my daughter, Rachel Hyman, gathered research and provided insight into the effects of our food system on the environment and workers' rights. Thank you to Kaya Purohit for supporting our research team and conducting interviews. *Food Fix* would not have been possible without this all-star team. My deep gratitude goes to Stephen Zwick, a fountain of insight, knowledge, nuance, and science who helped me get the story right. And to Dr. Dariush Mozaffarian, a visionary thinker and leader doing the hard research and telling the whole story of food and its impact on everything and inspiring me with his advocacy linking food and policy— thanks to him as well for reviewing and helping with the final manuscript! And of course, my friend David Ludwig, whose rigorous science, public health advocacy, and political vision for a better future of health for all of us has guided my way for a long, long time.

Much gratitude to Scott Hatch for his thoughtful review of the manuscript, which hopefully kept me on mission and out of trouble, and for envisioning a campaign to fix our food system: FoodRx.

A special thank-you to everyone we interviewed and who contributed their wealth of knowledge to this project: Lisel Loy, Barry Popkin, Chris Kresser, Gunhild Stordalen, Congressman Tim Ryan, Congresswoman Chellie Pingree, Larry Summers, Dan Glickman, Ann Veneman, Michele Simon, Jerold Mande, Laura Schmidt, John Robbins, Lance Price, Aseem Malhotra, Vishen Lakhiani, Steven Druker, Kelly Brownell, Nina Teicholz, John Ioannidis, Vani Hari, Pamela Koch, Hawk Newsome, Navina Khanna, Dr. David Montgomery, Paul Hawken, Walter Robb, William Li, Leah Penniman, Kimbal Musk, Danielle Niernberg, Kavita Shulka, Mark Bittman, Dan Barber, Tom Colicchio, David Wallace-Wells, Sonia Angell, Marco Canora, David Bouley, Thomas Newmark, Rain Henderson, Chilean senator Guido Girardi, Stephen Ritz, Robert Egger, and Ben Simon—thank you for all that you do and allowing us to share it with the world.

I'd also like to thank my teams at the UltraWellness Center and the Cleveland Clinic Center for Functional Medicine. A special thank-you to Liz Boham, Todd Lepine, George Papanicolaou, Gerry Doherty, and the entire UWC staff, and at CCFM thank you to Toby Cosgrove, Tawny Jones, Patrick Hanaway, Michele Beidelschies, Elizabeth Bradley, Mary Curran, Tomislav Mihaljevic, Adam Myers, Nazleen Bharmal, and Jim Young. These teams are dedicated to transforming health care, and I am so grateful to get to work with every single one of these folks in our joint mission.

A huge thank-you to the Hyman Digital Team: Dhru Purohit, Kaya Purohit, Ronit Menashe, Yali Menashe, Jennifer Sanders, Farrell Feighan, Ailsa Cowell, Melanie Haraldson, Lauren Feighan, Ben Tseitlin, Darci Gross, Audria Brumberg, Courtney McNary, Alex Gallegos, and Hema Shah. Thank you for making my life so much easier and for nurturing and expanding our platform so that we can spread our message far and wide. And a special thank-you to Meredith Jones, who helps me keep all of my projects and life in order so that I get to do what I love to do every single day.

All of my success over the last 20 years would not have been possible without the support and guidance of my publishing team, which believed in me and gave me the chance to publish so many books. My editor, Tracy Behar, makes every word and story better and is beyond patient with me. Richard Pine, my agent, has made all my dreams come true. My team at Little, Brown is fabulously talented at getting my books out in the world. Without them, my hopes and dreams would still be in my head and not making the impact they are. Thank you.

And finally, I'd like to thank my family, and my wife, Mia, for bringing so much joy, laughter, and adventure to my life, and for being my greatest friend and confidante.

Notes

CHAPTER 1

1. Chen S, Kuhn M, Prettner K, Bloom DE. "The Macroeconomic Burden of Noncommunicable Diseases in the United States: Estimates and Projections." *PLoS One*. 2018 Nov 1;13(11):e0206702.

2. Ng M, Fleming T, Robinson M, et al. "Global, Regional, and National Prevalence of Overweight and Obesity in Children and Adults during 1980–2013: A Systematic Analysis for the Global Burden of Disease Study 2013." *Lancet*. 2014 Aug 30;384(9945):766–81.

3. Schnabel L, Kesse-Guyot E, Allès B, et al. "Association between Ultraprocessed Food Consumption and Risk of Mortality among Middle-Aged Adults in France." *JAMA Intern Med*. 2019 Feb 11.

4. Waters H, Graf M. "The Cost of Chronic Diseases in the U.S.: Executive Summary." Milken Institute. May 2018. https://assets1c.milkeninstitute.org/assets/Publication/Viewpoint/PDF/Chronic-Disease-Executive-Summary-r2.pdf.

5. Waters H, Graf M. "America's Obesity Crisis: The Health and Economic Costs of Excess Weight." Milken Institute. October 2018. https://assets1c.milkeninstitute.org/assets/Publication/ResearchReport/PDF/Mi-Americas-Obesity-Crisis-WEB.pdf.

6. GBD 2015 Obesity Collaborators, Murray CJL, et al. "Health Effects of Overweight and Obesity in 195 Countries over 25 Years." *N Engl J Med*. 2017 Jul 6;377(1):13-27.

7. Levit MR, Austin DA, Stupak JM. "Mandatory Spending Since 1962." Congressional Research Service. March 18, 2015. https://fas.org/sgp/crs/misc/RL33074.pdf.

8. US Government Accountability Office. "The Nation's Fiscal Health: Action Is Needed to Address the Federal Government's Fiscal Future." GAO-19-314SP. April 2019. https://www.gao.gov/assets/700/698368.pdf.

9. Bloom DE, Cafiero ET, Jané-Llopis E, et al. "The Global Economic Burden of Noncommunicable Diseases." Geneva, World Economic Forum. Retrieved May 25, 2016, from http://www3.weforum.org/docs/WEF_Harvard_HE_GlobalEconomicBurdenNonCommunicableDiseases_2011.pdf.

10. Dobbs R, Sawers C, Thompson F, et al. "Overcoming Obesity: An Initial Economic Analysis." McKinsey Global Institute. November 2014. https://www.mckinsey.com/~/media/McKinsey/Business%20Functions/Economic%20Studies%20TEMP/Our%20Insights/How%20the%20world%20could%20better%20fight%20obesity/MGI_Overcoming_obesity_Full_report.ashx.

11. Ibid.

12. New York State Assembly bill A8419. June 16, 2019. https://nyassembly.gov/leg/?default_fld=&leg_video=&bn=A08419&term=2019&Summary=Y&Memo=Y&Text=Y.

13. Bureau of Labor Statistics. (2017). "Occupational Employment and Wages, May 2017." https://www.bls.gov/oes/2017/may/oes353031.htm.

14. Sustainable Food Trust. "The True Cost of American Food: Conference Proceedings." San Francisco, April 2016. http://sustainablefoodtrust.org/wp-content/uploads/2013/04 /TCAF-report.pdf.

15. Patel S, Sangeeta S. "Pesticides As the Drivers of Neuropsychotic Diseases, Cancers, and Teratogenicity among Agro-Workers As Well As General Public." *Environ Sci Pollut Res Int.* 2019 Jan;26(1):91–100.

16. Wood TJ, Goulson D. "The Environmental Risks of Neonicotinoid Pesticides: A Review of the Evidence Post 2013." *Environ Sci Pollut Res Int.* 2017 Jul;24(21):17285–325.

17. Food and Agriculture Organization of the United Nations. "What Is Happening to Agrobiodiversity?" Retrieved May 25, 2019, from http://www.fao.org/3/y5609e/y5609e 02.htm.

18. Mozaffarian D, Rogoff KS, Ludwig DS. "The Real Cost of Food: Can Taxes and Subsidies Improve Public Health?" *JAMA.* 2014;312(9):889–90.

19. Plumer B. "How Much of the World's Cropland Is Actually Used to Grow Food?" *Vox.* December 16, 2014. https://www.vox.com/2014/8/21/6053187/cropland-map-food-fuel -animal-feed.

20. Lehner P. "The Hidden Costs of Food." *HuffPost.* August 16, 2017. https://www.huff post.com/entry/the-hidden-costs-of-food_b_11492520.

21. United Nations. "United Nations Decade: For Deserts and the Fight against Desertification." https://www.un.org/en/events/desertification_decade/value.shtml.

22. Alavanja MC. "Introduction: Pesticides Use and Exposure Extensive Worldwide." *Rev Environ Health.* 2009;24(4):303–9.

23. Thomas D. "A Study on the Mineral Depletion of the Foods Available to US As a Nation Over the Period 1940 to 1991." *Nutr Health* 2003;17:85–115.

24. Garris A. "Industrial Methane Emissions Are Underreported, Study Finds." *Cornell Chronicle.* June 6, 2019. https://news.cornell.edu/stories/2019/06/industrial-methane-emi ssions-are-underreported-study-finds.

25. Lehner P. "The Hidden Costs of Food." *HuffPost.* August 16, 2017. https://www.huff post.com/entry/the-hidden-costs-of-food_b_11492520.

26. Khokhar T. (2017). "Chart: Globally, 70% of Freshwater Is Used for Agriculture." *Data Blog.* World Bank. March 22, 2017. https://blogs.worldbank.org/opendata/chart-glob ally-70-freshwater-used-agriculture.

27. Frankel J. "Crisis on the High Plains: The Loss of America's Largest Aquifer—the Ogallala." *U Denv Water L Rev.* May 17, 2018. http://duwaterlawreview.com/crisis-on-the-high -plains-the-loss-of-americas-largest-aquifer-the-ogallala/.

28. Majendie A, Parija Pratik. "How to Halt Global Warming for $300 Billion." *Bloomberg.* October 23, 2019. https://www.bloomberg.com/news/articles/2019-10-23/how-to-halt -global-warming-for-300-billion.

29. Canning P, Charles A, Huang S, et al. "Energy Use in the U.S. Food System." US Department of Agriculture. Economic Research Report Number 94. March 2010. http://web.mit.edu/dusp/dusp_extension_unsec/reports/polenske_ag_energy.pdf.

30. Food and Agriculture Organization of the United Nations. (2015). "Fertilizer Use to Surpass 200 Million Tonnes in 2018." http://www.fao.org/news/story/en/item/277488/icode/.

31. Prior R. (2019). "An Ohio City Has Voted to Grant Lake Erie the Same Rights As a Person." CNN. https://www.cnn.com/2019/02/21/us/ohio-city-lake-erie-rights-trnd/index.html.

32. Biello D. (2008). "Oceanic Dead Zones Continue to Spread." *Scientific American*. https://www.scientificamerican.com/article/oceanic-dead-zones-spread/.

33. Sobota DJ, Compton JE, McCrackin ML, Singh S. "Cost of Reactive Nitrogen Release from Human Activities to the Environment in the United States." *Environ Res Lett*. 2015 Feb 17;10(2):025006.

34. Temkin A, Evans S, Manidis T, Campbell C, Naidenko OV. "Exposure-Based Assessment and Economic Valuation of Adverse Birth Outcomes and Cancer Risk Due to Nitrate in United States Drinking Water." *Environ Res*. 2019 Jun 11:108442.

35. Davis W. (2018). "Overflowing Hog Lagoons Raise Environmental Concerns in North Carolina." National Public Radio. https://www.npr.org/2018/09/22/650698240/hurricane-s-aftermath-floods-hog-lagoons-in-north-carolina.

36. Lennerz BS, Alsop DC, Holsen LM, et al. "Effects of Dietary Glycemic Index on Brain Regions Related to Reward and Craving in Men." *Am J Clin Nutr*. 2013 Sep;98(3):641–47.

37. Lehner P. "The Hidden Costs of Food." *HuffPost*. August 16, 2017. https://www.huffpost.com/entry/the-hidden-costs-of-food_b_11492520.

38. Gustavsson J, Cederberg C, Sonesson U, van Otterdijk R, Meybeck A. "Global Food Losses and Food Waste: Extent, Causes and Prevention." Food and Agriculture Organization of the United Nations. 2011. http://www.fao.org/3/a-i2697e.pdf.

39. Watts N, Amann M, Arnell N, et al. "The 2018 Report of the *Lancet* Countdown on Health and Climate Change: Shaping the Health of Nations for Centuries to Come." *Lancet*. 2018 Dec 8;392(10163):2479–514.

40. IPSNews.net. "Climate Migrants Might Reach One Billion by 2050." August 11, 2017. United Nations University. https://unu.edu/media-relations/media-coverage/climate-migrants-might-reach-one-billion-by-2050.html.

41. Watts N, Amann M, Arnell N, et al. "The 2018 Report of the *Lancet* Countdown on Health and Climate Change: Shaping the Health of Nations for Centuries to Come." *Lancet*. 2018 Dec 8;392(10163):2479–514.

42. Intergovernmental Panel on Climate Change. (2019). "Land Is a Critical Resource, IPCC Report Says." https://www.ipcc.ch/2019/08/08/land-is-a-critical-resource_srccl/.

43. Midwest Center for Investigative Reporting. (2014). "Growing Influence: Lobbying and the 2014 Farm Bill." https://investigatemidwest.org/series/growing-influence-lobbying-and-the-2014-farm-bill/.

44. Sustainable Food Trust. (2016). "The Trust Cost of American Food." https://sustainablefoodtrust.org/events/the-true-cost-of-american-food/.

45. Malik VS, Popkin BM, Bray GA, Després JP, Hu FB. "Sugar-Sweetened Beverages, Obesity, Type 2 Diabetes Mellitus, and Cardiovascular Disease Risk." *Circulation*. 2010 Mar 23;121(11):1356–64.

46. Malik VS, Li Y, Pan A, et al. "Long-Term Consumption of Sugar-Sweetened and Artificially Sweetened Beverages and Risk of Mortality in US Adults." *Circulation*. 2019 Mar 18.

47. Ibid.

48. Bleich SN, Vercammen KA. "The Negative Impact of Sugar-Sweetened Beverages on Children's Health: An Update of the Literature." *BMC Obes*. 2018 Feb 20;5:6.

doi:10.1186/s40608-017-0178-9; Harvard University. "Sugary Drinks." *Nutrition Source*. Retrieved May 27, 2019, from https://www.hsph.harvard.edu/nutritionsource/healthy-drinks/sugary-drinks/.

49. Waters H, Graf M. "The Cost of Chronic Diseases in the U.S.: Executive Summary." Milken Institute. May 2018. https://assets1b.milkeninstitute.org/assets/Publication/Viewpoint/PDF/Chronic-Disease-Executive-Summary-r2.pdf.

50. Evans S, Idicula I. "Food Marking Institute v. Argus Leader Media." *LII Supreme Court Bulletin*. https://www.law.cornell.edu/supct/cert/18-481.

51. Guttmann A. "Food Advertising: Statistics and Facts." Statista. November 28, 2017. https://www.statista.com/topics/2223/food-advertising/.

CHAPTER 2

1. Afshin A, Sur PJ, Fay K, et al. "Health Effects of Dietary Risks in 195 Countries, 1990–2017: A Systematic Analysis for the Global Burden of Disease Study 2017." *Lancet*. 2019 Apr 4. https://www.thelancet.com/journals/lancet/article/PIIS0140-6736(19)30041-8/fulltext.

2. Christakis NA, Fowler JH. "The Spread of Obesity in a Large Social Network Over 32 Years." *N Engl J Med*. 2007 Jul 26;357(4):370–79; Powell K, et al. "The Role of Social Networks in the Development of Overweight and Obesity among Adults: A Scoping Review." *BMC Public Health*. 2015 Sep 30;15:996.

3. Ludwig J, Sanbonmatsu L, Gennetian L, et al. "Neighborhoods, Obesity, and Diabetes—a Randomized Social Experiment." *N Engl J Med*. 2011 Oct 20;365(16):1509–19.

4. State of Obesity. (2017). "Obesity Rates by Age Group." Robert Wood Johnson Foundation. https://www.stateofobesity.org/obesity-by-age/.

5. Baraldi LG, Martinez SE, Cannella DS, Monteiro CA. "Consumption of Ultra-Processed Foods and Associated Sociodemographic Factors in the USA between 2007 and 2012: Evidence from a Nationally Representative Cross-Sectional Study." *BMJ Open*. 2018;8:e020574.

6. Bird JK, Murphy RA, Ciappio ED, McBurney MI. "Risk of Deficiency in Multiple Concurrent Micronutrients in Children and Adults in the United States." *Nutrients*. 2017 Jun 24;9(7).

7. Via M. "The Malnutrition of Obesity: Micronutrient Deficiencies That Promote Diabetes." *ISRN Endocrinol*. 2012:103472. doi:10.5402/2012/103472.

8. "Food and Grocery Retail Market Analysis Report by Type, by Region and Segment Forecasts, 2011–2020." July 2018. https://www.reportbuyer.com/product/5491690/food-and-grocery-retail-market-analysis-report-by-type-by-region-and-segment-forecasts-2011-2020.html.

9. The World Bank. "Agriculture and Food." Retrieved May 27, 2018, from https://www.worldbank.org/en/topic/agriculture/overview.

10. Holt-Gimenez E. "We Already Grow Enough Food for 10 Billion People—and Still Can't End Hunger." *HuffPost*. December 18, 2014. https://www.huffpost.com/entry/world-hunger_n_1463429?guccounter=1&guce_referrer=aHR0cHM6Ly93d3cuZ29vZ2xlLmNvbS8&guce_referrer_sig=AQAAAELCC2gLn0PZ0iumxHsDxS-AR26P9mHpi5MlGPpClfVjp7oy_8XA7QsKDtMQ-5f6utCOyK-Kaj6pzdZWyYADBNh53aI6dB42wMHJG4Cio_zuLc3x43Rrjqylgz5zIAoCArC5Yfy93nc3XokYjY6JgbpIQr44IWc5owHvTHmROF3Y.

11. US Department of Agriculture. "Key Statistics & Graphics." Economic Research Service. https://www.ers.usda.gov/topics/food-nutrition-assistance/food-security-in-the-us/key-statistics-graphics.aspx.

12. Coleman-Jensen A, Rabbitt MP, Gregory CA, Singh A. "Household Food Security in the United States in 2017." US Department of Agriculture. September 2018. https://www.ers.usda.gov/webdocs/publications/90023/err256_summary.pdf?v=0.

13. Seligman HK, Bindman AB, Vittinghoff E, Kanaya AM, Kushel MB. "Food Insecurity Is Associated with Diabetes Mellitus: Results from the National Health Examination and Nutrition Examination Survey (NHANES) 1999–2002." *J Gen Intern Med.* 2007;22:1018–23.

14. Drewnowski A, Specter SE. "Poverty and Obesity: The Role of Energy Density and Energy Costs." *Am J Clin Nutr.* 2004;79:6–16.

15. Institute for Health Metrics and Evaluation (IHME). Findings from the Global Burden of Disease Study 2017. http://www.healthdata.org/sites/default/files/files/policy_report/2019/GBD_2017_Booklet.pdf

16. Schnabel L, Kesse-Guyot E, Allès B, et al. "Association between Ultraprocessed Food Consumption and Risk of Mortality among Middle-Aged Adults in France." *JAMA Intern Med.* 2019 Feb 11.

17. Park A. "Why Food Could Be the Best Medicine of All." *Time.* February 21, 2019. http://time.com/longform/food-best-medicine/.

18. Feinberg AT, Hess A, Passaretti M, Coolbaugh S, Lee TH. "Prescribing Food as a Specialty Drug." *NJEM Catalyst.* April 10, 2018. https://catalyst.nejm.org/prescribing-fresh-food-farmacy/.

19. Lock K, Pomerleau J, Causer L, Altmann DR, McKee M. "The Global Burden of Disease Attributable to Low Consumption of Fruit and Vegetables: Implications for the Global Strategy on Diet." *Bull World Health Organ.* 2005 Feb;83(2):100–108.

20. Siegel KR, Ali MK, Srinivasiah A, Nugent RA, Narayan KM. "Do We Produce Enough Fruits and Vegetables to Meet Global Health Need?" *PLoS One.* 2014 Aug 6;9(8):e104059.

21. Bahadur K, Dias GM, Veeramani A, et al. "When Too Much Isn't Enough: Does Current Food Production Meet Global Nutritional Needs?" *PLoS One.* 2018 Oct 23;13(10):e0205683.

22. Siegel KR, McKeever Bullard K, Imperatore G, et al. "Association of Higher Consumption of Foods Derived from Subsidized Commodities with Adverse Cardiometabolic Risk among US Adults." *JAMA Intern Med.* 2016 Aug 1;176(8):1124–32.

23. US Department of Health and Human Services. "Mortality Dashboard." National Center for Health Statistics. https://www.cdc.gov/nchs/nvss/vsrr/mortality-dashboard.htm.

24. Dwyer-Lindgren L, Bertozzi-Villa A, Stubbs RW, et al. "Inequalities in Life Expectancy among US Counties, 1980 to 2014: Temporal Trends and Key Drivers." *JAMA Intern Med.* 2017 Jul 1;177(7):1003–11.

25. Manzel A, Muller DN, Hafler DA, et al. "Role of 'Western Diet' in Inflammatory Autoimmune Diseases." *Curr Allergy Asthma Rep.* 2014 Jan;14(1):404.

26. Li Y, Lv MR, Wei YJ, et al. "Dietary Patterns and Depression Risk: A Meta-Analysis." *Psychiatry Res.* 2017 Jul;253:373–82.

27. Firth J, Marx W, Dash S, et al. "The Effects of Dietary Improvement on Symptoms of Depression and Anxiety: A Meta-Analysis of Randomized Controlled Trials." *Psychosom Med.* 2019 Apr;81(3):265–80.

28. Thorbecke M, Dettling J. "Carbon Footprint Evaluation of Regenerative Grazing at White Oak Pastures." February 25, 2019. https://blog.whiteoakpastures.com/hubfs/WOP -LCA-Quantis-2019.pdf.

29. Health Resource Institute Laboratories report no. S00004900-2019-05-06. May 6, 2019. https://d3n8a8pro7vhmx.cloudfront.net/yesmaam/pages/8069/attachments/original /1557958339/COA_S0004900_Impossible_Burger_and_Beyond_Meat_patty_-_glyph osate.pdf?1557958339.

30. Shehata AA, Schrödi W, Aldin AA, et al. "The Effect of Glyphosate on Potential Patho-gens and Beneficial Members of Poultry Microbiota in Vitro." *Curr Microbiol.* 2013 Apr;66(4):350–8.

31. Regenetarianism. (2016). "Understanding Water Footprint Numbers." July 4. https:// lachefnet.wordpress.com/2016/07/04/la-chef-editorial-understanding-numbers/.

32. Berkowitz SA, Terranova J, Hill C, et al. "Programs Reduce the Use of Costly Health Care in Dually Eligible Medicare and Medicaid Beneficiaries." *Health Aff.* 2018 Apr; University of North Carolina at Chapel Hill School of Medicine. (2018). "Medically Tai-lored Meal Delivery Service Reduces Costs for High Utilizers of Health Care." April 4. Press release. https://medicalxpress.com/news/2018-04-medically-tailored-meal-delivery -high.html.

33. Gurvey J, Rand K, Daugherty S, et al. "Examining Health Care Costs among MANNA Clients and a Comparison Group." *J Prim Care Community Health.* 2013 Oct;4(4):311–17.

34. Cohen SB, Yu W. "Statistical Brief #354: The Concentration and Persistence in the Level of Health Expenditures over Time: Estimates for the U.S. Population, 2008–2009." Agency for Healthcare Research and Quality. January 2012. https://meps.ahrq.gov /data_files/publications/st354/stat354.shtml.

35. Food Is Medicine Coalition. (2019). "Who We Are." https://calfimc.org/.

36. Food Is Medicine Coalition. (2019). "Research." http://www.fimcoalition.org/new-page/.

37. Mozaffarian D, Angell SY, Lang T, Rivera JA. "Role of Government Policy in Nutrition—Barriers to and Opportunities for Healthier Eating." *BMJ.* 2018;361:k2426.

38. Berkowitz SA, Terranova J, Randall L, et al. "Association between Receipt of a Medi-cally Tailored Meal Program and Health Care Use." *JAMA Intern Med.* 2019 Apr 22.

39. Gurvey J, Rand K, Daugherty S, et al. "Examining Health Care Costs among MANNA Clients and a Comparison Group." *J Prim Care Community Health.* 2013 Oct;4(4):311–17.

40. Senior A. "John Hancock Leaves Traditional Life Insurance Model behind to Incentivize Longer, Healthier Lives." John Hancock. September 19, 2018. https://www.johnhan cock.com/news/insurance/2018/09/john-hancock-leaves-traditional-life-insurance -model-behind-to-incentivize-longer—healthier-lives.html.

41. Feinberg AT, Hess A, Passaretti M, Coolbaugh S, Lee TH. "Prescribing Food as a Spe-cialty Drug." *NEJM Catalyst.* April 10, 2018. https://catalyst.nejm.org/prescribing-fresh -food-farmacy/.

42. Jim McGovern, Congressman for the Second District of Massachusetts. "Bipartisan Members of Congress Launch Food Is Medicine Working Group to Highlight Impacts of Hunger on Health." Press release. January 17, 2018. https://mcgovern.house.gov/news /documentsingle.aspx?DocumentID=397179.

43. Beidelschies M, et al. Association of the Functional Medicine Model of Care With Patient-Reported Health-Related Quality-of-Life Outcomes. *JAMA* Netw Open. 2019 Oct 2; 2(10).

44. Virta Health. (2019). "Virta Reverses Type 2 Diabetes." https://www.virtahealth.com/.

45. Pothering J. "Investors Wake Up to a \$2.3 Trillion Opportunity in Sustainable Food and Agriculture." *Impact Alpha.* February 1, 2018. https://impactalpha.com/investors-wake-up-to-a-2-3-trillion-opportunity-in-sustainable-food-and-agriculture-ef10f3566fd9/.

CHAPTER 3

1. Jacobs A, Richtel M. "How Big Business Got Brazil Hooked on Junk Food." *New York Times.* September 16, 2017.

2. Dhanjal SS, Tandon S. "With Sapphire Foods Franchisee, Yum Reorganizes India Business." *LiveMint.* September 29, 2015.

3. Pereira MA, Kartashov AI, Ebbeling CB, et al. "Fast-Food Habits, Weight Gain, and Insulin Resistance (the CARDIAstudy): 15-Year Prospective Analysis." *Lancet.* 2005 Jan 1–7;365(9453):36–42.

4. Seeking Alpha. "Yum! Brands, Inc. (YUM) CEO Greg Creed Hosts 2018 Investor and Analyst Day Conference (Transcript)." December 7, 2018. https://seekingalpha.com/article/4227124-yum-brands-inc-yum-ceo-greg-creed-hosts-2018-investor-analyst-day-conference-transcript.

5. State of Obesity. (2019). "Childhood Obesity Trends." Robert Wood Johnson Foundation. https://www.stateofobesity.org/childhood-obesity-trends/.

6. Ng M, Fleming T, Robinson M, et al. "Global, Regional, and National Prevalence of Overweight and Obesity in Children and Adults during 1980–2013: A Systematic Analysis for the Global Burden of Disease Study 2013." *Lancet.* 2014 Aug 30;384(9945):766–81.

7. Doak CM, Adair LS, Bentley M, et al. "The Dual Burden Household and the Nutrition Transition Paradox." *Int J Obes (Lond).* 2005 Jan;29(1):129–36.

8. Khan M. "The Dual Burden of Overweight and Underweight in Developing Countries." Population Reference Bureau. March 1, 2006.

9. International Diabetes Federation. "IDF Diabetes Atlas—8th Edition." https://diabetesatlas.org/resources/2017-atlas.html.

10. Shrivastav S. "Heart, Lung Diseases Now Leading Killers in India." *Times of India.* April 8, 2015.

11. World Health Organization. "Diabetes: The Situation in China." http://www.wpro.who.int/china/mediacentre/factsheets/diabetes/en/.

12. Abuvassin B, Laher I. "Diabetes Epidemic Sweeping the Arab World." *World J Diabetes.* 2016 Apr 25;7(8):165–74.

13. Jacobs A, Richtel M. "A Nasty, Nafta-Related Surprise: Mexico's Soaring Obesity." *New York Times.* December 11, 2017. https://www.nytimes.com/2017/12/11/health/obesity-mexico-nafta.html.

14. Cochrane L, Vimonsuknopparat S. "Thai Buddhist Monks' Health Suffering from Sugary Drinks." ABC News Australia. May 27, 2018.

15. Jacobs A, Richtel M. "How Big Business Got Brazil Hooked on Junk Food." *New York Times.* September 16, 2017.

16. Jacobs A, Richtel M. "She Took on Colombia's Soda Industry. Then She Was Silenced." *New York Times.* November 13, 2017.

17. Rodríguez OL, Pizarro QT. "Food Labeling and Advertising Law: Chile Innovating in Public Nutrition Once Again." *Rev Chil Pediatr.* 2018 Oct;89(5):579–81. https://www

.ncbi.nlm.nih.gov/pubmed/?term=Food+Labeling+and+Advertising+Law%3A+Chile +innovating+in+public+nutrition+once+again; Jacobs A. "In Sweeping War on Obesity, Chile Slays Tony the Tiger." *New York Times.* February 7, 2018.

18. Swinburn BA, Kraak V, Allender S, et al. "The Global Syndemic of Obesity, Undernutrition, and Climate Change: The Lancet Commission Report." The Lancet Commissions. January 27, 2019.

19. "FAO Awards." Food and Agriculture Organization of the United Nations. http://www .fao.org/fao-awards/conference-awards/jacques-diouf/en/.

20. Cardello H. "Food Companies Need to Change Before Doomsday Package Labels Kill Them." *Forbes.* November 30, 2018.

CHAPTER 4

1. Centers for Medicare and Medicaid Services. "National Health Expenditure Data." December 11, 2018. https://www.cms.gov/research-statistics-data-and-systems/statistics -trends-and-reports/nationalhealthexpenddata/nationalhealthaccountshistorical.html.

2. Sawyer N. "Soda Tax Starts Paying Off." *SF Weekly.* May 29, 2018.

3. Patel AI, Schmidt LA. "Water Access in the United States: Health Disparities Abound and Solutions Are Urgently Needed." *Am J Public Health.* 2017 Sep;107(9):1354–56.

4. Diet Doctor. "Tax Sugary Foods to Reverse Type 2 Diabetes Epidemic within 3 Years." Press release. 2018. https://www.dietdoctor.com/wp-content/uploads/2018/05/Press-Re lease-Tax-Sugary-Food-To-Reverse-Type-2-Diabetes.pdf.

5. Ludwig DS, Ebbeling CB. The Carbohydrate-Insulin Model of Obesity: Beyond "Calories In, Calories Out." *JAMA* Intern Med. 2018 Aug 1;178(8):1098–1103. Review.

6. Falbe J, Thompson HR, Becker CM, et al. "Impact of the Berkeley Excise Tax on Sugar-Sweetened Beverage Consumption." *Am J Public Health.* 2016 Oct;106(10):1865–71.

7. O'Connor A. "Mexican Soda Tax Followed by Drop in Sugary Drink Sales." *New York Times.* January 6, 2016.

8. Colchero MA, Molina M, Guerrero-López CM. "After Mexico Implemented a Tax, Purchases of Sugar-Sweetened Beverages Decreased and Water Increased: Difference by Place of Residence, Household Composition and Income Level." *J Nutr.* 2017 Aug;147(8):1552–57.

9. Sánchez-Romero LM, Penko J, Coxson PG, et al. "Projected Impact of Mexico's Sugar-Sweetened Beverage Tax Policy on Diabetes and Cardiovascular Disease: A Modeling Study." *PLoS Med.* 2016 Nov 1;13(11):e1002158. https://www.ncbi.nlm.nih.gov/pubmed /27802278.

10. Langellier BA, Lê-Scherban F, Purtle J, et al. "Funding Quality Pre-Kindergarten Slots with Philadelphia's New 'Sugary Drink Tax': Simulating Effects of Using an Excise Tax to Address a Social Determinant of Health." *Public Health Nutr.* 2017 Sep;20(13):2450–58.

11. Spector K. (2010). "Sugar-Sweetened Food, Beverages No Longer Will Be Sold at the Cleveland Clinic." *Cleveland.* https://www.cleveland.com/healthfit/2010/07/sugar-sweet ened_food_beverages.html.

CHAPTER 5

1. O'Connor A. "In the Shopping Cart of a Food Stamp Household: Lots of Soda." *New York Times.* January 13, 2017.

2. Hyman M. (2018). "Our Food System: An Invisible Form of Oppression." DrHyman .com. April 9. https://drhyman.com/blog/2018/04/09/our-food-system-an-invisible-form -of-oppression/.

3. Conrad Z, Rehm CD, Wilde P, Mozaffarian D. "Cardiometabolic Mortality by Supplemental Nutrition Assistance Program Participation and Eligibility in the United States." *Am J Public Health.* 2017;107(3):466–74.

4. US Department of Agriculture, Food and Nutrition Service. *Supplemental Nutrition Assistance Program (SNAP). Characteristics of Supplemental Nutrition Assistance Program Households: Fiscal Year 2014.* 2014.

5. Andreyeva T, Tripp AS, Schwartz MB. "Dietary Quality of Americans by Supplemental Nutrition Assistance Program Participation Status." *Am J Prev Med.* 2015 Oct;49(4):594–604; Leung CW, Ding EL, Catalano PJ, et al. "Dietary Intake and Dietary Quality of Low-Income Adults in the Supplemental Nutrition Assistance Program." *Am J Clin Nutr.* 2012 Nov;96(5):977–88.

6. Leung CW, Blumenthal SJ, Hoffnagle EE, et al. "Associations of Food Stamp Participation with Dietary Quality and Obesity in Children." *Pediatrics.* 2013 Mar;131(3):463–72.

7. US Department of Agriculture, Food and Nutrition Service. *Diet Quality of Americans by SNAP Participation Status: Data from the National Health and Nutrition Survey 2007–2010.* 2015. fns-prod.azureedge.net/sites/default/files/ops/NHANES-SNAP07-10.pdf.

8. Moran AJ, Musicus A, Gorski Findling MT, et al. "Increases in Sugary Drink Marketing during Supplemental Nutrition Assistance Program Benefit Issuance in New York." *Am J Prev Med.* 2018 Jul;55(1):55–62.

9. Dewey C. "Soda Ad Blitzes Conspicuously Match Food Stamp Schedules, Study Says." *Washington Post.* June 7, 2018.

10. Tufts University. (2017). "Americans in the Supplemental Nutrition Assistance Program (SNAP) Have Higher Mortality." Tufts Now. https://now.tufts.edu/news-releases/ameri cans-supplemental-nutrition-assistance-program-snap-have-higher-mortality.

11. Mozaffarian D, Liu J, Sy S, et al. "Cost-Effectiveness of Financial Incentives and Disincentives for Improving Food Purchases and Health through the U.S. Supplemental Nutrition Assistance Program (SNAP)." *PLoS Med.* 2018 Oct 2;15(10):e1002661.

12. "What Can SNAP Buy?" US Department of Agriculture. Retrieved May 4, 2019, from https://www.fns.usda.gov/snap/eligible-food-items.

13. Ibid.

14. Center for Responsive Politics. "Rep. David Scott—Georgia District 13." (2018). https:// www.opensecrets.org/members-of-congress/contributors?cid=N00024871&cycle =2018&type=I.

15. Center for Responsive Politics. "Rep. Roger Marshall—Kansas District 01." (2018). https:// www.opensecrets.org/members-of-congress/contributors?cid=N00037034&cycle=2018.

16. Merlin M. "Farm Bill Still Hanging: More Than 70 Groups Lobby on Food Stamps." Center for Responsive Politics. OpenSecrets.org. December 3, 2012.

17. Sessa-Hawkins M. "Congress Could Cut Soda and Candy from SNAP, but Big Sugar Is Pushing Back." *Civil Eats.* August 28, 2017.

18. Harnack L, Oakes JM, Elbel B, et al. "Effects of Subsidies and Prohibitions on Nutrition in a Food Benefit Program: A Randomized Clinical Trial." *JAMA Intern Med.* 2016 Nov 1;176(11):1610–18.

19. Shemkus S. "The Healthy Incentives Program Is So Popular, Its Future Is Now in Doubt." *Boston Globe*. April 2, 2018.

20. Virginia Farmers Market Association. "Virginia Fresh Match: A Statewide Network to Help Farmers Markets Serve Low-Income Shoppers." https://vafma.org/programs/vir ginia-fresh-match/.

21. Double Up National Network. "Bring Double Up to Your Community!" http://www .doubleupfoodbucks.org/national-network/.

22. Tufts University. (2019). "Prescribing Healthy Food in Medicare/Medicaid Is Cost Effective, Could Improve Health Outcomes." https://now.tufts.edu/news-releases/pres cribing-healthy-food-medicaremedicaid-cost-effective-could-improve-health -outcomes.

23. Bipartisan Policy Center. "Leading with Nutrition: Leveraging Federal Programs for Better Health: Recommendations from the BPC SNAP Task Force." 2018. https:// bipartisanpolicy.org/wp-content/uploads/2018/03/BPC-Health-Leading-With -Nutrition.pdf.

24. Stern D, Mazariegos M, Ortiz-Panozo E, et al. "Sugar-Sweetened Soda Consumption Increases Diabetes Risk among Mexican Women." *J Nutr.* 2019 May 1;149(5):795–803.

25. Harnack L, Oakes JM, Elbel B, et al. "Effects of Subsidies and Prohibitions on Nutrition in a Food Benefit Program: A Randomized Clinical Trial." *JAMA Intern Med.* 2016 Nov 1;176(11):1610–18.

26. Bartlett S, Klerman J, Wilde P, et al. "Healthy Incentives Pilot (HIP) Interim Report." US Department of Agriculture. July 2013. https://fns-prod.azureedge.net/sites/default /files/ops/HIP_Interim.pdf.

27. Cohn DJ, Waters DB. "Food As Medicine." February 2013. https://www.hungercenter .org/wp-content/uploads/2013/07/Community-Servings-Food-as-Medicine -Cohn.pdf.

CHAPTER 6

1. University of Rochester. "Campaign Contributions Influence Public Policy, Finds Study of 50 State Legislatures." 2012. http://www.rochester.edu/news/show.php?id=4060.

2. Bernick Jr B, Davidson L. "No End to Lobbyists' Gifts?" *Deseret News*. January 12, 2008.

3. Gerstein J. "How Obama Failed to Shut Washington's Revolving Door." *Politico*. December 31, 2015. https://www.politico.com/story/2015/12/barack-obama-revolving-door -lobbying-217042.

4. Kotch A. "Corn Syrup Lobbyist Is Helping Set USDA Dietary Guidelines." *International Business Times*. February 2, 2018.

5. McGahn II DF. "Limited Waiver of Paragraph 7 of the Ethics Pledge." White House memorandum. August 25, 2017. https://www.foodpolitics.com/wp-content/uploads/Tkacz _Ethics_Pledge_Waiver.pdf.

6. Office of Government Ethics. "Agency Ethics Pledge Waivers." https://www.oge.gov /web/oge.nsf/Agency+Ethics+Pledge+Waivers+(EO+13770).

7. Office of Government Ethics. "Agency Ethics Pledge Waivers." https://www.oge.gov /web/oge.nsf/0/385A180F619D3AE9852582490069D586/$FILE/USDA%20-%20 Appleton%20(002)%205.pdf.

8. Ibid.

9. Drutman L. "How Corporate Lobbyists Conquered American Democracy." *The Atlantic*. April 20, 2015.

10. Fang L. "The Shadow Lobbying Complex." *Type Investigations*. February 20, 2014.

11. Evers-Hillstrom K. "Lobbying Spending Reaches $3.4 Billion in 2018, Highest in 8 Years." Opensecrets.org. January 25, 2019. https://www.opensecrets.org/news/2019/01/lobbying-spending-reaches-3-4-billion-in-18/.

12. Aaron DG, Siegel MB. "Sponsorship of National Health Organizations by Two Major Soda Companies." *Am J Prev Med*. 2017 Jan;52(1):20–30.

13. Prins GS, Patisaul HB, Belcher SM, Vandenberg LN. "CLARITY-BPA Academic Laboratory Studies Identify Consistent Low-Dose Bisphenol A Effects on Multiple Organ Systems." *Basic Clin Pharmacol Toxicol*. 2018 Sep 12.

14. Bardelline J. "BPA Ban Blocked from Food Safety Bill." *Green Biz*. November 19, 2010.

15. Guo J. "These 26 States Won't Let You Sue McDonald's for Making You Fat. The Surprising Consequence of Banning Obesity Lawsuits." *Washington Post*. May 28, 2015.

16. Meier CF. "Keller, Kraft Weigh in on Obesity." The Heartland Institute. August 1, 2003.

17. Simon M. *Appetite for Profit: How the Food Industry Undermines Our Health and How to Fight Back*. New York: Bold Type Books, 2006.

18. Cassidy E. "EPA Watchdog to Investigate Monsanto GMOs and Superweeds." *AgMag*. March 28, 2016; Center for Biological Diversity. "California Becomes First State to Declare Glyphosate Causes Cancer." *EcoWatch*. March 30, 2017.

19. Guest Contributor. "If GMOs Are Safe, Why Not Label Them? (64 Other Countries Do)." *EcoWatch*. May 22, 2015.

20. Robertson K. "Independent Study: Why Label Changes Don't Affect Food Prices." Just Label It. September 11, 2013.

21. Foley L. "Big Food Companies Spend Millions to Defeat GMO Labeling." Environmental Working Group. August 4, 2015.

22. Kopicki A. "Strong Support for Labeling Modified Foods." *New York Times*. July 27, 2013.

23. Simon M. "Fighting GMO Labeling in California Is Food Lobby's 'Highest Priority.'" *HuffPost*. July 30, 2012.

24. Peeples L. "Prop 37 GMO Labeling Law Defeated by Corporate Dollars and Deception, Proponents Say." *HuffPost*. November 7, 2012.

25. State of Washington Thurston County Supreme Court. "State of Washington v. Grocery Manufacturers Association." October 16, 2013. Docket No. 13-2-02156-8. https://agportal-s3bucket.s3.amazonaws.com/uploadedfiles/Complaint-20131016-Conformed.pdf.

26. Ibid.

27. Connelly J. "Grocery Lobby Must Pay $18M for Laundering Campaign Money." *Seattle PI*. November 2, 2016.

28. Washington State Office of the Attorney General. (2016). "AG: Grocery Manufacturers Assoc. to Pay $18M, Largest Campaign Finance Penalty in US History." Retrieved from https://www.atg.wa.gov/news/news-releases/ag-grocery-manufacturers-assoc-pay-18m-largest-campaign-finance-penalty-us.

29. Brunner J. "Grocery Group Fined $18M in Fight against GMO Food-Labeling Initiative." *Seattle Times*. November 2, 2016.

30. Strom S. "Danone of France to Buy WhiteWave in $10 Billion Deal to Bolster U.S. Portfolio." *New York Times*. July 17, 2016.

31. Peters A. "Get Ready for a Meatless Meat Explosion, As Big Food Gets on Board." *Fast Company*. December 18, 2017; Bennett C. "Flesh and Blood: What's the Future of Fake Meat?" *Drovers*. August 13, 2018.

32. Blythman J. "How Vegan Evangelists Are Propping Up the Ultra-Processed Food Industry." *Mouthy Money*. January 26, 2019. https://www.mouthymoney.co.uk/how-vegan -evangelists-are-propping-up-the-ultra-processed-food-industry/.

33. Mayer J. *Dark Money: The Hidden History of the Billionaires behind the Rise of the Radical Right*. New York: Anchor Books, 2017.

34. Lee MYH. "Eleven Donors Have Plowed $1 Billion into Super PACs Since They Were Created." *Washington Post*. October 26, 2018. https://www.washingtonpost.com/politics /eleven-donors-plowed-1-billion-into-super-pacs-since-2010/2018/10/26/31a07510 -d70a-11e8-aeb7-ddcad4a0a54e_story.html?noredirect=on.

35. Wiener-Bronner D. "How to Solve the World's Plastics Problem: Bring Back the Milk Man." CNN. January 14, 2019.

36. Grossman E. "Will Trump Revive COOL and Make American Meat Great Again?" *Civil Eats*. April 6, 2017.

37. Drutman L. "A Better Way to Fix Lobbying." *Issues in Governance Studies*. June 2011.

CHAPTER 7

1. Union of Concerned Scientists. (2019). "The Farm Bill." https://www.ucsusa.org/food _and_agriculture/solutions/strengthen-healthy-farm-policy/the-farm-bill.html.

2. Kearns CE, Schmidt LA, Glantz SA. "Sugar Industry and Coronary Heart Disease Research: A Historical Analysis of Internal Industry Documents." *JAMA Intern Med*. 2016;176(11):1680–85.

3. The Editors. "For a Healthier Country, Overhaul Farm Subsidies." *Scientific American*. May 1, 2012.

4. Mercola J. "Soybean Oil: One of the Most Harmful Ingredients in Processed Foods." *Mercola*. January 27, 2013.

5. Nestle M. "The Farm Bill Drove Me Insane." *Politico*. March 17, 2016.

6. Russo M, Smith D. "Apples to Twinkies 2013: Comparing Taxpayer Subsidies for Fresh Produce and Junk Food." US PIRG. July 2013. https://uspirg.org/reports/usp/apples -twinkies-2013.

7. Siegel KR. "Association of Higher Consumption of Foods Derived from Subsidized Commodities with Adverse Cardiometabolic Risk among US Adults." *JAMA Intern Med*. 2016 Aug 1;176(8):1124–32.

8. US Department of Agriculture. "Specialty Crops." February 25, 2019. https://www.ers.usda .gov/agriculture-improvement-act-of-2018-highlights-and-implications/specialty-crops/.

9. O'Connor A. "How the Government Supports Your Junk Food Habit." *New York Times*. July 19, 2016.

10. Union of Concerned Scientists. "The Healthy Farmland Diet: How Growing Less Corn Would Improve Our Health and Help America's Heartland (2013)." October 2013. https://www.ucsusa.org/food_and_agriculture/solutions/expand-healthy-food-access /the-healthy-farmland-diet.html.

11. Nestle M. "The Farm Bill Drove Me Insane." *Politico*. March 17, 2016.
12. Bittman M, Pollan M, Salvador R, De Schutter O. "How a National Food Policy Could Save Millions of American Lives." *Washington Post*. November 7, 2014.
13. Bottemiller Evich H. "Bipartisan Nutrition Group Kicks Off in House." *Politico*. January 22, 2018; US Congressman Jim McGovern. (2018). "Bipartisan Members of Congress Launch Food Is Medicine Working Group to Highlight Impacts of Hunger on Health." Press release. January 17, 2018. https://mcgovern.house.gov/news/documentsingle.aspx?DocumentID=397179.

CHAPTER 8

1. Centers for Disease Control and Prevention. (2019). "Childhood Obesity Facts." https://www.cdc.gov/healthyschools/obesity/facts.htm.
2. May AL, Kuklina EV, Yoon PW. "Prevalence of Cardiovascular Disease Risk Factors among US Adolescents, 1999–2008." *Pediatrics*. 2012 Jun;129(6):1035–41.
3. Kitahara CM, Flint AJ, Berrington de Gonzalez A, et al. "Association between Class III Obesity (BMI of 40–59 kg/m) and Mortality: A Pooled Analysis of 20 Prospective Studies." *PLoS Med*. July 8, 2014.
4. Center for Responsive Politics. "Clients Lobbying on S.3307: Healthy, Hunger-Free Kids Act of 2010." https://www.opensecrets.org/lobby/billsum.php?id=s3307-111.
5. Green E, Piccoli S. "Trump Administration Sued Over Rollback of School Lunch Standards." *New York Times*. April 3, 2019. https://www.nytimes.com/2019/04/03/us/politics/trump-school-lunch-standards.html.
6. Park A. "The Food Industry Lobby Groups behind the New School Nutrition Standards." *Mother Jones*. July 18, 2014.
7. Bottemiller Evich H. "Behind the School Lunch Fight." *Politico*. June 4, 2014.
8. Jacobs E. "Klobuchar Explains Why She Fought for Pizza Sauce to Be Classified As a Vegetable." *New York Post*. April 23, 2019. https://nypost.com/2019/04/23/klobuchar-explains-why-she-fought-for-pizza-sauce-to-be-classified-as-a-vegetable/.
9. Butler K. "Yes, Cheetos, Funnel Cake, and Domino's Are Approved School Lunch Items." *Mother Jones*. July 16, 2014.
10. Siegel BA. "Under Betti Wiggins, Houston ISD Signs $8 Million Contract for Domino's 'Smart Slice' Pizza." *The Lunch Tray*. August 2, 2018.
11. Alexander R, Lincoff N. "Battle Intensifies to Keep Junk Food Out of School Lunch Rooms." *Healthline*. August 30, 2016.
12. American Psychological Association. (2019). "The Impact of Food Advertising on Childhood Obesity." https://www.apa.org/topics/kids-media/food.
13. GBD 2017 Diet Collaborators. "Health Effects of Dietary Risks in 195 Countries, 1990–2017: A Systematic Analysis for the Global Burden of Disease Study 2017." *Lancet*. 2019 May 11;393(10184):1958–72.
14. McGinnis JM, Gootman JA, Kraak VI, eds. *Food Marketing to Children and Youth: Threat or Opportunity?* Washington, DC: National Academies Press, 2006.
15. Nestle M. "Food Marketing and Childhood Obesity—a Matter of Policy." *N Engl J Med*. 2006 Jun 15;354(24):2527–29.
16. Federal Trade Commission. "A Review of Food Marketing to Children and Adolescents." December 2012.

17. UConn Rudd Center for Food Policy and Obesity. *Increasing Disparities in Unhealthy Food Advertising Targeted to Hispanic and Black Youth.* 2019. http://uconnruddcenter.org/files/Pdfs/TargetedMarketingReport2019.pdf.

18. American Psychological Association. (2019). "The Impact of Food Advertising on Childhood Obesity." https://www.apa.org/topics/kids-media/food.

19. Cheyne AD, Dorfman L, Bukofzer E, Harris JL. "Marketing Sugary Cereals to Children in the Digital Age: A Content Analysis of 17 Child-Targeted Websites." *J Health Commun.* 2013;18(5):563–82.

20. Weatherspoon LJ, Quilliam ET, Paek HJ, et al. "Consistency of Nutrition Recommendations for Foods Marketed to Children in the United States, 2009–2010." *Prev Chronic Dis.* 2013 Sep 26;10:E165.

21. Story M, French S. "Food Advertising and Marketing Directed at Children and Adolescents in the US." *Int J Behav Nutr Phys Act.* 2004;1(1):3. Published February 10, 2004.

22. Borzekowski DL, Robinson TN. "The 30-Second Effect: An Experiment Revealing the Impact of Television Commercials on Food Preferences of Preschoolers." *J Am Diet Assoc.* 2001 Jan;101(1):42–46.

23. American Psychological Association. *The Impact of Food Advertising on Childhood Obesity.* https://www.apa.org/topics/kids-media/food.

24. Reichelt AC, Rank MM. "The Impact of Junk Foods on the Adolescent Brain." *Birth Defects Res.* 2017 Dec 1;109(20):1649–58.

25. McClure AC, Tanski SE, Gilbert-Diamond D, et al. "Receptivity to Television Fast-Food Restaurant Marketing and Obesity among U.S. Youth." *Am J Prev Med.* 2013 Nov;45(5):560–68.

26. Burrows D. "Barrage of Junk Food Ads Fueling Teenage Obesity." *Food Navigator.* March 19, 2018.

27. Lardieri A. "Study: Teens Exposed to More Junk Food Ads Eat More Junk Food." *U.S. News & World Report.* May 22, 2018.

28. Skinner AC, Ravanbakht SN, Skelton JA, et al. "Prevalence of Obesity and Severe Obesity in US Children, 1999–2016." *Pediatrics.* 2018 Mar;141(3).

29. O'Connor A. "Threat Grows from Liver Illness Tied to Obesity." *New York Times.* June 13, 2014.

30. Layton L, Eggen D. "Industries Lobby against Voluntary Nutrition Guidelines for Food Marketed to Kids." *Washington Post.* July 9, 2011.

31. IHS Consulting. "Assessing the Economic Impact of Restricting Advertising for Products That Target Young Americans." 2011. https://www.foodpolitics.com/wp-content/uploads/Global-Insight-Report.pdf.

32. Federal Trade Commission. (2011). "What's on the Table." https://www.ftc.gov/news-events/blogs/business-blog/2011/07/whats-table.

33. Neuman W. "Ad Rules Stall, Keeping Cereal a Cartoon Staple." *New York Times.* July 23, 2010.

34. UConn Rudd Center for Food Policy and Obesity. "Food Industry Self-Regulation After 10 Years." http://www.uconnruddcenter.org/files/Pdfs/FACTS-2017_Final.pdf.

35. Gallagher J. "Stop Junk Food Ads on Kids' Apps—WHO." BBC News. November 4, 2016.

36. Constine J. "Pokémon GO Reveals Sponsors Like McDonald's Pay It Up to $0.50 Per Visitor." *TechCrunch.* May 31, 2017.

37. World Health Organization. *Tackling Food Marketing to Children in a Digital World: Trans-Disciplinary Perspectives.* 2016. http://www.euro.who.int/__data/assets/pdf_file/0017/322226 /Tackling-food-marketing-children-digital-world-trans-disciplinary-perspectives-en .pdf?ua=1.

38. Shah Family Foundation. "Boston Public Schools Focus on Children My Way Café." https://www.shahfoundation.org/grantbostonpublicschool.

39. Gross SJ. "Hub and Spoke Thrives in Eastie School Cafeterias." *Metro.* January 22, 2018.

40. City of Boston. (2018). "Fresh Food Program Expanded at Boston Public Schools." Press release. https://www.boston.gov/news/fresh-food-program-expanded-boston-public -schools.

41. Ludwig DS, Willett WC. "Three Daily Servings of Reduced-Fat Milk: An Evidence-Based Recommendation?" *JAMA Pediatr.* 2013 Sep;167(9):788–89.

42. Tucker J. "Chocolate Milk Booted Off the Menu at SF School Cafeterias." *San Francisco Chronicle.* July 10, 2017.

43. Strasburger VC. "Policy Statement—Children, Adolescents, Obesity, and the Media." *Pediatrics.* 2011 Jul;128(1):201–8.

44. Musemeche C. "Ban on Advertising to Children Linked to Lower Obesity Rates." *New York Times.* July 13, 2012.

45. Cordes R. "Swedish Call for Ban on TV Advertising to Children Faces Defeat." *Politico.* October 18, 2000.

46. BBC News. "First Ads Banned Under New Junk Food Rules." July 4, 2018.

47. Bowles N. "Silicon Valley Nannies Are Phone Police for Kids." *New York Times.* October 26, 2018. https://www.nytimes.com/2018/10/26/style/silicon-valley-nannies.html?module =inline.

48. Tamana SK, Ezeugwu V, Chikuma J, et al. "Screen-Time Is Associated with Inattention Problems in Preschoolers: Results from the CHILD Birth Cohort Study." *PLoS One.* 2019 Apr 17;14(4):e0213995.

49. Fang K, Mu M, Liu K, He Y. "Screen Time and Childhood Overweight/Obesity: A Systematic Review and Meta-Analysis." *Child Care Health Dev.* 2019 Jul 3.

CHAPTER 9

1. Food and Drug Administration. (2006). "FDA's Approach to the GRAS Provision: A History of Processes." https://www.fda.gov/food/ingredientspackaginglabeling/gras/ucm 094040.htm.

2. Cronin J. "FDA Food Ingredient Approval Process Violates Law, Says CSPI." Center for Science in the Public Interest. April 15, 2015.

3. Neltner TG, Alger HM, O'Reilly JT, et al. "Conflicts of Interest in Approvals of Additives to Food Determined to Be Generally Recognized As Safe: Out of Balance." *JAMA Intern Med.* 2013 Dec 9–23;173(22):2032–36.

4. Ibid.; US Government Accountability Office. (2010). *Food Safety: FDA Should Strengthen Its Oversight of Food Ingredients Determined to Be Generally Recognized as Safe (GRAS).* https://www.gao.gov/products/GAO-10-246.

5. FDA. (2018). "FDA Removes 7 Synthetic Flavoring Substances from Food Additives List." https://www.fda.gov/food/cfsan-constituent-updates/fda-removes-7-synthetic-flavor ing-substances-food-additives-list.

6. Food Babe. "Subway: Stop Using Dangerous Chemicals in Your Bread." February 2014. https://foodbabe.com/subway/.

7. Electronic Code of Federal Regulations. (2019). "e-CFR Data Is Current as of June 14, 2019." https://www.ecfr.gov/cgi-bin/text-idx?SID=3ee286332416f26a91d9e6d786a604 ab&mc=true&tpl=/ecfrbrowse/Title21/21tab_02.tpl.

8. Arnold LE, Lofthouse N, Hurt E. "Artificial Food Colors and Attention-Deficit/Hyper-activity Symptoms: Conclusions to Dye For." *Neurotherapeutics*. 2012;9(3):599–609. doi:10.1007/s13311-012-0133-x.

9. Brandt EJ, Myerson R, Perraillon MC, Polonsky TS. "Hospital Admissions for Myocar-dial Infarction and Stroke before and after the Trans-Fatty Acid Restrictions in New York." *JAMA Cardiol*. 2017 Jun 1;2(6):627–34.

10. Strom S. "Social Media as a Megaphone to Pressure the Food Industry." *New York Times*. December 30, 2013.

11. Food Babe. "A 'Food Babe Investigates' Win—Chipotle Posts Ingredients." February 2015. https://foodbabe.com/a-food-babe-investigates-win-chipotle-posts-ingredients/.

12. Associated Press. "Kraft to Remove Artificial Dyes from Three Macaroni and Cheese Varieties." October 31, 2013. https://www.theguardian.com/business/2013/oct/31/kraft -remove-artificial-dyes-macaroni-and-cheese.

13. Chamlee V. "Subway Wasn't the Only Chain to Use the 'Yoga Mat Chemical' in Its Bread." *Eater*. August 8, 2016.

14. Andrade MJ, Jayaprakash C, Bhat S, et al. "Antibiotics-Induced Obesity: A Mitochon-drial Perspective." *Public Health Genomics*. 2017;20(5):257–73; Turta O, Rautava S. "Antibiotics, Obesity and the Link to Microbes—What Are We Doing to Our Chil-dren?" *BMC Med*. 2016 Apr 19;14:57.

15. O'Brien M. "Global Antibiotic Overuse Is Like a 'Slow Motion Train Wreck.'" *PBS Newshour*. March 28, 2018.

16. "Making the World Safe from Superbugs." *Consumer Reports*. November 18, 2015.

17. Moyer MW. "How Drug-Resistant Bacteria Travel from the Farm to Your Table." *Scien-tific American*. December 1, 2016.

18. Jechalke S, Heuer H, Siemens J, et al. "Fate and Effects of Veterinary Antibiotics in Soil." *Trends Microbiol*. 2014 Sep;22(9):536–45.

19. "Making the World Safe from Superbugs." *Consumer Reports*. November 18, 2015.

20. RAND Corporation. "Estimating the Economic Costs of Antimicrobial Resistance." Retrieved May 27, 2019, from https://www.rand.org/randeurope/research/projects/anti microbial-resistance-costs.html.

21. Gurian-Sherman D. "CAFOs Uncovered: The Untold Costs of Confined Animal Feed-ing Operations." Union of Concerned Scientists. April 2008. https://www.ucsusa.org/sites /default/files/legacy/assets/documents/food_and_agriculture/cafos-uncovered .pdf.

22. US Food and Drug Administration. "Summary Report on Antimicrobials Sold or Dis-tributed for Use in Food-Producing Animals." Department of Health and Human Ser-vices. September 2014. https://www.fda.gov/downloads/ForIndustry/UserFees/Animal DrugUserFeeActADUFA/UCM231851.pdf.

23. Landers TF, Cohen B, Wittum TE, Larson EL. "A Review of Antibiotic Use in Food Animals: Perspective, Policy, and Potential." *Public Health Rep*. 2012 Jan–Feb;127(1):4–22.

24. "Making the World Safe from Superbugs." *Consumer Reports.* November 18, 2015.

25. World Health Organization. (2018). "Antibiotic Resistance." https://www.who.int/news-room/fact-sheets/detail/antibiotic-resistance.

26. World Health Organization. (2018). "Antibiotic Resistance." https://www.who.int/news-room/fact-sheets/detail/antibiotic-resistance; US PIRG. *Weak Medicine: Why the FDA's Guidelines Are Inadequate to Curb Antibiotic Resistance and Protect Public Health.* September 10, 2014. https://uspirg.org/reports/usf/weak-medicine.

27. Center for Science in the Public Interest. (2010). "Food Labeling Chaos." https://cspinet.org/resource/food-labeling-chaos.

CHAPTER 10

1. Applebaum, RS. "Balancing the Debate. The Food Industry: Trends & Opportunities." 29th International Sweetener Symposium. PowerPoint presentation. 2012. http://www.phaionline.org/wp-content/uploads/2015/08/Rhona-Applebaum.pdf.

2. Hagstrom Report. (2012). "Coca-Cola Exec: Sugar Growers Need to Fight Off Detractors." August 17. http://www.hagstromreport.com/2012news_files/2012_0817_coke.html.

3. Ibid.

4. Katzmarzyk P. E-mails to Rhona Applebaum, vice president, Coca-Cola. January 15, 2014. UCSF Food Industry Documents Library. https://www.industrydocuments.ucsf.edu/food/docs/#id=jjvy0227.

5. Ludwig DS, Ebbeling CB. "The Carbohydrate-Insulin Model of Obesity: Beyond 'Calories In, Calories Out.'" *JAMA Intern Med.* 2018;178(8):1098–103.

6. Pennington Biomedical Research Center. (2015). "Pennington Biomedical Research Study Shows Lack of Physical Activity Is a Major Predictor of Childhood Obesity." Press release. August 3, 2015. https://www.pbrc.edu/news/press-releases/?ArticleID=284.

7. Serôdio PM, McKee M, Stuckler D. "Coca-Cola—a Model of Transparency in Research Partnerships? A Network Analysis of Coca-Cola's Research Funding (2008–2016)." *Public Health Nutr.* 2018 Jun;21(9):1594–607.

8. Fabbri A, Holland TJ, Bero LA. "Food Industry Sponsorship of Academic Research: Investigating Commercial Bias in the Research Agenda." *Public Health Nutr.* 2018 Dec;21(18):3422–30.

9. Peters JC, Wyatt HR, Foster GD, et al. "The Effects of Water and Non-Nutritive Sweetened Beverages on Weight Loss during a 12-Week Weight Loss Treatment Program." *Obesity.* 2014 Jun;22(6):1415–21.

10. Litman EA, Gortmaker SL, Ebbeling CB, Ludwig DS. "Source of Bias in Sugar-Sweetened Beverage Research: A Systematic Review." *Public Health Nutr.* 2018 Aug;21(12):2345–50.

11. Fischer K. "Nutritionists Outraged by Study Touting Diet Soda for Weight Loss." *Parade.* May 30, 2014.

12. Olinger D. "CU Nutrition Expert Accepts $550,000 from Coca-Cola for Obesity Campaign." *Denver Post.* December 26, 2015.

13. Choi C. "Emails Reveal Coke's Role in Anti-Obesity Group." Associated Press. November 24, 2015.

14. Ebbeling CB, Feldman HA, Klein GL, et al. "Effects of a Low Carbohydrate Diet on Energy Expenditure during Weight Loss Maintenance: Randomized Trial." *BMJ.* 2018 Nov 14;363:k4583.

15. Stone K. "Internal Documents Show Coke Had Profits in Mind When It Funded Nutrition 'Science.'" HealthNewsReview.org. March 28, 2018.

16. O'Connor A. "Coke's Chief Scientist, Who Orchestrated Obesity Research, Is Leaving." *New York Times.* November 24, 2015.

17. Steele S, Ruskin G, McKee M, Stuckler D. "Always Read the Small Print: A Case Study of Commercial Research Funding, Disclosure and Agreements with Coca-Cola." *J Public Health Policy.* 2019 May 8.

18. Brownell KD, Warner KE. "The Perils of Ignoring History: Big Tobacco Played Dirty and Millions Died. How Similar Is Big Food?" *Milbank Q.* 2009 Mar;87(1):259–94.

19. Center for Consumer Freedom. (2019). "Obesity Hype." https://www.consumerfree dom.com/print-ad/obesity-hype/.

20. Wikipedia, s.v. "Personal Responsibility in Food Consumption Act." Last edited August 5, 2018. https://en.wikipedia.org/wiki/Personal_Responsibility_in_Food_Consumption _Act.

21. Ludwig DS, Peterson KE, Gortmaker SL. "Relation between Consumption of Sugar-Sweetened Drinks and Childhood Obesity: A Prospective, Observational Analysis." *Lancet.* 2001 Feb 17;357(9255):505–8.

22. Lesser LI, Ebbeling CB, Goozner M, et al. "Relationship between Funding Source and Conclusion among Nutrition-Related Scientific Articles." *PLoS Med.* 2007 Jan;4(1):e5.

23. Litman EA, Gortmaker SL, Ebbeling CB, Ludwig DS. "Source of Bias in Sugar-Sweetened Beverage Research: A Systematic Review." *Public Health Nutr.* 2018 Aug;21(12):2345–50.

24. Mandrioli D, Kearns CE, Bero LA. "Relationship between Research Outcomes and Risk of Bias, Study Sponsorship, and Author Financial Conflicts of Interest in Reviews of the Effects of Artificially Sweetened Beverages on Weight Outcomes: A Systematic Review of Reviews." *PLoS One.* 2016 Sep 8;11(9):e0162198. doi:10.1371/journal.pone .0162198. eCollection 2016. Review.

25. Mozaffarian D. "Conflict of Interest and the Role of the Food Industry in Nutrition Research." *JAMA.* 2017;317(17):1755–56.

26. O'Neill CE, Fulgoni VL III, Nicklas TA. "Association of Candy Consumption with Body Weight Measures, Other Health Risk Factors for Cardiovascular Disease, and Diet Quality in US Children and Adolescents: NHANES 1999–2004." *Food Nutr Res.* 2011;55. doi: 10.3402/fnr.v55i0.5794.

27. Choi C. "AP Exclusive: How Candy Makers Shape Nutrition Science." Associated Press. June 2, 2016.

28. O'Neil CE, Fulgoni VL III, Nicklas TA. "Candy Consumption Was Not Associated with Body Weight Measures, Risk Factors for Cardiovascular Disease, or Metabolic Syndrome in US Adults: NHANES 1999–2004." *Nutr Res.* 2011 Feb;31(2):122–30.

29. Erickson J, Sadeghirad B, Lytvyn L, et al. "The Scientific Basis of Guideline Recommendations on Sugar Intake: A Systematic Review." *Ann Intern Med.* 2017;166:257–67.

30. Mohamed HJJ, Loy SL, Taib MN, et al. "Characteristics Associated with the Consumption of Malted Drinks among Malaysian Primary School Children: Findings from the Mybreakfast Study." *BMC Public Health.* 2015 Dec 30;15:1322.

31. O'Connor A. "Sugar Industry Long Downplayed Potential Harms." *New York Times*. November 21, 2017.

32. Stare, FJ. *Adventures in Nutrition*. Hanover, MA: Christopher Publishing House, 1991.

33. Lipton E. "Rival Industries Sweet-Talk the Public." *New York Times*. February 11, 2014.

34. Rippe JM, Sievenpiper JL, Lê KA, et al. "What Is the Appropriate Upper Limit for Added Sugars Consumption?" *Nutr Rev*. 2017 Jan;75(1):18–36; Lowndes J, Sinnett SS, Rippe JM. "No Effect of Added Sugar Consumed at Median American Intake Level on Glucose Tolerance or Insulin Resistance." *Nutrients*. 2015 Oct 23;7(10):8830–45; Lowndes J, Sinnett S, Yu Z, Rippe J. "The Effects of Fructose-Containing Sugars on Weight, Body Composition and Cardiometabolic Risk Factors When Consumed at Up to the 90th Percentile Population Consumption Level for Fructose." *Nutrients*. 2014 Aug 8;6(8):3153–68.

35. Kelly SA. "Wholegrain Cereals for Coronary Heart Disease." *Cochrane Database Syst Rev*. 2007 Apr 18;2.

36. Mozaffarian D. "Conflict of Interest and the Role of the Food Industry in Nutrition Research." *JAMA*. 2017;317(17):1755–56.

37. Zhong VW, Van Horn L, Cornelis MC, et al. "Associations of Dietary Cholesterol or Egg Consumption with Incident Cardiovascular Disease and Mortality." *JAMA*. 2019;321(11):-1081–95.

38. Archer E, Pavela G, Lavie CJ. "The Inadmissibility of What We Eat in America and NHANES Dietary Data in Nutrition and Obesity Research and the Scientific Formulation of National Dietary Guidelines." *Mayo Clin Proc*. 2015 Jul;90(7):911–26.

39. Archer E, Marlow ML, Lavie CJ. "Controversy and Debate: Memory-Based Methods Paper 1: The Fatal Flaws of Food Frequency Questionnaires and Other Memory-Based Dietary Assessment Methods." *J Clin Epidemiol*. 2018 Dec;104:113–24.

40. Sinha R, Cross AJ, Graubard BI, et al. "Meat Intake and Mortality: A Prospective Study of Over Half a Million People." *Arch Intern Med*. 2009 Mar 23;169(6):562–71.

41. Ebbeling CB, Feldman HA, Klein GL, et al. "Effects of a Low Carbohydrate Diet on Energy Expenditure during Weight Loss Maintenance: Randomized Trial." *BMJ*. 2018 Nov 14;363:k4583.

CHAPTER 11

1. Confessore N. "Minority Groups and Bottlers Team Up in Battles Over Soda." *New York Times*. March 12, 2013.

2. Erbentraut J. "People of Color Bear the Brunt of Fast-Food Explosion." *HuffPost*. April 29, 2017.

3. Olson S. "Unhealthy Food Ads Target Minorities, Possibly Contributing to Childhood Obesity." *Medical Daily*. August 12, 2015.

4. Dewey C. "'We're Losing More People to the Sweets Than to the Streets': Why Two Black Pastors Are Suing Coca-Cola." *Washington Post*. July 13, 2017.

5. Ibid.

6. Lowe A, Hacker G. "Selfish Giving: How the Soda Industry Uses Philanthropy to Sweeten Its Profits." Center for Science in the Public Interest. https://cspinet.org/sites/default/files/attachment/cspi_soda_philanthropy_online.pdf.

7. Neuman W. "Save the Children Breaks with Soda Tax Effort." *New York Times*. December 14, 2010.

8. Warner M. "Beverage Lobby's New Weapon in the War against Soda Taxes: Cold Hard Cash." CBS News. March 16, 2011.

9. Zhong Y, Auchincloss AH, Lee BK, et al. "The Short-Term Impacts of the Philadelphia Beverage Tax on Beverage Consumption." *Am J Prev Med*. 2018 Jul;55(1):26–34.

10. Roberto CA, Lawman HG, LeVasseur MT, et al. "Association of a Beverage Tax on Sugar-Sweetened and Artificially Sweetened Beverages with Changes in Beverage Prices and Sales at Chain Retailers in a Large Urban Setting." *JAMA*. 2019;321(18):1799–810.

11. Jacobs A. "Tuesday Could Be the Beginning of the End of Philadelphia's Soda Tax." *New York Times*. May 20, 2019. https://www.nytimes.com/2019/05/20/health/soda-tax-phila delphia.html.

12. O'Connor A. "Coca-Cola Funds Scientists Who Shift Blame for Obesity Away from Bad Diets." *New York Times*. August 9, 2015.

13. Long MW, Gortmaker SL, Ward ZJ, et al. "Cost Effectiveness of a Sugar-Sweetened Beverage Excise Tax in the U.S." *Am J Prev Med*. 2015 Jul;49(1):112–23.

14. O'Connor A, Sanger-Katz M. "California, of All Places, Has Banned Soda Taxes. How a New Industry Strategy Is Succeeding." *New York Times*. June 27, 2018. https://www .nytimes.com/2018/06/27/upshot/california-banning-soda-taxes-a-new-industry-strategy -is-stunning-some-lawmakers.html.

15. Crosbie E, Schillinger D, Schmidt LA. "State Preemption to Prevent Local Taxation of Sugar-Sweetened Beverages." *JAMA Intern Med*. Published online January 22, 2019;179(3): 291–92.

16. Santora M. "In Diabetes Fight, Raising Cash and Keeping Trust." *New York Times*. November 25, 2006.

17. Shearer J, Swithers SE. "Artificial Sweeteners and Metabolic Dysregulation: Lessons Learned from Agriculture and the Laboratory." *Rev Endocr Metab Disord*. 2016 Jun;17(2):179–86.

18. Suez J, Korem T, Zilberman-Schapira G, et al. "Non-Caloric Artificial Sweeteners and the Microbiome: Findings and Challenges." *Gut Microbes*. 2015;6(2):149–55.

19. O'Connor A. "Coke Spends Lavishly on Pediatricians and Dietitians." *New York Times*. September 28, 2015.

20. Husten L. "Coca-Cola, the Olympic Torch and the American College of Cardiology." *Cardio Brief*. July 9, 2012. Retrieved February 15, 2013, from http://cardiobrief.org /2012/07/09/coca-cola-the-olympic-torch-and-the-american-college-of-cardiology/.

21. Ioannidis JPA. "Professional Societies Should Abstain from Authorship of Guidelines and Disease Definition Statements." *Circ Cardiovasc Qual Outcomes*. 2018 Oct;11(10):e004889.

22. Chowdhury R, Warnakula S, Kunutsor S, et al. "Association of Dietary, Circulating, and Supplement Fatty Acids with Coronary Risk: A Systematic Review and Meta-Analysis." *Ann Intern Med*. 2014 Mar 18;160(6):398–406.

23. Nutrition Coalition. 2018–19. "The Disputed Science on Saturated Fats." www.nutri tioncoalition.us/saturated-fats-do-they-cause-heart-disease/.

24. Simon M. "And Now a Word from Our Sponsors: Are America's Nutrition Professionals in the Pocket of Big Food?" January 23, 2013. Eat Drink Politics. http://www.eatdrink politics.com/2013/01/22/and-now-a-word-from-our-sponsors-new-report-from-eat -drink-politics/.

25. Ibid.

26. Ludwig DS, Willett WC. "Three Daily Servings of Reduced-Fat Milk: An Evidence-Based Recommendation?" *JAMA Pediatr.* 2013 Sep;167(9):788–89.

27. Ibid.

28. Strom S. "A Cheese 'Product' Gains Kids' Nutrition Seal." *New York Times.* March 12, 2015.

29. Strom S. "Dietitians Group Negotiating to End Labeling Deal With Kraft Singles." *New York Times.* March 30, 2015. https://www.nytimes.com/2015/03/31/business/dietitians-group-negotiating-to-end-labeling-deal-with-kraft-singles.html.

30. Strom S. "A Cheese 'Product' Gains Kids' Nutrition Seal." *New York Times.* March 12, 2015.

31. Choi C. "Coke As a Sensible Snack? Coca-Cola Works with Dietitians Who Suggest Cola As Snack." *Star Tribune.* March 16, 2015; Pfister K. "Is Coke Paying Dietitians to Tweet against the Soda Tax?" *Observer.* October 7, 2016. https://observer.com/2016/10/is-coke-paying-dietitians-to-tweet-against-the-soda-tax/.

32. Pfister K. "Is Coke Paying Dietitians to Tweet against the Soda Tax?" *Observer.* October 7, 2016. https://observer.com/2016/10/is-coke-paying-dietitians-to-tweet-against-the-soda-tax/; Nestle M. *Unsavory Truth: How Food Companies Skew the Science of What We Eat.* New York: Basic Books, 2018.

33. Pfister K. "Coke Is Running for President of the National Academy of Nutrition & Dietetics." *Medium.* February 20, 2017; Swerdloff A. "America's Largest Group of Dietitians Was Almost Run by Big Soda." *Munchies.* March 1, 2017.

34. Swerdloff A. "America's Largest Group of Dietitians Was Almost Run by Big Soda." *Munchies.* March 1, 2017.

35. Weaver CM, Dwyer J, Fulgoni VL III, et al. "Processed Foods: Contributions to Nutrition." *Am J Clin Nutr.* 2014 Jun;99(6):1525–42.

36. Nestle M. *Unsavory Truth: How Food Companies Skew the Science of What We Eat.* New York: Basic Books, 2018.

37. Center for Media and Democracy. "American Council on Science and Health." https://www.sourcewatch.org/index.php/American_Council_on_Science_and_Health#Funding.

38. Hogan B. (2019). "Paging Dr. Ross." *Mother Jones.* https://www.motherjones.com/politics/2005/11/paging-dr-ross/.

39. Ioannidis JPA. "Professional Societies Should Abstain from Authorship of Guidelines and Disease Definition Statements." *Circ Cardiovasc Qual Outcomes.* 2018 Oct;11(10):e004889.

40. Dietitians for Professional Integrity. "Ethical Sponsorship." https://integritydietitians.org/practice-area/sponsorship-rubric/.

41. Ibid.

42. Pew Charitable Trusts. "Conflicts-of-Interest Policies for Academic Medical Centers." December 18, 2013.

CHAPTER 12

1. Schulz LO, Chaudhari LS. "High-Risk Populations: The Pimas of Arizona and Mexico." *Curr Obes Rep.* 2015;4(1):92–98. doi: 10.1007/s13679-014-0132-9.

2. Phippen JW. "'Kill Every Buffalo You Can! Every Buffalo Dead Is an Indian Gone.'" *The Atlantic.* May 13, 2016. https://www.theatlantic.com/national/archive/2016/05/the-buffalo-killers/482349/.

3. Centers for Disease Control and Prevention. (2019). "National Vital Statistics System." https://www.cdc.gov/nchs/nvss/deaths.htm.

4. Centers for Disease Control and Prevention. (2019). "Deaths and Mortality." https://www.cdc.gov/nchs/fastats/deaths.htm.

5. Read about Paul Farmer in the book *Mountains beyond Mountains* (New York: Random House, 2003) by Tracy Kidder.

6. New England Journal of Medicine. (2017). "Social Determinants of Health (SDOH)." https://catalyst.nejm.org/social-determinants-of-health/.

7. Elnahas AI, Jackson TD, Hong D. "Management of Failed Laparoscopic Roux-en-Y Gastric Bypass." *Bariatr Surg Pract Patient Care.* 2014;9(1):36–40.

8. Chetty R, Stepner M, Abraham S, et al. "The Association between Income and Life Expectancy in the United States, 2001–2014." *JAMA.* 2016;315(16):1750–66.

9. US Census Bureau. "Income and Poverty in the United States: 2018." September 10, 2019. https://www.census.gov/library/publications/2019/demo/p60-266.html; "Poverty Facts: The Population of Poverty USA." Poverty USA. 2019. https://www.povertyusa.org/facts.

10. Gonzales S, Sawyer B. (2017). "How Does Infant Mortality in the U.S. Compare to Other Countries?" Kaiser Family Foundation. https://www.healthsystemtracker.org/chart-collection/infant-mortality-u-s-compare-countries/#item-start.

11. Hauck FR, Tanabe KO, Moon RY. "Racial and Ethnic Disparities in Infant Mortality." *Semin Perinatol.* 2011 Aug;35(4):209–20.

12. Mayer-Davis EJ, Lawrence JM, Dabelea D, et al. "Incidence Trends of Type 1 and Type 2 Diabetes among Youths, 2002–2012." *N Engl J Med.* 2017 Apr 13;376(15):1419–29.

13. Wheeler SM, Bryant AS. "Racial and Ethnic Disparities in Health and Health Care." *Obstet Gynecol Clin North Am.* 2017 Mar;44(1):1–11.

14. Cooksey-Stowers K, Schwartz M, Brownell K. "Food Swamps Predict Obesity Rates Better Than Food Deserts in the United States." *Int J Environ Res Public Health.* 2017 Nov 14;14(11):1366.

15. Schlosser E. *Fast Food Nation: The Dark Side of the All-American Meal.* Boston: Houghton Mifflin Harcourt, 2012.

16. Block JP, Scribner RA, DeSalvo KB. "Fast Food, Race/Ethnicity, and Income: A Geographic Analysis." *Am J Prev Med.* 2004 Oct 1;27(3):211–17.

17. Luna GT. "The New Deal and Food Insecurity in the Midst of Plenty." *Drake J Agric L.* 2004;9:213.

18. Nutrition and Well-Being A to Z. (2019). "Diet and African Americans." http://www.faqs.org/nutrition/A-Ap/African-Americans-Diet-of.html.

19. Freeman A. "Fast Food: Oppression through Poor Nutrition." *Calif L Rev.* 2007;95:2221.

20. Businessroundtable.org. Accessed November 4, 2019. https://opportunity.businessroundtable.org/ourcommitment/.

21. McCoy-Harms S, Tokunaga J, Wolin J, Wongking S. "Housing, Pregnancy & Preterm Birth in San Francisco." San Francisco State University Health Equity Institute. https://view.publitas.com/ucsf/benioff-community-innovators-assessment-report-2017/page/1.

22. Hunter S, Harvey M, Briscombe B, Cefalu M. "Evaluation of Housing for Health Permanent Supportive Housing Program." Santa Monica, CA: RAND Corporation, 2017. https://www.rand.org/pubs/research_reports/RR1694.html.

23. Hartline-Grafton H, Dean O. "The Impact of Poverty, Food Insecurity, and Poor Nutrition on Health and Well-Being." Food Research and Action Center. December 7, 2017. http://frac.org/wp-content/uploads/hunger-health-impact-poverty-food-insecurity-health-well-being.pdf.

24. Seligman HK, Bindman AB, Vittinghoff E, Kanaya AM, Kushel MB. "Food Insecurity Is Associated with Diabetes Mellitus: Results from the National Health Examination and Nutrition Examination Survey (NHANES) 1999–2002." *J General Intern Med.* 2007 Jul 1;22(7):1018–23.

25. Cook JT, Poblacion AP. *Estimating the Health-Related Costs of Food Insecurity and Hunger. The Nourishing Effect: Ending Hunger, Improving Health, Reducing Inequality (2016 Hunger Report).* Bread for the World Institute. Washington, DC. 2016.

26. Harris JL, Frazier W, Kumanyika S, Ramirez AG. "Increasing Disparities in Unhealthy Food Advertising Targeted to Hispanic and Black Youth." UConn Rudd Center for Food Policy and Obesity. 2019. http://uconnruddcenter.org/files/Pdfs/TargetedMarketingReport2019.pdf=.

27. Appiah O. "It Must Be the Cues: Racial Differences in Adolescents' Responses to Culturally Embedded Ads." In *Advertising and Consumer Psychology. Diversity in Advertising: Broadening the Scope of Research Directions*, ed. Williams JD, Lee WN, Haugtvedt CP, 319–39. Mahwah, NJ: Lawrence Erlbaum Associates Publishers, 2004; Pereira MA, Kartashov AI, Ebbeling CB, et al. "Fast-Food Habits, Weight Gain, and Insulin Resistance (the CARDIA Study): 15-Year Prospective Analysis." *Lancet.* 2005 Jan 1;365(9453):36–42.

28. Edwards C. "Empowering Citizens to Monitor Federal Spending." Cato Institute. 2006. https://object.cato.org/sites/cato.org/files/pubs/pdf/tbb_0718-38.pdf.

29. Food Tank. (2016). "20 Organizations Fighting for Food Justice." https://foodtank.com/news/2016/11/twenty-organizations-fighting-for-food-justice/.

30. Schillinger D, Huey N. "Messengers of Truth and Health—Young Artists of Color Raise Their Voices to Prevent Diabetes." *JAMA.* 2018 Mar 20;319(11):1076–78; see also http://www.thebiggerpictureproject.org.

31. Ibid.

CHAPTER 13

1. Nasim S, Naeini AA, Najafi M, Ghazvini M, Hassanzadeh A. "Relationship between Antioxidant Status and Attention Deficit Hyperactivity Disorder among Children." *Int J Prev Med.* 2019;10.

2. Bender A, Hagan KE, Kingston N. "The Association of Folate and Depression: A Meta-Analysis." *J Psychiatr Res.* 2017 Dec 1;95:9–18.

3. Sarris J, Logan AC, Akbaraly TN, et al. "Nutritional Medicine As Mainstream in Psychiatry." *Lancet Psychiatry.* 2015 Mar 1;2(3):271–74.

4. World Health Organization. "World Health Statistics 2016: Monitoring Health for the SDGs, Sustainable Development Goals." World Health Organization. June 8, 2016.

5. Banta JE, Segovia-Siapco G, Crocker CB, Montoya D, Alhusseini N. "Mental Health Status and Dietary Intake among California Adults: A Population-Based Survey." *Int J Food Sci Nutr.* 2019 Feb 8:1–2.

6. Marx W, Moseley G, Berk M, Jacka F. "Nutritional Psychiatry: The Present State of the Evidence." *Proc Nutr Soc.* 2017 Nov;76(4):427–36.

7. Facts Maps. (2019). "PISA Worldwide Ranking—Average Score of Math, Science and Reading." http://factsmaps.com/pisa-worldwide-ranking-average-score-of-math-science-reading/.

8. Centers for Disease Control and Prevention. (2019). "Attention-Deficit/Hyperactivity Disorder (ADHD)." https://www.cdc.gov/ncbddd/adhd/data.html.

9. Hair NL, Hanson JL, Wolfe BL, Pollak SD. "Association of Child Poverty, Brain Development, and Academic Achievement." *JAMA Pediatr.* 2015 Sep 1;169(9):822–29.

10. Reardon SF. "The Widening Academic Achievement Gap between the Rich and the Poor: New Evidence and Possible Explanations." In *Whither Opportunity*, ed. Duncan GJ, Murnane RJ, 91–116. New York: Russell Sage Foundation, 2011.

11. Centers for Disease Control and Prevention. "Health and Academic Achievement." 2014. https://www.cdc.gov/healthyyouth/health_and_academics/pdf/health-academic-achievement.pdf.

12. Basch CE. "Breakfast and the Achievement Gap among Urban Minority Youth." *J Sch Health.* 2011 Oct;81(10):635–40.

13. Kleinman RE, Murphy JM, Little M, et al. "Hunger in Children in the United States: Potential Behavioral and Emotional Correlates." *Pediatrics.* 1998 Jan 1;101(1):e3.

14. Lustig RH, Schmidt LA, Brindis CD. "Public Health: The Toxic Truth about Sugar." *Nature.* 2012 Feb 1;482(7383):27–29.

15. Jones TW, Borg WP, Boulware SD, et al. "Enhanced Adrenomedullary Response and Increased Susceptibility to Neuroglycopenia: Mechanisms Underlying the Adverse Effects of Sugar Ingestion in Healthy Children." *J Pediatr.* 1995 Feb 1;126(2):171–77.

16. Kennedy M. "Special Education Costs Weigh Down San Diego–Area Districts." *American School and University.* 2019. https://www.asumag.com/funding/special-education-costs-weigh-down-san-diego-area-districts.

17. Pollitt E. "Iron Deficiency and Cognitive Function." *Annu Rev Nutr.* 1993 Jul;13(1):521–37.

18. Chenoweth WL. "Vitamin B Complex Deficiency and Excess." In *Nelson Textbook of Pediatrics*, ed. Kliegman RM, Behrman RE, Jenson HB, Stanton BMD, 246–51. Amsterdam: Elsevier, 2007.

19. Zahedi H, Kelishadi R, Heshmat R, et al. "Association between Junk Food Consumption and Mental Health in a National Sample of Iranian Children and Adolescents: The CASPIAN-IV Study." *Nutrition.* 2014 Nov 1;30(11–12):1391–97.

20. Strang S, Hoeber C, Uhl O, et al. "Impact of Nutrition on Social Decision Making." *Proc Natl Acad Sci.* 2017 Jun 20;114(25):6510–14.

21. Hibbeln JR. "From Homicide to Happiness—A Commentary on Omega-3 Fatty Acids in Human Society." *Nutr Health.* 2007 Jul;19(1–2):9–19.

22. Bentley J. "U.S. Trends in Food Availability and a Dietary Assessment of Loss-Adjusted Food Availability, 1970–2014." US Department of Agriculture. 2017. http://mhaia.org/wp-content/uploads/002_Misc_Files/ERS_Paper_US_Trends_Food_Availability.pdf.

23. Gesch CB, Hammond SM, Hampson SE, Eves A, Crowder MJ. "Influence of Supplementary Vitamins, Minerals and Essential Fatty Acids on the Antisocial Behavior of Young Adult Prisoners: Randomized, Placebo-Controlled Trial." *Brit J Psychiatry.* 2002 Jul;181(1):22–28.

24. Schoenthaler S, Amos S, Doraz W, et al. "The Effect of Randomized Vitamin-Mineral Supplementation on Violent and Non-Violent Antisocial Behavior among Incarcerated Juveniles." *J Nutr Environ Med.* 1997 Jan 1;7(4):343–52.

25. Centers for Disease Control and Prevention. (2019). "WISQARS Leading Causes of Death Reports, National and Regional, 1999–2015." http://webappa.cdc.gov/sasweb/ncipc /leadcaus10_us.html.

26. Schoenthaler SJ. "The Northern California Diet-Behavior Program: An Empirical Examination of 3,000 Incarcerated Juveniles in Stanislaus County Juvenile Hall." *International Journal of Biosocial Research*. 1983.

27. Schoenthaler SJ, Bier ID. "The Effect of Vitamin-Mineral Supplementation on Juvenile Delinquency Among American Schoolchildren: A Randomized, Double-Blind Placebo-Controlled Trial." *J of Alt and Comp Med*. 2000 Feb 1;6(1):7–17.

28. Benton D. "The Impact of Diet on Anti-Social, Violent and Criminal Behavior." *Neuroscience & Biobehavioral Reviews*. 2007 Jan 1;31(5):752–74.

29. Jackson DB. "The link between poor quality nutrition and childhood antisocial behavior: A genetically informative analysis." *J of Crim Jus*. 2016 Mar 1;44:13–20.

30. Ramsbotham LD, Gesch B. "Crime and Nourishment: Cause for a Rethink?" *Prison Serv J*. 2009 Mar 1;182:3–9.

31. Ibid.

32. Council for a Strong America. (2018). "Unhealthy and Unprepared: National Security Depends on Promoting Healthy Lifestyles from an Early Age." https://www.strongnation.org/articles/737-unhealthy-and-unprepared.

33. Selhub E. (2015). "Nutritional Psychiatry: Your Brain on Food." https://www.health.harvard.edu/blog/nutritional-psychiatry-your-brain-on-food-201511168626; American Psychological Association. (2017). "The Link between Food and Mental Health." https://www.apa.org/monitor/2017/09/food-mental-health.

34. Hollar D, Messiah SE, Lopez-Mitnik G, et al. "Effect of a Two-Year Obesity Prevention Intervention on Percentile Changes in Body Mass Index and Academic Performance in Low-Income Elementary School Children." *Am J Public Health*. 2010 Apr;100(4):646–53.

35. Brigaid. (2019). "About Us." https://www.chefsbrigaid.com/.

CHAPTER 14

1. DeNavas-Walt C, Procter BD, Smith JC. "Income, Poverty, and Health Insurance Coverage in the United States: 2012." September 2013. https://www.census.gov/prod/2013pubs/p60-245.pdf.

2. Elsheikh E, Barhoum N. "Structural Racialization and Food Insecurity in the United States." University of California, Berkeley. September 2013. https://haasinstitute.berkeley.edu/sites/default/files/Structural%20Racialization%20%20%26%20Food%20Insecurity%20in%20the%20US-%28Final%29.pdf.

3. Kurtzleben D. "The 10 Lowest-Paid Jobs in America." *U.S. News & World Report*. March 29, 2013. https://www.usnews.com/news/articles/2013/03/29/the-10-lowest-paid-jobs-in-america.

4. Jacobs K, Perry I, and MacGillvary J. "The High Public Cost of Low Wages." Research brief. UC Berkeley Center for Labor Research and Education. April 2015. http://laborcenter.berkeley.edu/pdf/2015/the-high-public-cost-of-low-wages.pdf.

5. Sustainable Food Trust. "The True Cost of American Food." April 2016. http://sustainablefoodtrust.org/wp-content/uploads/2013/04/TCAF-report.pdf.

6. US Department of Labor. (2019). "Wage and Hour Division: Minimum Wages for Tipped Employees." https://www.dol.gov/whd/state/tipped.htm.

7. Ramchandi A. "There's a Sexual Harassment Epidemic on America's Farms." *The Atlantic*, January 29, 2018. https://www.theatlantic.com/business/archive/2018/01/agri culture-sexual-harassment/550109/.

8. *Proceso*. (2019). "'Desaparecen': 80 jornaleros indígenas en Chihuahua tras denuncia de abuso laboral." *Proceso*. https://www.proceso.com.mx/488517/desaparecen-80-jornaleros -indigenas-en-chihuahua-tras-denuncia-abuso-laboral.

9. Kahn C. (2018). "Blood Avocados No More: Mexican Farm Town Says It's Kicked Out Cartels." National Public Radio. https://www.npr.org/sections/parallels/2018/02/02 /582086654/mexicos-avocado-capital-says-it-s-kicked-cartels-off-the-farm.

10. Patel S, Sangeeta S. "Pesticides as the Drivers of Neuropsychotic Diseases, Cancers, and Teratogenicity among Agro-Workers as Well as General Public." *Environ Sci Pollut Res Int*. 2019 Jan;26(1):91–100.

11. Priyadarshi A, Khuder SA, Schaub EA, Shrivastava S. "A Meta-Analysis of Parkinson's Disease and Exposure to Pesticides." *Neurotoxicology*. 2000 Aug;21(4):435–40.

12. Bale R. "5 Pesticides Used in US Are Banned in Other Countries." *Reveal*. October 23, 2014. https://www.revealnews.org/article-legacy/5-pesticides-used-in-us-are-banned-in -other-countries/.

13. Davoren MJ, Schiestl RH. "Glyphosate-Based Herbicides and Cancer Risk: A Post-IARC Decision Review of Potential Mechanisms, Policy and Avenues of Research." *Carcinogenesis*. 2018 Oct 8;39(10):1207–15.

14. Heindel JJ, Blumberg B. "Environmental Obesogens: Mechanisms and Controversies." *Ann Rev Pharmacol Toxicol*. 2019 Jan 6;59:89–106.

15. University of California, Berkeley. "CHAMACOS Study." Retrieved May 27, 2019, from https://cerch.berkeley.edu/research-programs/chamacos-study.

16. Bellinger DC. "A Strategy for Comparing the Contributions of Environmental Chemicals and Other Risk Factors to Neurodevelopment of Children." *Environ Health Perspect*. 2012 Apr;120(4):501–7.

17. Filippelli C, Verso MG, Amicarelli V, et al. "Food service workers and cooks: occupational risk assessment" (in Italian). *Ann Ig*. 2008 Jan–Feb;20(1):57–67.

18. Newman KL, Leon JS, Newman LS. "Estimating Occupational Illness, Injury, and Mortality in Food Production in the United States: A Farm-to-Table Analysis." *J Occup Environ Med*. 2015 Jul;57(7):718–25.

19. Fair Food Program. *Fair Food 2017 Annual Report*. 2018. http://www.fairfoodprogram .org/wp-content/uploads/2018/06/Fair-Food-Program-2017-Annual-Report-Web.pdf.

20. HEAL Food Alliance. (2019). "Our Platform for Real Food." https://healfoodalliance .org/strategy/the-real-food-platform/.

CHAPTER 15

1. Huntington E. "Climatic Change and Agricultural Exhaustion As Elements in the Fall of Rome." *Q J Econ*. 1917 Feb 1;31(2):173–208.

2. Montgomery, DR. *Dirt: The Erosion of Civilizations*. Berkeley: University of California Press; 2012.

3. Food and Agriculture Organization of the United Nations. (2015). "Status of the World's Resources." http://www.fao.org/policy-support/resources/resources-details/en/c/435200/.

4. Food and Agriculture Organization of the United Nations. (2015). "Soils Are Endangered, but the Degradation Can Be Rolled Back." http://www.fao.org/news/story/en/item/357059/icode/.

5. Eco Nexus. "Agropoly: A Handful of Corporations Control World Food Production." 2013. https://www.econexus.info/sites/econexus/files/Agropoly_Econexus_BerneDeclaration.pdf.

6. Hubbard K. (2019). "The Sobering Details behind the Latest Seed Monopoly." *Civil Eats*. https://civileats.com/2019/01/11/the-sobering-details-behind-the-latest-seed-monopoly-chart/.

7. De Schutter O. "Towards a Common Food Policy for the European Union." iPES Food. 2019. http://www.ipes-food.org/_img/upload/files/CFP_FullReport.pdf.

8. Food and Agriculture Organization of the United Nations. (2019). "What Is Happening to Agrobiodiversity?" http://www.fao.org/3/y5609e/y5609e02.htm.

9. Ibid.; Barker D. "History of Seed in the U.S.: The Untold American Revolution." August 2012. https://www.centerforfoodsafety.org/files/seed-report-for-print-final_25743.pdf.

10. Huffstutter PJ and Pamuk H. "Exclusive: More Than 1 Million Acres of U.S. Cropland Ravaged by Floods." Reuters. March 29, 2019. https://www.reuters.com/article/us-usa-weather-floods-exclusive/exclusive-more-than-1-million-acres-of-u-s-cropland-ravaged-by-floods-idUSKCN1RA2AW.

11. Testimony of Mike Peterson. "Reviewing the State of the Farm Economy." May 9, 2019. https://docs.house.gov/meetings/AG/AG16/20190509/109416/HHRG-116-AG16-Wstate-PetersonM-20190509.pdf.

12. US Commission on Agricultural Workers. *Report of the Commission on Agricultural Workers.* 1992.

13. US Department of Agriculture, Economic Research Service. (2017). "Food Dollar Application." https://data.ers.usda.gov/reports.aspx?ID=17885.

14. Frerick A. "To Revive Rural America, We Must Fix Our Broken Food System." *The American Conservative*. February 27, 2019. https://www.theamericanconservative.com/articles/to-revive-rural-america-we-must-fix-our-broken-food-system/; *The Economic Viability of Farming in the United States.* Report of the Commission on Agricultural Workers. November 1992, 38; US Department of Agriculture. *What Is the Cost of Marketing the Farm Commodities Contained in a Typical $1 Food Purchase?* March 14, 2019. https://data.ers.usda.gov/reports.aspx?ID=17885.

15. Concentration Crisis. (2018). "Meat Processing Industry." https://concentrationcrisis.openmarketsinstitute.org/industry/meat-processing/.

16. Frerick A. "To Revive Rural America, We Must Fix Our Broken Food System." *The American Conservative*. February 27, 2019. https://www.theamericanconservative.com/articles/to-revive-rural-america-we-must-fix-our-broken-food-system/; IBISWorld. "Meat Processing Industry." 2019; Concentration Crisis. (2018). "Meat Processing Industry." https://concentrationcrisis.openmarketsinstitute.org/industry/meat-processing/.

17. US Department of Agriculture. (2018). "Adoption of Genetically Engineered Crops in the United States, 1996–2018." https://www.ers.usda.gov/webdocs/charts/58020/biotechcrops_d.html?v=7149.

18. US Right to Know. (2019). "Monsanto Roundup Trial Tracker." https://usrtk.org/mon santo-roundup-trial-tracker-index/.

19. MacDonald JM, Hoppe RA, Newton D. "Three Decades of Consolidation in U.S. Agriculture." US Department of Agriculture. March 2018. https://www.ers.usda.gov/web docs/publications/88057/eib-189.pdf?v=43172.

20. MacDonald JM, Hoppe RA. (2018). "By the Numbers: A Look at Consolidation in U.S. Agriculture." https://www.alternet.org/2018/03/consolidation-us-agriculture/.

21. Lusk J. (2016). "The Evolution of American Agriculture." http://jaysonlusk.com/blog /2016/6/26/the-evolution-of-american-agriculture.

22. Hakim D. "Doubts About the Promised Bounty of Genetically Modified Crops." *New York Times.* October 29, 2016. https://www.nytimes.com/2016/10/30/business/gmo-pro mise-falls-short.html.

23. Montgomery D. "3 Big Myths About Modern Agriculture." *Scientific American.* April 5, 2017. https://www.scientificamerican.com/article/3-big-myths-about-modern-agriculture1/.

24. Haspel T. "Monocrops: They're a Problem, but Farmers Aren't the Only Ones Who Can Solve It." *Washington Post.* May 9, 2014. https://www.washingtonpost.com/lifestyle/food /monocrops-theyre-a-problem-but-farmers-arent-the-ones-who-can-solve-it/2014 /05/09/8bfc186e-d6f8-11e3-8a78-8fe50322a72c_story.html.

25. Environmental Working Group. (2019). "Farm Subsidy Primer." https://farm.ewg.org /subsidyprimer.php.

26. University of Minnesota. "Norman Borlaug: The Researcher." (2019). https://borlaug .cfans.umn.edu/about-borlaug/researcher.

27. Tierney, John. "Greens and Hunger." Tierney Lab—Putting Ideas in Science to the Test. *New York Times.* May 19, 2008.

28. Pepper D. "The Toxic Consequences of the Green Revolution." *US News & World Report.* July 7, 2008. https://www.usnews.com/news/world/articles/2008/07/07/the-toxic-con sequences-of-the-green-revolution.

29. Bittman M. "How to Feed the World." *New York Times.* October 15, 2013. https://www .nytimes.com/2013/10/15/opinion/how-to-feed-the-world.html.

30. Perroni E. "Can We Feed the World without Destroying It?" *Civil Eats.* January 10, 2019. https://civileats.com/2019/01/10/feeding-the-world-without-destroying-it/.

31. UN Food and Agricultural Organization. *Livestock's Long Shadow.* Rome, Italy: FAO; 2006.

32. GM Watch. (2018). "'Father of Green Revolution in India' Slams GM Crops as Unsustainable and Unsafe." https://www.gmwatch.org/en/news/latest-news/18623-father-of -green-revolution-in-india-slams-gm-crops-as-unsustainable-and-unsafe.

33. Kesavan PC, Swaminathan MS. "Modern Technologies for Sustainable Food and Nutrition Security." *Curr Sci.* 2018 Nov 25;115(10):1876. http://www.currentscience.ac.in /Volumes/115/10/1876.pdf.

34. Daigle K. "Warming Climate Pushing Desperate India Farmers to Suicide." *Chicago Tribune.* July 31, 2017. https://www.chicagotribune.com/news/environment/ct-india-farmers -suicide-climate-change-20170731-story.html.

35. Bowden J. (2019). "PepsiCo Sues Indian Farmers for Growing Trademarked Potatoes." *The Hill.* https://thehill.com/policy/international/440773-pepsico-sues-indian-farmers -for-growing-trademarked-potatoes.

36. Hakim D. "Doubts about the Promised Bounty of Genetically Modified Crops." *New York Times*. October 30, 2016. https://www.nytimes.com/2016/10/30/business/gmo-promise-falls-short.html.

37. Strom S. "National Biotechnology Panel Faces New Conflict of Interest Questions." *New York Times*. December 27, 2016. https://www.nytimes.com/2016/12/27/business/national-academies-biotechnology-conflicts.html?rref=collection%2Fbyline%2Fstephanie-strom&action=click&contentCollection=undefined&region=stream&module=stream_unit&version=latest&contentPlacement=1&pgtype=collection&_r=0.

38. Bellinger DC. "A Strategy for Comparing the Contributions of Environmental Chemicals and Other Risk Factors to Neurodevelopment of Children." *Environ Health Perspect*. 2012 Apr;120(4):501–7.

39. Benbrook CM. "Trends in Glyphosate Herbicide Use in the United States and Globally." *Environ Sci Eur*. 2016 Dec;28(1):3.

40. Formuzis A. "Tests Reveal More Weed Killer Than Some Vitamins in Kids' Cereals." Environmental Working Group. October 31, 2018. https://www.ewg.org/release/tests-reveal-more-weed-killer-some-vitamins-kids-cereals.

41. Berg CJ, King HP, Delenstarr G, et al. "Glyphosate Residue Concentrations in Honey Attributed through Geospatial Analysis to Proximity of Large-Scale Agriculture and Transfer Off-Site by Bees." *PLoS One*. 2018 Jul 11;13(7):e0198876.

42. International Agency for Research on Cancer. March 1, 2016. "IARC Monograph on Glyphosate." www.iarc.fr/featured-news/media-centre-iarc-news-glyphosate/.

43. Aitbali Y, Ba-M'hamed S, Elhidar N, et al. "Glyphosate Based-Herbicide Exposure Affects Gut Microbiota, Anxiety and Depression-Like Behaviors in Mice." *Neurotoxicol Teratol*. 2018 May–Jun;67:44–49.

44. Kubsad D, Nilsson EE, King SE, et al. "Assessment of Glyphosate Induced Epigenetic Transgenerational Inheritance of Pathologies and Sperm Epimutations: Generational Toxicology." *Sci Rep*. 2019 Apr 23;9(1):6372.

45. Helander M, Saloniemi I, Omacini M, et al. "Glyphosate Decreases Mycorrhizal Colonization and Affects Plant-Soil Feedback." *Sci Total Environ*. 2018 Nov 15;642:285–91.

46. Kubsad D, Nilsson EE, King SE, et al. "Assessment of Glyphosate Induced Epigenetic Transgenerational Inheritance of Pathologies and Sperm Epimutations: Generational Toxicology." *Sci Rep*. 2019 Apr 23;9(1):6372.

47. Maixner E, Wyant S. (2019). "Big Changes Ahead in Land Ownership and Farm Operators." https://www.agri-pulse.com/articles/11869-big-changes-ahead-in-land-ownership-and-farm-operators.

48. Economics of Ecosystems and Biodiversity. "TEEB for Agriculture & Food." http://teebweb.org/agrifood/.

49. United Nations (2013). "Wake Up before It Is Too Late: Make Agriculture Truly Sustainable Now for Food Security in a Changing Climate." Conference on Trade and Development. United Nations. https://unctad.org/en/PublicationsLibrary/ditcted2012d3_en.pdf; Grain (2014). "How Much of World's Greenhouse Gas Emissions Come from Agriculture?" https://www.grain.org/article/entries/5272-howmuch-of-world-s-greenhouse-gas-emissions-come-from-agriculture.

50. Economist Intelligence Unit. (2019). "Fixing Food 2016: Towards a More Sustainable Food System." http://foodsustainability.eiu.com/whitepaper/.

51. The Office of US Representative Earl Blumenauer. (2017). "Growing Opportunities: Reforming the Farm Bill for Every American." https://blumenauer.house.gov/sites/blu menauer.house.gov/files/documents/GrowingOpportunities.pdf.

52. US Department of Agriculture. (2012). "Census of Agriculture." https://www.nass.usda .gov/Publications/AgCensus/2012/Online_Resources/Typology/.

53. Environmental Working Group. (2019). "Commodity Subsidies in the United States Totaled 205.4 Billion from 1995–2017." https://farm.ewg.org/progdetail.php?fips=0000 0&progcode=totalfarm&page=conc&regionname=theUnitedStates.

54. Coleman R. (2016). "The Rich Get Richer: 50 Billionaires Got Federal Farm Subsidies." Environmental Working Group. https://www.ewg.org/agmag/2016/04/rich-get -richer-50-billionaires-got-federal-farm-subsidies.

CHAPTER 16

1. United Nations Food and Agriculture Organization. (2019). "Every 5 seconds the equivalent of one soccer pitch is eroded..." https://twitter.com/FAO/status/1128607546447683585.

2. Arsenault C. (2019). "Only 60 Years of Farming Left If Soil Degradation Continues." *Scientific American*. https://www.scientificamerican.com/article/only-60-years-of-farming -left-if-soil-degradation-continues/.

3. Crawford J. (2012). "What If Soil Runs Out?" We Forum. https://www.weforum.org /agenda/2012/12/what-if-soil-runs-out/.

4. Batjes NH. "Total Carbon and Nitrogen in the Soils of the World." *Eur J Soil Sci*. 2014 Jan;65(1):10–21. https://onlinelibrary.wiley.com/doi/abs/10.1111/j.1365-2389.1996 .tb01386.x.

5. Davis DR. "Declining Fruit and Vegetable Nutrient Composition: What Is the Evidence?" *Hort Science*. 2009 Feb 1;44(1):15–19.

6. Harvard T.H. Chan School of Public Health. (2018). "As CO2 Levels Continue to Climb, Millions at Risk of Nutritional Deficiencies." Phys.org. https://phys.org/news/2018 -08-co2-climb-millions-nutritional-deficiencies.html.

7. Sanderman J, Hengl T, Fiske GJ. "Soil Carbon Debt of 12,000 Years of Human Land Use." *Proc Natl Acad Sci USA*. 2017 Sep 5;114(36):9575–80. https://www.pnas.org/con tent/pnas/early/2017/08/15/1706103114.full.pdf.

8. Bafana B. (2017). "The High Price of Desertification: 23 Hectares of Land a Minute." Inter Press Service. https://reliefweb.int/report/world/high-price-desertification-23-hec tares-land-minute.

9. National Science and Technology Council. *The State and Future of U.S. Soils: Framework for a Federal Strategic Plan for Soil Science*. December 2016. https://obamawhitehouse. archives.gov/sites/default/files/microsites/ostp/ssiwg_framework_december_2016 .pdf.

10. Shcherbak I, Millar N, Robertson GP. "Global Metaanalysis of the Nonlinear Response of Soil Nitrous Oxide (N_2O) Emissions to Fertilizer Nitrogen." *Proc Natl Acad Sci USA*. 2014 Jun 24;111(25):9199–204.

11. Mulvaney RL, Khan SA, Ellsworth TR. "Synthetic Nitrogen Fertilizers Deplete Soil Nitrogen: A Global Dilemma for Sustainable Cereal Production." *J Environ Qual*. 2009 Nov 1;38(6):2295–314.

12. Gullap M, Erkovan HI, Koç A. "The Effect of Bovine Saliva on Growth Attributes and Forage Quality of Two Contrasting Cool Season Perennial Grasses Grown in Three Soils of Different Fertility." *Rangeland J.* 2011;33(3):307–13.

13. Lal R. "Soil Carbon Sequestration Impacts on Global Climate Change and Food Security." *Science.* 2004 Jun 11;304(5677):1623–27.

14. Rodale Institute. "Regenerative Organic Agriculture and Climate Change." 2014. https://rodaleinstitute.org/wp-content/uploads/rodale-white-paper.pdf.

15. Majendie, Adam, and Pratik Parija. "These U.N. Climate Scientists Think They Can Halt Global Warming for $300 Billion. Here's How." *Time.* October 24, 2019.

16. Gelski J. "Nestle, Kellogg Among Companies Forming Biodiversity Initiative." *Food Business News.* September 23, 2019. https://www.foodbusinessnews.net/articles/14556 -nestle-kellogg-among-companies-forming-biodiversity-initiative.

17. Byck P. "Soil Carbon Cowboys." Vimeo video, 12:21. 2014. https://vimeo.com/ 80518559.

18. World Economic Forum. (2019). *The Global Risks Report 2019.* http://www3.wefo rum.org/docs/WEF_Global_Risks_Report_2019.pdf.

19. Alexander C. (2019). "Cape Town's 'Day Zero' Water Crisis, One Year Later." City Lab. https://www.citylab.com/environment/2019/04/cape-town-water-conservation-south -africa-drought/587011/.

20. Mekonnen MM, Hoekstra AY. "Four Billion People Facing Severe Water Scarcity." *Sci Adv.* 2016 Feb 1;2(2):e1500323.

21. Plumer B. (2015). "Saudi Arabia Squandered Its Groundwater and Agriculture Collapsed. California, Take Note." *Vox.* https://www.vox.com/2015/9/14/9323379/saudi -arabia-squandered-its-groundwater-and-agriculture-collapsed.

22. Little JB. "The Ogallala Aquifer: Saving a Vital U.S. Water Source." *Scientific American.* March 1, 2009. https://www.scientificamerican.com/article/the-ogallala-aquifer/.

23. Hiel MP, Barbieux S, Pierreux J, et al. "Impact of Crop Residue Management on Crop Production and Soil Chemistry after Seven Years of Crop Rotation in Temperate Climate, Loamy Soils." *PeerJ.* 2018 May 23;6:e4836.

24. Union of Concerned Scientists. (2008). "CAFOs Uncovered: The Untold Costs of Confined Animal Feeding Operations." https://www.ucsusa.org/food_and_agriculture/our -failing-food-system/industrial-agriculture/cafos-uncovered.html.

25. Adams A. (2018). "Scaling Grassfed Beef by Allen Williams." HMI. https://holisticman agement.org/featured-blog-posts/scaling-grassfed-beef-by-allen-williams/.

26. Baron V. (2018). "Before Florence, EPA Weakened Protections for CAFO Neighbors." NRDC. https://www.nrdc.org/experts/valerie-baron/florence-epa-weakened-protections -cafo-neighbors.

27. Surrusco EK. (2019). "The Storm Moved on, but North Carolina's Hog Waste Didn't." Earth Justice. https://earthjustice.org/blog/2019-january/hog-waste-creates-problems -for-north-carolina-residents.

28. Watts C. (2010). "Gulf of Mexico Dead Zone: Mitigating the Damage." Gulf of Mexico Hypoxia. https://gulfhypoxia.net/gulf-of-mexico-dead-zone-mitigating-the-damage/; Rose KA, Gutiérrez D, Levin LA, et al. "Declining Oxygen in the Global Ocean and Coastal Waters." *Science.* January 5, 2018.

29. Kolpin DW, Furlong ET, Meyer MT, et al. "Pharmaceuticals, Hormones, and Other Organic Wastewater Contaminants in US Streams, 1999–2000: A National Reconnaissance." *Environ Sci Technol.* 2002 Mar 15;36(6):1202–11.

30. Lebreton L, Slat B, Ferrari F, et al. "Evidence that the Great Pacific Garbage Patch Is Rapidly Accumulating Plastic." *Sci Rep.* 2018 Mar 22;8(1):4666.

31. IPBES. "IPBES Global Assessment Summary for Policy Makers." May 6, 2019. https://www.ipbes.net/news/ipbes-global-assessment-summary-policymakers-pdf.

32. Living Planet Index. (2014). "Living Plant Index (LPI) Project." http://livingplanetindex.org/home/index.

33. Costanza R, de Groot R, Sutton P, et al. "Changes in the Global Value of Ecosystem Services." *Glob Environ Change.* 2014 May 1;26:152–58.

34. United Nations. (2019). "Nature's Dangerous Decline 'Unprecedented'; Species Extinction Rates 'Accelerating.'" https://www.un.org/sustainabledevelopment/blog/2019/05/nature-decline-unprecedented-report/.

35. Hoff M. "As Insect Populations Decline, Scientists Are Trying to Understand Why." *Scientific American.* November 1, 2018. https://www.scientificamerican.com/article/as-insect-populations-decline-scientists-are-trying-to-understand-why/.

36. Graham K. (2018). "Beyond Honey Bees: Wild Bees Are Also Key Pollinators, and Some Species Are Disappearing." The Conversation. https://theconversation.com/beyond-honey-bees-wild-bees-are-also-key-pollinators-and-some-species-are-disappearing-89214.

37. Hallmann CA, Sorg M, Jongejans E, et al. "More Than 75 Percent Decline Over 27 Years in Total Flying Insect Biomass in Protected Areas." *PLoS One.* 2017;12(10).

38. Ramanujan K. (2012). "Insect Pollinators Contribute $29 Billion to U.S. Farm Income." Cornell University. http://news.cornell.edu/stories/2012/05/insect-pollinators-contribute-29b-us-farm-income.

39. Thorpe D. "How Investing in Regenerative Agriculture Can Help Stem Climate Change Profitably." *Forbes.* December 12, 2018. https://www.forbes.com/sites/devinthorpe/2018/12/12/how-investing-in-regenerative-agriculture-can-help-stem-climate-change-profitably/#538149f03e5c.

40. Seachrist KF. (2018). "Longtime Soil-Driven Innovators Ready to Provide Regenerative Ag System Expertise." FarmProgress. https://www.farmprogress.com/soil-health/soil-health-pro-team.

41. Main Street Project. (2019). "Our Story." mainstreetproject.org.

42. EcoWatch. (2016). "Tyson Foods Dumps More Pollution into Waterways Each Year Than Exxon." https://www.ecowatch.com/tyson-foods-dumps-more-pollution-into-waterways-each-year-than-exxon-1882169913.html.

43. Spiegel B. "General Mills Aims to Drive Regenerative Agriculture on 1 Million Acres by 2030." *Successful Farming.* March 4, 2019. https://www.agriculture.com/news/crops/general-mills-aims-to-drive-regenerative-agriculture-on-1-million-acres-by-2030.

44. Bio-Integrity Growers Australia. "Biological Farming and Ecological Farming in Australia." YouTube, 4:44. February 17, 2016. https://www.youtube.com/watch?v=lljYXVli3X8&feature=youtu.be.

45. Farmland LP. (2019). "About Us." http://www.farmlandlp.com/.

46. Pretty J, Benton T, Bharucha ZP, et al. "Global Assessment of Agricultural System Redesign for Sustainable Intensification." *Nat Sustain.* 2018 Aug;1(8):441.

47. UPenn. (2019). "With Unprecedented Threats to Nature at Hand, How to Turn the Tide." *Penn Today.* https://penntoday.upenn.edu/news/unprecedented-threats-nature-hand-how-turn-tide.

48. Bittman M, Pollan M, Salvador R, De Schutter O. (2015). "A National Food Policy for the 21st Century." *Medium.* https://medium.com/food-is-the-new-internet/a-national-food-policy-for-the-21st-century-7d323ee7c65f.

49. Faust DR, Kumar S, Archer DW, et al. (2017). "Potential Water Quality Outcomes from Integrated Crop-Livestock Systems in the Northern Great Plains." Managing Global Resources for a Secure Future Annual Meeting. https://scisoc.confex.com/crops/2017am/webprogram/Paper105136.html.

50. St. Clair, T. (2014). "Farming without Subsidies—a Better Way. Why New Zealand Agriculture Is a World Leader." *Politico.* https://www.politico.eu/article/viewpoint-farming-without-subsidies-a-better-way-why-new-zealand-agriculture-is-a-world-leader/.

51. Mumm RH, Goldsmith PD, Rausch KD, and Stein HH. "Land Usage Attributed to Corn Ethanol Production in the United States: Sensitivity to Technological Advances on Corn Grain Yield, Ethanol Conversion, and Co-product Utilization." *Biotechnol Biofuels.* 2014;7:61.

52. "Ethanol Fuel From Corn Faulted as 'Unsustainable Subsidized Food Burning' in Analysis by Cornell Scientist." *Cornell Chronicle.* August 6, 2001. http://news.cornell.edu/stories/2001/08/ethanol-corn-faulted-energy-waster-scientist-says.

53. Wikipedia, s.v. "Payment for Ecosystem Services." Last edited October 2, 2019. https://en.wikipedia.org/wiki/Payment_for_ecosystem_services.

54. Union of Concerned Scientists. (2019). "Infographic: Plant the Plate." https://www.ucsusa.org/food_and_agriculture/solutions/expand-healthy-food-access/plant-the-plate.html#.VhMWTxNViko.

55. Union of Concerned Scientists. "The Healthy Farmland Diet: How Growing Less Corn Would Improve Our Health and Help America's Heartland." October 2013. Retrieved June 2019 from https://www.ucsusa.org/sites/default/files/legacy/assets/documents/food_and_agriculture/healthy-farmland-diet.pdf.

56. Mitchell S. "6 Ways to Rein in Today's Toxic Monopolies." *The Nation.* February 16, 2018. https://www.thenation.com/article/six-ways-to-rein-in-todays-toxic-monopolies/; Ikerd J. "Corporatization of Agricultural Policy." *Small Farm Today.* 2010. http://web.missouri.edu/ikerdj/papers/SFT-Corporatization%20of%20Fm%20Pol%20%289-10%29.htm.

57. Regenerative Organic Alliance. (2019). "ROC Pilot Program & Participants." https://regenorganic.org/pilot/.

58. Mariposa Ranch Meats. (2019). "Quarter Beef." https://mariposaranchmeats.com/product/14-beef/.

59. Centers for Disease Control and Prevention. (2010). "Community Gardens." https://www.cdc.gov/healthyplaces/healthtopics/healthyfood/community.htm.

60. Carbon Underground. (2019). "White Papers." https://thecarbonunderground.org/the-science/resources/white-papers/.

61. Intentional Endowments Network. (2019). "Farm Animal Investment Risk and Return (FAIRR)." http://www.intentionalendowments.org/farm_animal_investment_risk_and _return.

62. Desilver D. (2018). "U.S. Trails Most Developed Countries in Voter Turnout." Pew Research Center. https://www.pewresearch.org/fact-tank/2018/05/21/u-s-voter-turnout -trails-most-developed-countries/.

63. Food Policy Action. (2014). "An Eater's Guide to Congress." https://foodpolicyaction .org/an-eaters-guide-to-congress/.

64. Harper A, Alkon A, Shattuck A, Holt-Giménez E, Lambrick F. (2009). "Food Policy Councils: Lessons Learned." Food First. https://foodfirst.org/publication/food-policy -councils-lessons-learned/.

65. Clark L. (2016). "Why Farm-to-Institution Sourcing Is the Sleeping Giant of Local Food." *Civil Eats.* https://civileats.com/2016/08/29/forget-farm-to-table-its-farm-to -institution-sourcing-that-could-make-a-real-dent-the-food-system/.

66. HEAL. (2019). "News." https://healfoodalliance.org.

CHAPTER 17

1. Saxifrage B. "Global Warming Increasing by 400,000 Atomic Bombs Every Day." *Vancouver Observer.* May 15, 2012. https://www.vancouverobserver.com/blogs/climate snapshot/2012/05/15/global-warming-increasing-400000-atomic-bombs-every-day.

2. The Foster Lab. (2019). "415 ppm CO2 Threshold Crossed May 2019." http://www .thefosterlab.org/blog/2019/5/14/415-ppm-co2-threshold-crossed-may-2019.

3. Wallace-Wells D. (2019). "The Uninhabitable Earth, Annotated Edition." *New York.* http://nymag.com/intelligencer/2017/07/climate-change-earth-too-hot-for-humans -annotated.html?gtm=bottom.

4. Fourth National Climate Assessment. (2019). "Volume II: Impacts, Risks, and Adaptation in the United States." https://nca2018.globalchange.gov.

5. IPCC. (2019). "Global Warming of 1.5°C." https://www.ipcc.ch/sr15/.

6. Marvel K. (2019). "What I'm Going to Tell Congress Today: A Thread…" Twitter. https://twitter.com/DrKateMarvel/status/1128650655151919104.

7. Dorward LJ. "Where Are the Best Opportunities for Reducing Greenhouse Gas Emissions in the Food System (Including the Food Chain)? A Comment." *Food Policy.* 2012 Aug 1;37(4):463–66. https://www.sciencedirect.com/science/article/abs/pii/S03069192 10001132.

8. "Ruminations: Methane Math and Context." Regenetarianism. May 4, 2018. https:// lachefnet.wordpress.com/2018/05/04/ruminations-methane-math-and-context/.

9. IPCC. "Mitigating of Climate Change." Cambridge University. 2014. https://www .ipcc.ch/site/assets/uploads/2018/02/ipcc_wg3_ar5_frontmatter.pdf.

10. Mottett A, Steinfeld H. (2018). "Cars or Livestock: Which Contribute More to Climate Change?" Thomas Reuters Foundation. http://news.trust.org/item/20180918083629 -d2wf0/.

11. Gerber PJ, Steinfeld H, Henderson B, et al. *Tackling Climate Change through Livestock: A Global Assessment of Emissions and Mitigation Opportunities.* Rome: Food and Agriculture Organization of the United Nations (FAO), 2013.

12. Basche A. (2016). "Why the Loss of Grasslands Is a Troubling Trend for Agriculture, in 11 Maps and Graphs." Union of Concerned Scientists. https://blog.ucsusa.org/andrea -basche/why-the-loss-of-grasslands-is-a-troubling-trend-for-agriculture-in-11-maps -and-graphs.

13. Belsie L. "Habitat Meets Profit as Ranchers Restore Native Prairies." *Christian Science Monitor*. June 14, 2019. https://www.csmonitor.com/Environment/2019/0614/Habitat -meets-profit-as-ranchers-restore-native-prairies.

14. Grain. (2018). "Emissions Impossible: How Big Meat and Dairy Are Heating Up the Planet." https://www.grain.org/article/entries/5976-emissions-impossible-how-big-meat -and-dairy-are-heating-up-the-planet.

15. Garnett T, Godde C, Muller A, et al. *Grazed and Confused? Ruminating on Cattle, Grazing Systems, Methane, Nitrous Oxide, the Soil Carbon Sequestration Question—and What It All Means for Greenhouse Gas Emissions.* Food Climate Research Network. 2017. https://www .fcrn.org.uk/sites/default/files/project-files/fcrn_gnc_report.pdf.

16. Horwath R. (2017). "Is the Global Spike in Methane Emissions Caused by the Natural Gas Industry or Animal Agriculture? Reconciling the Conflicting Views." UN Climate Change. https://unfccc.cloud.streamworld.de/webcast/dr-robert-howarth-is-the-global -spike-in-methane-e.

17. Rowntree, J. (2017). "Amazing Grazing: Why Grass-Fed Beef Isn't to Blame in the Climate Change Debate." Sustainable Dish. https://sustainabledish.com/beef-isnt-to-blame/.

18. Sustainable Food Trust. (2017). "Grazed and Confused—An Initial Response from the Sustainable Food Trust." https://sustainablefoodtrust.org/articles/grazed-and-confused -an-initial-response-from-the-sustainable-food-trust/?utm_source=SFT+Newsletter &utm_campaign=12987e6aef-Newsletter_07_10_2014&utm_medium=email&utm _term=0_bf20bccf24-12987e6aef-90447153.

19. Stanley PL, Rowntree JE, Beede DK, DeLonge MS, Hamm MW. "Impacts of Soil Carbon Sequestration on Life Cycle Greenhouse Gas Emissions in Midwestern USA Beef Finishing Systems." *Agric Syst.* 2018 May 1;162:249–58.

20. Itzkan S. "Regarding Holechek and Briske, and Rebuttals by Teague, Gill & Savory Correcting Misconceptions About the Supposed Discrediting of Savory's Approach." Planet-TECH Associates. June 2011. https://planet-tech.com/sites/default/files/Itzkan%20 2011,%20RegardingHolechekSavory%20v4_0.pdf.

21. Thorbecke M, Dettling J. "Carbon Footprint Evaluation of Regenerative Grazing at White Oak Pastures." February 25, 2019. https://blog.whiteoakpastures.com/hubfs/WOP -LCA-Quantis-2019.pdf.

22. PR Newswire. (2019). "Study; White Oak Pastures Beef Reduces Atmospheric Carbon." https://www.prnewswire.com/news-releases/study-white-oak-pastures-beef-reduces -atmospheric-carbon-300841416.html.

23. University of Oxford. "Climate Metrics for Ruminant Livestock." Oxford Martin School. 2018. https://www.oxfordmartin.ox.ac.uk/downloads/reports/Climate-metrics -for-ruminant-livestock.pdf; Fairlie S. (2019). "A Convenient Untruth." Resilience. https://www.resilience.org/stories/2019-05-10/a-convenient-untruth/.

24. DeLonge MS, Owen JJ, Silve WL. "Greenhouse Gas Mitigation Opportunities in California Agriculture: Review of California Rangeland Emissions and Mitigation Potential."

University of California, Berkeley. 2014. https://nicholasinstitute.duke.edu/sites/default/files/ni_ggmoca_r_4.pdf.

25. Stanley PL, Rowntree JE, Beede DK, DeLonge MS, Hamm MW. "Impacts of Soil Carbon Sequestration on Life Cycle Greenhouse Gas Emissions in Midwestern USA Beef Finishing Systems." *Agric Syst.* 2018 May 1;162:249–58.

26. Niman NH. *Defending Beef: The Case for Sustainable Meat Production.* White River Junction, VT: Chelsea Green Publishing, 2014.

27. Silvestri S, Osana P, Leeuw J de, et al. "Greening Livestock: Assessing the Potential of Payment for Environmental Services in Livestock Inclusive Agricultural Production Systems in Developing Countries." International Livestock Research Institute. 2012.

28. Capper JL. "Is the Grass Always Greener? Comparing the Environmental Impact of Conventional, Natural and Grass-Fed Beef Production Systems." *Animals (Basel).* 2012 Apr 10;2(2):127–43.

29. Thorbecke M, Dettling J. "Carbon Footprint Evaluation of Regenerative Grazing at White Oak Pastures." February 25, 2019. https://blog.whiteoakpastures.com/hubfs/WOP-LCA-Quantis-2019.pdf.

30. Williams A. (2016). "Can We Produce Grass Fed Beef at Scale?" Grassfed Exchange. https://grassfedexchange.com/blog/can-we-produce-grass-fed-beef-at-scale.

31. Fischer B, Lamey A. "Field Deaths in Plant Agriculture." *Journal of Agricultural and Environmental Ethics,* 2018.

32. Harcombe Z. (2019). "The EAT Lancet Diet Is Nutritionally Deficient." http://www.zoeharcombe.com/2019/01/the-eat-lancet-diet-is-nutritionally-deficient/.

33. World Business Council for Sustainable Development. (2019). "Our Members." https://www.wbcsd.org/Overview/Our-members.

34. Rees T. (2019). "The EAT/Lancet Backers: Definitely NOT in It for the Good of the Planet." Nutritional Therapy Online. https://nutritionaltherapyonline.com/definitely-not-in-it-for-the-good-of-the-planet/.

35. Shiva V. (2019). "A New Report Sustains Unsustainable Food Systems." Seed Freedom. https://seedfreedom.info/poison-cartel-toxic-food-eat-report/.

36. Ibid.

37. Sinha R, Cross AJ, Graubard BI, Leitzmann MF, Schatzkin A. "Meat Intake and Mortality: A Prospective Study of Over Half a Million People." *Arch Intern Med.* 2009;169(6):562–71.

38. Dehghan M, Mente A, Zhang X, et al. "Associations of Fats and Carbohydrate Intake with Cardiovascular Disease and Mortality in 18 Countries from Five Continents (PURE): A Prospective Cohort Study." *Lancet.* 2017 Nov 4;390(10107):2050–62.

39. Grasgruber P, Sebera M, Hrazdira E, et al. "Food Consumption and the Actual Statistics of Cardiovascular Diseases: An Epidemiological Comparison of 42 European Countries." *Food Nutr Res.* 2016 Jan 1;60(1):31694.

40. Key TJ, Thorogood M, Appleby PN, Burr ML. "Dietary Habits and Mortality in 11,000 Vegetarians and Health Conscious People: Results of a 17 Year Follow Up." *BMJ.* 1996 Sep 28;313(7060):775–79.

41. Daley CA, Abbott A, Doyle PS, Nader GA, Larson S. "A Review of Fatty Acid Profiles and Antioxidant Content in Grass-Fed and Grain-Fed Beef." *Nutr J.* 2010 Dec;9(1):10.

42. Kresser C. (2019). "Why Eating Meat Is Good for You." https://chriskresser.com/why-eating-meat-is-good-for-you/.

43. Hawken P, ed. *Drawdown: The Most Comprehensive Plan Ever Proposed to Reverse Global Warming.* New York: Penguin, 2017.

44. Conrad Z, Niles M, Neher D, et al. "Relationship between Food Waste, Diet Quality, and Environmental Sustainability." *PLoS One.* 2018 Apr 18;13(4):e0195405.

45. Food Loss and Waste Protocol. "Food Loss and Waste Accounting and Reporting Standard." 2019. https://www.theconsumergoodsforum.com/wp-content/uploads/2017/10/The-Consumer-Goods-Forum-Food-Waste-FLW-Standard.pdf.

46. FiBL. "Food Wastage Costs the World 2.6 Trillion Dollars Each Year." October 1, 2014. https://www.fibl.org/fileadmin/documents/en/news/2014/mr-fao-food-waste141001.pdf.

47. United Nations. (2019). "Sustainable Development Goals." https://sustainabledevelopment.un.org/topics/sustainabledevelopmentgoals.

48. Sustainable Brands. (2019). "This Startup Is Giving Ugly Watermelons a Refreshing Purpose." https://sustainablebrands.com/read/product-service-design-innovation/this-startup-is-giving-ugly-watermelons-a-refreshing-purpose.

49. US Department of Agriculture. (2019). "Food Waste Challenges: Frequently Asked Questions." https://www.usda.gov/oce/foodwaste/faqs.htm.

50. Natural Resources Defense Council. "Wasted: How America Is Losing up to 40 Percent of Its Food from Farm to Fork to Landfill." 2017. https://www.nrdc.org/sites/default/files/wasted-2017-report.pdf.

51. ReFED. "A Roadmap to Reduce U.S. Food Waste by 20 Percent." 2016. https://www.refed.com/downloads/ReFED_Report_2016.pdf.

52. Natural Resources Defense Council. (2019). "Food Waste." https://www.nrdc.org/issues/food-waste.

53. Toti E, Di Mattia C, Serafini M. "Metabolic Food Waste and Ecological Impact of Obesity in FAO World's Region." *Front Nutr.* 2019;6.

54. Beardsley E. (2018). "French Food Waste Law Changing How Grocery Stores Approach Excess Food." National Public Radio. https://www.npr.org/sections/thesalt/2018/02/24/586579455/french-food-waste-law-changing-how-grocery-stores-approach-excess-food.

55. Phat Beets Produce. (2018). "The Ugly Truth of Ugly Produce." https://www.phatbeetsproduce.org/uglyproduce/.

56. Ryals R, Silver WL. "Effects of Organic Matter Amendments on Net Primary Productivity and Greenhouse Gas Emissions in Annual Grasslands." *Ecol Appl.* 2013 Jan 1;23(1):46–59.

EPILOGUE

1. Beacons of Hope. 2019. https://foodsystemstransformations.org/.

Index

About the Author

DR MARK HYMAN has devoted his life to helping others discover optimal health and address the root causes of chronic disease through the power of functional medicine. Dr Hyman is an internationally recognized leader, speaker, educator, and advocate in the fields of functional medicine and nutrition. He is the founder and director of the UltraWellness Center, the head of strategy and innovation for the Cleveland Clinic Center for Functional Medicine, a twelve-time *New York Times* bestselling author, and board president for clinical affairs at the Institute for Functional Medicine. He is the host of one of the leading health podcasts, *The Doctor's Farmacy*. Dr Hyman is a regular medical contributor on several television shows and networks, including *CBS This Morning*, *Today*, *Good Morning America*, *The View*, and CNN. He is also an adviser and guest cohost on *The Dr Oz Show*.

Through his work to change policy for the betterment of public health, Dr Hyman has testified before the Senate Working Group on Health Care Reform on Functional Medicine. He has consulted with the surgeon general on diabetes prevention and participated in the 2009 White House Forum on Prevention and Wellness. Senator Tom Harkin of Iowa nominated Dr Hyman for the President's Advisory Group on Prevention, Health Promotion, and Integrative and Public Health.

Dr Hyman has presented at the Clinton Foundation's Health Matters, Achieving Wellness in Every Generation conference and the Clinton Global Initiative, as well as with the World Economic Forum on global health issues, TEDMED, TEDx, and the Vatican. He is the winner of the Linus Pauling Award and the Nantucket Project Award. Dr Hyman received the Christian Book of the Year Award for his work on *The Daniel Plan*, a faith-based initiative that helped the Saddleback Church collectively lose 250,000 pounds, which he created with Rick Warren, Dr Mehmet Oz, and Dr Daniel Amen. He was inducted into the Books for Better Life Hall of Fame.

With Dr Dean Ornish and Dr Michael Roizen, Dr Hyman crafted and helped introduce the Take Back Your Health Act of 2009 to the US Senate, which promotes reimbursement for lifestyle treatment of chronic disease. With Tim Ryan in 2015, he helped introduce the ENRICH Act to Congress to fund nutrition in medical education. Dr Hyman plays a substantial role in the major 2014 film *Fed Up*, produced by Laurie David and Katie Couric, which addresses childhood obesity. Please join him in celebrating the power of food as medicine at www.drhyman.com, follow him on Twitter, Facebook, and Instagram, and listen to his podcast, *The Doctor's Farmacy*, for conversations that matter around health, wellness, food, and politics.

BOOKS BY DR MARK HYMAN

Food: What the Heck Should I Cook? • *Food: WTF Should I Eat?* •
The Eat Fat, Get Thin Cookbook • *Eat Fat, Get Thin* • *The Blood Sugar Solution 10-Day Detox Diet Cookbook* • *The Blood Sugar Solution 10-Day Detox Diet* •
The Blood Sugar Solution Cookbook • *The Blood Sugar Solution* • *The Daniel Plan* • *The Daniel Plan Cookbook* • *UltraPrevention* • *UltraMetabolism* •
The Five Forces of Wellness (CD) • *The UltraMetabolism Cookbook* •
The UltraThyroid Solution • *The UltraSimple Diet* • *The UltraMind Solution* • *Six Weeks to an UltraMind* (CD)